D1559676

THE LAMBAS OF
NORTHERN RHODESIA

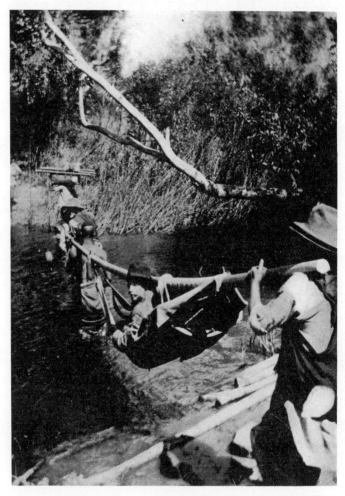

FIG. 1. THE LATE REV. J. J. DOKE CROSSING THE KAFULAFUTA RIVER
BY MACHILA ON THE JOURNEY IN 1913 WHICH COST HIM
HIS LIFE

Photo by Ç. M. Doke

THE LAMBAS OF
NORTHERN RHODESIA

A STUDY OF THEIR CUSTOMS
AND BELIEFS

BY

CLEMENT M. DOKE M.A. D.Litt.

SOMETIME MISSIONARY IN LAMBALAND PROFESSOR IN BANTU
PHILOLOGY UNIVERSITY OF THE WITWATERSRAND JOHANNESBURG
AUTHOR OF "GRAMMAR OF THE LAMBA LANGUAGE" "THE
PHONETICS OF THE ZULU LANGUAGE" "TEXT-BOOK OF ZULU
GRAMMAR" "LAMBA FOLK-LORE" "UNIFICATION OF THE SHONA
DIALECTS" ETC.

NEGRO UNIVERSITIES PRESS
WESTPORT, CONNECTICUT

DT
955
D6
1970

Originally published in 1931 by
G. G. Harrop & Co., Ltd., London

Reprinted 1970 by
Negro Universities Press
A Division of Greenwood Press, Inc.
Westport, Connecticut

SBN 8371-3751-9

Printed in United States of America

THIS BOOK IS
AFFECTIONATELY DEDICATED TO
THE MEMORY OF MY FATHER
THE LATE REV. J. J. DOKE
WHO GAVE HIS LIFE
IN FURTHERING THE WORK OF THE
GOSPEL AMONG THE LAMBAS
AND WHOSE LIFE AND EXAMPLE
HAVE EVER BEEN A STIMULUS TO
THAT WHICH IS HIGHEST AND
NOBLEST

NOTE ON THE ORTHOGRAPHY AND CHOICE OF NATIVE WORDS

THE symbol $ẇ$ represents the voiced bilabial fricative, a *b*-sound made with the lips not quite touching.

The symbol ŋ represents the sound of *ng* in the English word ' singing.'

In referring to the names of native tribes I have deleted all prefixes and used the stems as English words. Thus, instead of *umulamba* (' a Lamba person ') and *aẇalamba* (' Lamba people ') I have used the terms ' Lamba ' and ' Lambas '; similarly, such roots as ' Ẇemba,' ' Kaonde,' ' Lenje,' ' Ila,' are used in the plural as ' Ẇembas,' ' Kaondes,' ' Lenjes,' ' Ilas,' instead of being given the Bantu plural prefixes. This is analogous to the accepted use of such terms as ' the Zulus,' ' the Swazis,' instead of the Bantu forms *amazulu* and *amaswazi*.

PREFACE

THIS book makes no pretence to being an exhaustive survey of the Lamba people; it is mainly the record of observations made during the period of my missionary work on the staff of the South African Baptist Missionary Society during the years 1914–21. These observations I was enabled to check, correct, and elaborate during the years 1927 and 1928, when, through a grant made to me by the University of the Witwatersrand from funds for research in Bantu studies provided by the Union Government, two Lambas, Joshua Kamwendo and his wife, were brought to Johannesburg for nine months in order to assist me, more particularly with the Lamba dictionary.

It is my hope that the facts recorded in these pages will assist missionaries, Government officials, and others who have direct contact with the natives to understand better the people and their point of view. I have said nothing about the missionary work in the country—this is a record of the thoughts and lives of the people, as far as I could observe them, unaffected by Christianizing and the influences of Western civilization, which are now beginning to tell. I can only say that I wish I had had more knowledge of the significance of the native customs when I first went to work among the Lambas: I should have been saved from many a grievous mistake and many a misjudgment. The ability to see through Bantu eyes will give the missionary and the official better understanding and more sympathy with the people, and a greater ability to gain their confidence.

C. M. DOKE

CONTENTS

ILLUSTRATIONS

ILLUSTRATIONS

15

THE LAMBAS OF
NORTHERN RHODESIA

CHAPTER I

THE COUNTRY AND THE PEOPLE

Ilamba

THE country inhabited by the Lamba-speaking people is called by the missionaries Lambaland, but by the people themselves

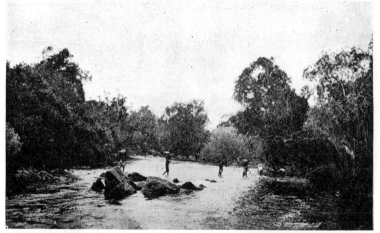

FIG. 2.   CROSSING THE UPPER KAFUE—DRY SEASON
Photo by Miss O. C. Doke

Ilamba.   It comprises a territory of some 25,000 square miles, partly in North-western Rhodesia and partly in that tongue of the Belgian Congo which forms the southernmost portion of the Katanga district.   As will be seen from the map, the railway from Livingstone to the Belgian Congo cuts through Ilamba from south to north, entering the territory some miles north of Broken Hill and leaving it a few miles south of Elisabethville.

The average altitude of the territory is a little over 4000 feet, the hills which really constitute the international boundary and the watershed between the Congo and the Zambesi systems rising not very much higher than the surrounding country. Apart from the Irume Range in the extreme east, Ilamba boasts no mountains. The whole country is flat and slightly undulating, with here and there isolated kopjes or low ranges of hills. In very recent times attention has been drawn to the central and northern area of Ilamba by the discovery and working of a number of copper-mines from Bwana M'Kubwa on the railway-line to Nchanga, north-westward. Copper is usually, though not always, located in the kopjes.

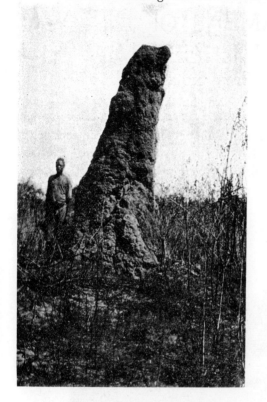

FIG. 3. AN UMUSHINJE, OR NEEDLE ANTHILL
Photo by C. M. Doke

Ilamba is distinctly forest-land. From east to west and north to south stretch seemingly interminable forests. The trees grow to a considerable height, but are not densely packed together, nor do their leaves afford much shelter from the midday summer sun. At intervals, almost mechanically regular intervals, the forests are broken by open glades, through which run the numerous streams which drain the country. So regular are these intervals that natives use them to describe the distance from one village to another. To "How far have we yet to travel?" the answer will usually be something like this: "There remain three forests." That is, three more stretches of forest-land, with a stream between each.

The glades between the forests increase in size proportionately

18

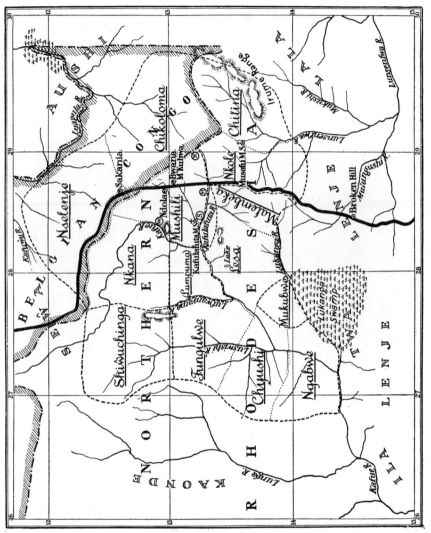

LAMBALAND

19

to the size of the stream which runs through them. The permanent rivers have wide plains on either side of them, while the beautiful parent river of Ilamba, the Kafue, is renowned for the far-stretching Kafue Flats which border its banks, at times for miles on either side. Directly, however, one reaches the higher ground, which is not subjected to the annual inundations, the forest once more commences.

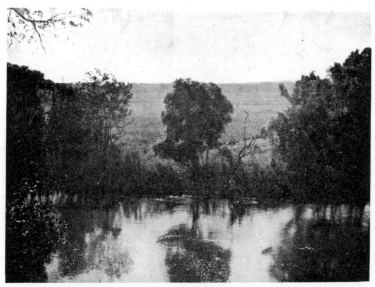

FIG. 4. A BEND IN THE UPPER KAFUE RIVER, THE LOW BANK-SIDE SHOWING
THE PLAIN WHICH BECOMES FLOODED
Photo by C. M. Doke

Ilamba is a land of streams and rivers. It is wonderfully well watered. With an annual rainfall averaging 50 inches, practically confined to the five months November to March, so level a country, with very slow drainage, constitutes to a great extent a vast sponge. From this sponge drain off into the Zambesi system the Luswishi, Lufwanyama, Kafulafuta, and Lukanga— all tributaries of the Kafue river, which is known to the Lambas as the Lufuŵu or Hippopotamus river—also, on the eastern side, the Lunsenfwa, 'Child of the Loangwa,' 'Child of the Zambesi'; while northward many streams, the largest of which is the Kafuŵu, feed the Luapula, one of the large tributaries of the Congo.

THE COUNTRY AND THE PEOPLE

The climate of Ilamba is, on the whole, delightful. In the winter months frost in the early morning gives a freshness and crispness to the air, while in the summer the oppressive heat of October is soon broken by the coming of the rains, which temper the hottest day. Two potent enemies, however, militate against the opening up and development of this fertile country—the mosquito and the tsetse. Owing to the swampy nature of much of the country during and immediately after the rains, malaria

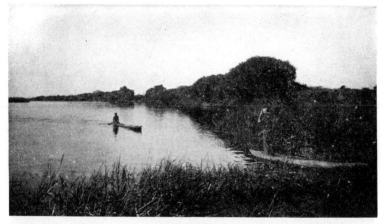

FIG. 5. VIEW ON THE CENTRAL KAFUE RIVER, WITH DUG-OUT CANOES
Author standing.
Photo by the late Rev. J. J. Doke

is extremely prevalent, and the natives themselves suffer much from this disease. Practically all of Ilamba is tsetse country. Belt after belt of tsetse is met as one travels, and this has a tremendous influence upon the habits and life of the people. There are no cattle, except in parts of Nkole's and Chitina's country on the south-east. Agriculture, food, mode of travelling, are all influenced by this lack of cattle.

In Ilamba one lives down on the level, pent up within the interminable forests. It is only when one climbs on to one of the scattered kopjes and gets a view over the rolling sea of trees, or visits the great Kafue Flats, that one becomes aware of the tremendous distances and enormous spaces which so characterize Africa.

Ilamba is rich hunting country. Game of almost every kind abounds, though with the advent of the white hunter and the

21

increase of muzzle-loading guns in the hands of the natives it is fast diminishing. In 1913, when I first visited the country, portions of the Kafue plains were still teeming with herds of big game, and one could stand on an anthill and choose one's breakfast from any of ten or more species feeding with apparent unconcern. The existence of the game, like the absence of the cattle, has constituted

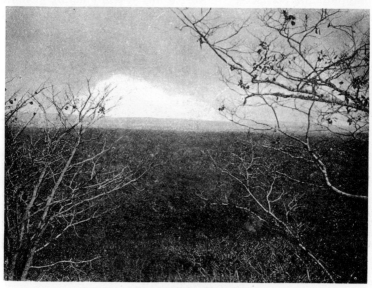

FIG. 6. THE INTERMINABLE FORESTS, WITH A GLIMPSE OF THE PLAINS
OF THE LUFWANYAMA IN THE DISTANCE
Photo by C. M. Doke

a strong deciding factor in the habits and mode of life of the Lamba-speaking peoples.

Neighbours

Ilamba is bounded on the north by the country of the Seŵa people in the Congo, the Kafuŵu (tributary of the Luapula) roughly constituting the boundary. The Seŵas are a buffer tribe between the Lambas and their northern neighbours, the Lubas; they understand *uŵulamba*, and might almost be termed Lamba-speaking. Few in numbers and lacking in influence and importance, they scarcely constitute a separate tribe. On the north-east the Lamba boundary reaches almost to the Luapula river, on either side of which live the Aushi people, undoubtedly of Ŵemba stock, acting as a buffer between the Lambas and the Ŵembas. Though speaking a dialect with individual peculiarities, these people really belong to the Ŵemba-speaking group. The eastern boundary of Ilamba is formed by the Irume Range and the watershed between the Mukushi and Lunsenfwa rivers. Beyond this boundary lies Ilala, the country of the Lala people. In speech the Lalas and the Lambas are closely akin; the languages may be regarded as

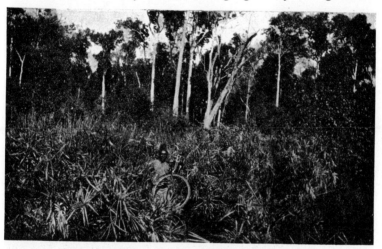

FIG. 7. SWAMP GROWTH ON THE EDGE OF AN UMUSHITU,
OR SWAMP FOREST

Joshua Kamwendo with bicycle.

Photo by Miss O. C. Doke

sister languages, and in fact were treated together as one by the late A. C. Madan.[1] The southern border of Ilamba is marked for the most part by the Lukanga river, which loses itself in the great Lukanga Swamp, extending in the rains over some 1600 square miles. In this swamp have lived, and still to a slight extent do live, that most interesting swamp people, the Twas.[2] Very few in numbers, degraded in the extreme, physically

[1] See his *Lala-Lamba Handbook* (Clarendon Press, Oxford, 1908). Madan even mixes up Lala, Lamba, and Ŵisa (eastward from the Lala country)—see his *Lala-Lamba-Ŵisa Dictionary* (Clarendon Press, Oxford, 1913). Ŵisa is as distinct from Lamba as is Ŵemba, though all belong to the same Central Bantu Group.

[2] The Lambas call these people Aŵatwa, and say that the term is derived from *twa, twila*, to pound and set fish-poison, to catch fish by poison. But it must be remembered that the 'inferior people' of the swamps of Bangweulu are so called by the Ŵembas, and those of the swamps of the Kafue by the Ilas;

23

and intellectually backward, the Twa people have made the Lukanga Swamp their refuge from stronger neighbours. They used to live entirely in little villages built on the floating sudd, maintaining a precarious existence on fish, water-lily roots, and what they could get by barter from the land folk living around them. Perhaps the best description we have of these interesting people is that given by J. M. Moubray.[1] As far as we know, the

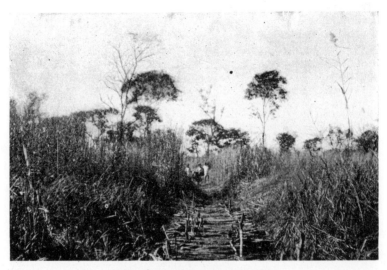

FIG. 8. LAMBA SWAMP BRIDGE
Author on bush-car.
Photo by the Rev. W. H. Doke

speech of these Twa people is a branch of Lenje. The real southern neighbours of the Lamba people are the Lenjes, or Bwene-mukuni, who are allied, linguistically and otherwise, with their southern and south-western neighbours, the Tonga and Ila peoples. A. C. Madan wrote a little handbook of Lenje,[2] and Father J. Torrend, S.J., has done considerable work on

while the pygmies (again inferior) of the Congo forests are called Twa by their neighbours, as are the Bushmen by the Zulus and Xosas. The same root is found in the Sotho and Chwana term for the Bushmen—Baroa. This root must have originally indicated outcast or inferior person, and the explanation given by the Lambas must be but a clever attempt at explaining what is not known to them. As a matter of fact, the Twa people seldom fish with poison ; they use the spear, *ukusumba*, not *ukutwa*.

[1] See *In South Central Africa* (Constable, London, 1912), chapter vi.
[2] *Lenje Handbook* (Clarendon Press, Oxford, 1908).

this language.[1] The Ila-speaking people, so ably described by E. W. Smith and the late A. M. Dale,[2] approach the Lamba boundary on the extreme south-west, where the Kafue river, after taking the waters drained from the Lukanga Swamp, turns westward to form the 'hook of the Kafue.' The western boundary of Ilamba is made by the watershed between the Luswishi and the

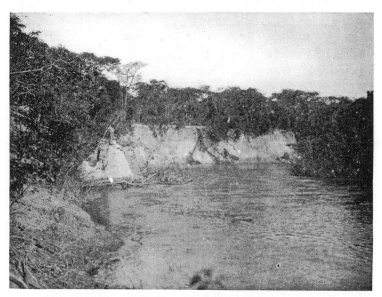

FIG. 9. A BEND IN THE UPPER KAFUE RIVER, THE HIGH BANK-SIDE
Photo by C. M. Doke

Lunga rivers. The western neighbours of the Lambas are the Kaonde people, an offshoot of the Lubas of the Congo. The Kaondes have been well described by F. H. Melland.[3]

Territorial Divisions of Ilamba

Ilamba is inhabited by certain sub-tribes in addition to the real Lambas. The territory occupied by all of these, however, is reckoned as belonging to Ilamba. These sub-tribes are the

[1] See his *Specimens of Bantu Folk-lore from Northern Rhodesia* (Kegan Paul, London, 1921).
[2] See *The Ila-speaking Peoples of Northern Rhodesia* (Macmillan, London, 1920).
[3] See *In Witch-bound Africa* (Seeley, Service, London, 1923).

Aŵenambonshi, under the headship of Shiŵuchinga, an intrusive Kaonde chief, and are comprised of mixed elements of Lamba, Seŵa, and Kaonde, though mostly of Lamba; the Ŵaŵulima, inhabiting a large tract of land south of the real Lamba district, and under the headship of five territorial chiefs, Lesa (the paramount), Malembeka, Fungulwe, Chyushi, and Ngabwe; the Aŵenamukuni, intrusive Lenje elements, under the chieftainship

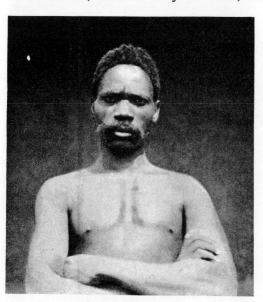

of Mukubwe, on the northern section of theLukanga Swamp in the Ŵulima area; and the Aŵenamaswaka, under two chiefs, Nkole and Chitina (the paramount), a buffer sub - tribe sharing much in common with the Lala and the real Lamba peoples. From a glance at the map (p. 19), it is quickly seen that the true Lambas are confined to a comparatively small area, about one half of Ilamba. This area again is divided in halves

FIG. 10. SANDAŴUNGA, HEIR TO THE CHIEFTAINSHIP OF KATANGA'S VILLAGE
Photo by C. M. Doke

between the great chiefs Nselenje in Congo Lambaland and Mushili in Rhodesian Lambaland. The relative positions of importance of these chiefs will be discussed in a subsequent chapter. It is but necessary here to note that there are two territorial chiefs in the Congo area, Nselenje and Chikoloma, and two in the Rhodesian area, Mushili and Nkana, and that their boundary practically coincides with the international border between the Belgian and British territories.

Although I have travelled over practically every part of Ilamba, this present study of the Lambas is for the most part confined to the people of Mushili's district, which I know best.

THE COUNTRY AND THE PEOPLE

The Lambas

The Lamba-speaking people may be described as hunting agriculturists. The lack of cattle has to a great extent determined their mode of life. They are typical exponents of hoe culture. The hoe is their most important implement, so much so that until recent times the marriage pledge was always made in hoes.

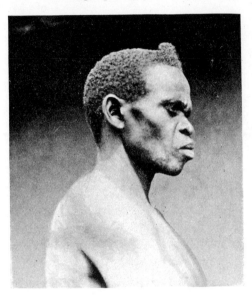

FIG. 11. KACHYASU, A MACHILA-CARRIER OF THE
1913 TREK
Photo by C. M. Doke

Throughout their vast territory the Lambas are scattered in numbers of small villages, each under its headman. Usually the villages contain from twenty to thirty circular huts, though some villages have many less and some a few more.

The people are divided into a number of exogamous clans, which only to a slight degree may be described as totemistic, and clan descent is matrilineal. This important feature of their social organization is seen to be interwoven with their religious and spiritual conceptions.

Physically the Lambas are of medium build, and though they do not as a whole show the physical proportions of such a tribe as the Zulus, they are remarkably robust and strong. The men

27

make very good carriers, and they stood up to the heavy war-load porterage to the East African theatre of war as well as any of the neighbouring tribes. The women too are able to carry enormous loads. I have repeatedly seen women coming from long distances with a baby on the back and an 8o-lb. load of thatching grass on the head. One day, for a wager, a Ŵulima man carried a huge load of corn twenty miles to Kafulafuta Mission Station; when

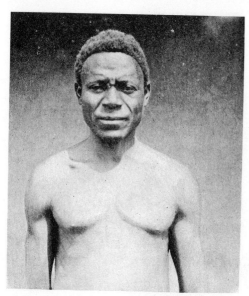

FIG. 12. MAŴETI, A MACHILA-CARRIER OF THE
1913 TREK
Photo by C. M. Doke

weighed the load turned the scale at 120 lb., and the carrier walked back home with his purchases the same day!

The Lambas have no tribal mark such as distinguishes the Ŵembas. They are a handsome folk, and their women generally are extremely comely, so much so that in the past Ilamba was repeatedly depopulated by Swahili slavers from the east and Mbundu traders from the west, so great was the demand for Lamba women. Their history reveals them to have been a peace-loving people, and, though they are roused to fight on various occasions, fighting is by no means one of their characteristics.

Linguistically the Lambas belong to the Central Bantu Group, of which *uŵulamba* is a typical example. Their language is remarkably rich in folk- and proverb-lore, and they take a great delight in talking. Practically every Lamba is a born orator, unafraid to voice his views, no matter what size the assembly may be. I estimate that the average man's vocabulary far exceeds

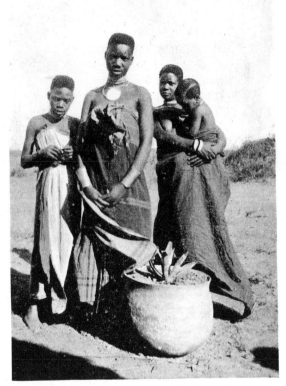

FIG. 13. LAMBA BELLES
Photo by C. M. Doke

10,000 words, an estimate which would not apply in many European communities.

From the moral point of view I do not consider the Lambas to be degraded as a people. Their standard of morals certainly differs greatly from that which we have inherited from centuries of Christian precept, but the standard which they have is not low, nor is its observance by the people lax. Of this I trust that the succeeding chapters will give some clear idea.

CHAPTER II

LAMBA LEGEND AND HISTORY

History and Myth

THE earliest reference which we can trace to the Lamba people is contained in the journal of Dr Francisco José Maria de Lacerda e Almeida,[1] who wrote on September 21, 1798:

> The Caffres say that on both sides of and near the high road are small villages. They also assured me that to northward lies the Uemba [2] nation, between the Muizas [3] and the Mussucuma,[4] who reach the banks of the Chire [5] or Nhanjà.[6] Also they assure us that the Uemba and the Mussucuma are mortal enemies to, never sparing, the Cazembe's [7] people; but they are equally so with the Muizas, whom they know by their combed heads. On the south are the Arambas [8] and the Ambos,[9] peaceful friends of the Cazembe, who trade, they declare, with the Caffres near Zumbo.[10]

Reliable Lamba history does not go very far back, and we are glad to have such a reference as this given by Lacerda. On questioning the old people one finds very quickly that historical data merge into legend, and legend into pure myth, and I therefore give an account of the generally accepted myths and legends of the past before recording the sparse historical data I have been able to collect.

Luchyele

If one asks a Lamba to speak of the beginnings of Lamba history he invariably goes back to the coming of Luchyele. In a later chapter [11] will be discussed Lamba beliefs in theism and cosmogony

---

[1] Cf. *The Lands of Cazembe, Lacerda's Journey to Cazembe in* 1798, translated by Captain R. F. Burton (John Murray, London, 1873), pp. 98 and 99.

[2] The Aŵaŵemba of North-eastern Rhodesia.

[3] The Aŵaŵisa of North-eastern Rhodesia.

[4] The Ŵasukuma of Tanganyika Territory.

[5] Shiré river.   [6] Lake Nyasa.

[7] Kazembe was chief of a section of the Lunda people living in the area between Lakes Mweru and Bangweulu.

[8] The Aŵalamba.

[9] Evidently the Aŵenambo or Aŵenambonshi.

[10] At the junction of the Loangwa and the Zambesi rivers. It is well known that the Lambas went on trading expeditions to the Nsenga country.

[11] Chapter XIV.

and their conception of Lesa, the deity. It is but necessary here to note that the Lambas believe that Lesa visited the earth in the beginning under the name of Luchyele.

Luchyele is said to have come from the east, 'arranging' the whole country, rivers, hills, anthills, trees, and grass. He came with numbers of people, planting the tribes and communities in their respective places, and passed on to the westward.[1] Curious markings on the sandstone in the Itabwa plain, not far from Chiwala's village and Ndola township, are pointed out as being the footprints of Luchyele and his people as they passed. It is said that the stones then were soft like mud, but that as soon as Luchyele had passed the mud hardened, and the marks have thus been preserved ever since.

Chipimpi

In those early days the people had no chief, and they were but few in number. But when they began to increase there came a superior man from the west country whose name was Chipimpi.[2] He was accompanied by his sister Kaŵunda Shimanjemanje, who is credited with having obtained seeds by stratagem. There were no seeds or cultivated vegetables in her country, and so she journeyed with her son to the Lualaba river [3] in the Luba country, and was well received by the chief there. The Luba people cultivated their gardens, and Kaŵunda used to go and do her share of the work. She let her hair grow very long, and after a while worked it up like a great pot hollowed inside, with a small opening on top. As she went out to plant the seeds in the chief's garden she would take seeds of every type, maize, sorghum, millet, pumpkin, etc., and throw them into her hollow headgear, until it was quite full. Her son did the same, and used to beg seeds to roast or fry, and store these in his headgear. They then returned to their own country.

So Chipimpi, with his sister and their households, came to the

[1] A recent addition to this account states that he instructed the communities to plant their corn and, when they had reaped a harvest, to follow after him. But they were too lazy, and stayed where they were. Those, however, who did obey reached a great river (? the sea), where Luchyele washed them white and gave them great wisdom and much wealth from out the water.

[2] See the interesting variant to this myth given by me in *Bantu Studies*, vol. i, No. 3. The name of Kaŵunda is attributed to several persons in early legend.

[3] There is one other reference in Lamba folklore to the Lualaba river; *cf.* my *Lamba Folk-lore* (American Folk-lore Society Memoir, No. XX, 1927), p. 165. These references to a river otherwise unknown to the Lamba people suggest that in the past they may have known that river, and that their route of migration may have lain in that direction.

THE LAMBAS OF NORTHERN RHODESIA

Lamba country, far superior in their knowledge of foodstuffs. The people of the country had no proper food; they ate what leaves and roots they could find in the bush.

Chipimpi and his sister prepared gardens and sowed the seeds they had brought. This so astonished the people that when the crops were reaped word went round, *Ifyakulya kwipanga! Twendeni, tukapoke kumfumu!* "There is food at the royal village!

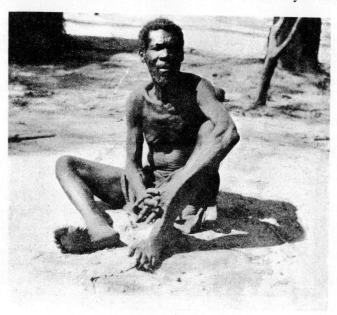

FIG. 14. TYPICAL OLD LAMBA
Photo by Miss O. C. Doke

Let us go and receive from the chief!" The possession of food had become the sign of chieftainship. Thereafter Chipimpi became known throughout the country as chief of the Lambas. He was also credited with introducing the fire-sticks (*ulushiko* and *ichipantu*).

Now Chipimpi had a son, whose name was Kaŵunda. One day, when Chipimpi's people were building a grain-store, every one was called upon to assist in the plastering. When the plastering was done *inshima* (porridge) was prepared by the chief for his people to eat. He also brought a goat (*imbushi*), so that his son and nephew might wash themselves in its blood. His nephew washed off the mud in the goat's blood, but Chipimpi's son,

32

Kaŵunda, refused to follow his example. He had set his heart on washing in the blood of a man, having been urged to do this by his mother. So Chipimpi gave him a slave, saying, "Here is a slave, he will help you with your work." Kaŵunda picked up his hoe, slew the slave, and bathed in his blood. Then he said, "Now we are *aŵenamishishi* [hair clan people], for we have killed a man with the hair on his head! But as for you [indicating his father and his

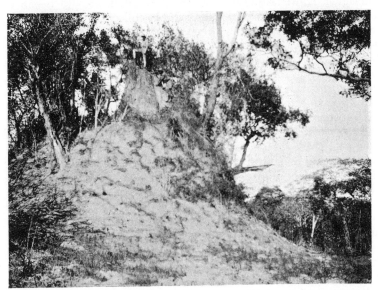

FIG. 15. AN ICHYULU ANTHILL
Photo by the Rev. W. H. Doke

cousin], you are *aŵenambushi* [goat clan people], for you bathed in the blood of a goat." And Kaŵunda slew Chipimpi and became chief.

Then Kaŵunda gave orders that the body of his father should be taken up and buried. After the burial the villagers returned home, and were amazed to find Chipimpi sitting outside his house. Kaŵunda then said, "Burn this chief!" Again, when they believed that they had successfully burned the body, on returning to the village they found the skull resting there. Kaŵunda then ordered the skull to be placed in a shrine and thus preserved. And the skull remained where it was put; so the people said, "This is what Chipimpi himself wants: he does not want to be buried, and he does not want to be burnt; he just wants to stay in a shrine."

33

THE LAMBAS OF NORTHERN RHODESIA

Some while after this Kaŵunda began to ill-treat the younger
relatives of Chipimpi who belonged to the goat clan, and their
anger was roused. "It is ours," they said, "which is the chief's
clan! Why should we be treated thus? Let us now kill ourselves! [1] Let us see what will remain! Kaŵunda himself can
remain and the kingdom be his!"

So they all arose and went to the lake of the Mofya clan—the
Akashiŵa Kaŵena-mofya [2]—where they sat down and began to
extract oil from castor-oil beans,[3] and to collect it into calabashes,
bowls, and baskets. They then took all their goods and chattels,
fowls, dogs, etc., and, tying themselves together with one long rope,
threw themselves into the lake. A member of the leopard clan
was the last on the line, and at the last moment he seized a knife,
severed the rope in front of his wife, and cast her on to the bank.
The woman screamed hysterically (so goes the native legend), but
her husband took her away to the village, and she became the
mother of all the present aŵenambushi. Thus did the human-
hair clan wrest the chieftainship from the goat clan.

But Chipimpi's head was not quite so easily disposed of. The
children of Chipimpi beat out new bark-cloth to wrap around
the head, to preserve it in its shrine, but in the morning they
found the cloth split. And one said, "Father's calico is already
perished! Let us go and beat another piece, that Father may
stay in it!" And this they did; and even in the present day it
is said that they still continue to beat out cloth for Chipimpi's
head.

The shrine with Chipimpi's head is said to be near Kashise's
village in the Congo, near the source of the Kafulafuta river. The
Lambas reverence the head very greatly, and look upon it as an
oracle of the tribe. If some evil is committed the head is said to
become annoyed, leave its shrine, and go bounding away into the
bush! The regular keeper [4] of the shrine, umwinamulenda, then
follows it out into the bush and calls for it, whereupon it appears

[1] Suicide is often preferred by Lambas to humiliation.
[2] Now often called the Akashiŵa Kaŵenambushi, 'Lake of the Goat Clan
People.' It is a beautiful rectangular lake, situated about 50 miles west of
Kashitu railway-station. The length is about 400 feet, the width 300 feet, and
the depth has recently been sounded at 350 feet. Apart from the legend given
here, the lake is shrouded in mystery and pregnant with native superstition.
An account of some of these beliefs is given in *Lambaland* for July 1917. The
term *mofya* is derived from the verb *ofya*, to entangle, as these people entangled
themselves with the rope.
[3] Castor-oil plants are to this day found growing around the lake. It is by
no means clear why the people extracted the castor-oil.
[4] Chyandashika is the present *umwinamulenda* of this shrine, and is living
at the village of Chyasoŵakana.

34

seated on a stump. On being assured that the evil will be dealt with, and on being presented with gifts, the head consents to return to its shrine.

History

It has been extremely difficult to collect accurate genealogical tables of the Lamba chiefs. Different informants give entirely

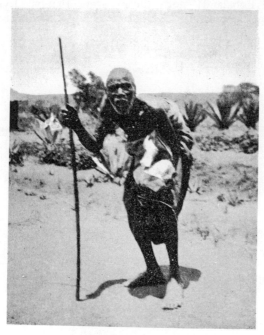

FIG. 16. OLD NSAKA
Photo by Miss O. C. Doke

different sets, and to add to the confusion various chiefs and members of their families have more than one name, being known by one in one area and by another in another. Absolute verification has been impossible in several cases. As an instance of this, Mulilakwenda, the mother of Mushili I, is also known as Kaŵalu and as Nkonde.

Despite their uncertainty in some details, the tables of Lamba and Ŵulima chiefs given (pp. 40 and 41) will not be without their interest and value. It will be seen at once from these that the succession is from chief to brother or to sister's son: this is

35

THE LAMBAS OF NORTHERN RHODESIA

necessary because of the matrilineal clan succession, which will be discussed in Chapter XII.

Chipimpi and Kaŵunda are regarded as the first Lamba chiefs; then there is a gap, no doubt of considerable length, before we come to the definitely historical names, though one informant [1] would run the lists continuously. The list of historical chiefs soon splits up into those reigning over Ilamba Lyachinkumba (Congo Lambaland) and those over Ilamba Lyaŵusenga (Rhodesian Lambaland). The list of chiefs, then, is as follows:

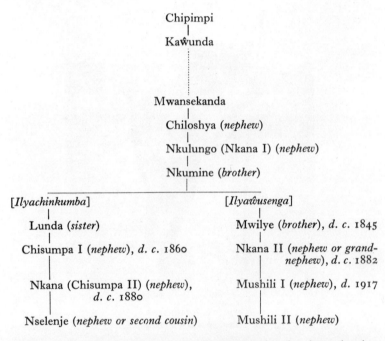

```
                         Chipimpi
                            |
                         Kaŵunda
                            ⋮

                        Mwansekanda
                            |
                      Chiloshya (nephew)
                            |
                   Nkulungo (Nkana I) (nephew)
                            |
                      Nkumine (brother)
                            |
```

[Ilyachinkumba]	[Ilyaŵusenga]
Lunda (sister)	Mwilye (brother), d. c. 1845
Chisumpa I (nephew), d. c. 1860	Nkana II (nephew or grand-nephew), d. c. 1882
Nkana (Chisumpa II) (nephew), d. c. 1880	Mushili I (nephew), d. 1917
Nselenje (nephew or second cousin)	Mushili II (nephew)

Some accounts attribute to Mwansekanda the introduction of seeds and cultivation, which is more properly put down to Chipimpi, the first chief. Chiloshya, Mwansekanda's nephew, who succeeded him, is credited with introducing weapons to the Lamba people.

Nkumine

Lamba remembrance of Nkumine as a chief is not very happy. They say that he would not cultivate, but continually seized the

---

[1] Old Nsaka, who knew Mwilye and Nkana very intimately.

36

foodstuffs of other people. Without any provocation he harassed his people, confiscated their food, and transferred it to his own grain-houses. Many of his people he sold as slaves to the Mbundu traders from the west coast for calico, guns, and powder. It was during his chieftainship that the true Lamba territories, at present those of Nselenje and Mushili, became divided. The story goes that the chief's sister Lunda married a *lumbwe* (consort) named Kalyaŵune. This man belonged to the honey-guide clan.

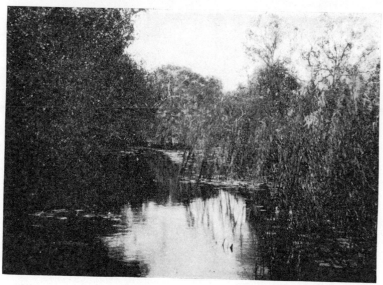

FIG. 17. THE ITABWA RIVER
Photo by C. M. Doke

Kalyaŵune slew Lunkeshi, an *umwinamishishi*, a member of the reigning clan. Thereupon Lunda fled by night with her consort to the present Congo Lambaland. She then tried to go to the Ŵemba territory across the Luapula, but Nkumine, usually referred to as Nkana, besought his sister to remain on the western side of the Luapula, within Lamba territory, and he, her younger brother, would pay the death-price for the murder committed by Kalyaŵune. Lunda thereafter became a great chieftainess, and Kombo, who had been chief of that country, became subservient to her. Thus it was that two great chiefs reigned in Ilamba at one and the same time, and the chieftainship has been divided ever since.

37

Chisumpa

The chieftainship of Chisumpa is marked by two events, the great famine which followed a visitation of locusts and the war with the Chikundas.

The people had sowed their foodstuffs, and when the pumpkins and maize were ripening there came great swarms of locusts, com-

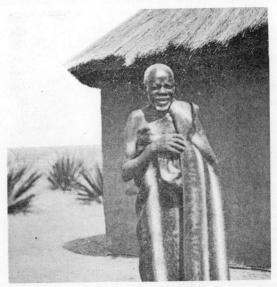

FIG. 18. KATANGA ARRAYED IN THE GLORY OF A NEW BLANKET
Photo by C. M. Doke

pletely destroying the crops, eating, so the people say, even the roots. Then came the *insala yachipumpula*, a terrible famine, when people boiled leaves of ordinary trees and tried to subsist thereby, some even trying to eat grass. Very many people perished. Chisumpa sent many people to buy food in the Aushi country, but the food was insufficient for those who went, and many of them died. It was principally those who remained in Ilamba who survived the famine.

When Chisumpa lived on the Chimeto river, a tributary of the Luapula, there came into the country Chikunda adventurers from the Lower Zambesi, elephant-hunting. It is said that they came to Chisumpa with guile, pretending to form a friendship (*uŵulunda*). But Chisumpa was more than equal to them in suave

38

dealing. Under cover of the friendship they induced Chisumpa to give a meal-offering to the spirits and pray for their success in elephant-hunting, "for," they said, "Chisumpa, these forests are your garden!" They were successful, and took back to their country much ivory. So impressed were they with Ilamba as an elephant country that they returned in force to stir up a quarrel with Chisumpa and take the land. They dug a trench around their camp and fortified the place, and then sent to Chisumpa demanding ten baskets of meal and ten slaves. Chisumpa refused, and said, "If you want war you will get it!" The Chikundas called on Chisumpa to come and hold a palaver. He sent a slave to speak with them. This roused the Chikundas, who left their fortification and went to attack Chisumpa's village. Chisumpa had had time to summon his men, whose guns outnumbered those of the attackers, and in the fight many Chikundas were killed. The remnant fled to those who had remained in camp and else-where, and again came to attack Chisumpa. This time Chisumpa did not wait for them. He poisoned water and foodstuffs; and the few who survived fled from the country. Chisumpa gained considerable spoil in guns and tusks.

There are still a few scattered families of Chikundas living in Ilamba. Mukakangoma, a half-caste Portuguese-Chikunda, now a petty village headman in Lesa's country, originally came to the country after these disturbances with goods to buy slaves, but owing to debts and eventually to the coming of the white man he remained in the country and lost all his slaves.

At the time of Chisumpa natives say that the Amapundi (Ngoni) fought with the Lala people, but did not get as far as Lambaland.

When Chisumpa was near to death, and suffering from lung trouble, Kalachilimuka, who afterward became Mushili I, then a youth, sent a man to Chisumpa to beg for some of the poison with which he had defeated the Chikundas. Chisumpa refused to give it unless Mushili came himself, but Mushili feared he might be killed, as he was an heir to the chieftainship and Chisumpa might want some one else to die with him. Shortly afterward Chisumpa died. This must have been about 1860.

Nkana

Chisumpa was succeeded by Nkana, whom he had nominated as his successor. He was often called by the name of Chisumpa, and was chief until about 1880.

LAMBA CHIEFS

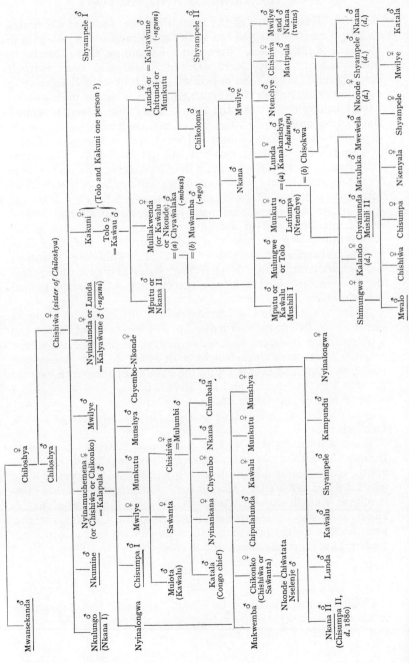

LAMBA LEGEND AND HISTORY

Meanwhile in Ilamba Lyaŵusenga another Nkana had succeeded the old chief Mwilye, who died about 1845. Old Nsaka used to call this Nkana *Nkana wachibwela*, "Nkana returned," meaning Nkana II.

ŴULIMA CHIEFS

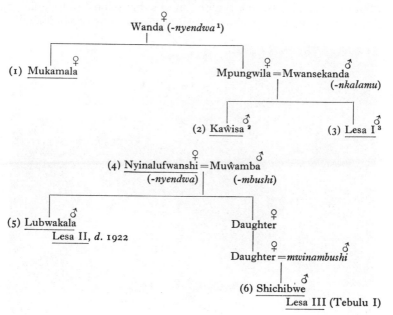

Mushili

Nkana II died about the year 1882, and was succeeded in the chieftainship by his nephew Mputu, otherwise known as Kalachilimuka and Kaŵalu. Mputu took the name of his predecessor Nkana, and kept that name until, out of courtesy to the Congo-despot, he took the title of Mushili.

About the year 1885 the great Yeke despot of the Garenganze, whose headquarters were at Mwenda, in the Belgian Congo, sent an expedition into Ilamba. The leader of the expedition was Chimfumpa. At that time many people fled from the country.

---

[1] Here and elsewhere I have indicated the roots of the clan names of certain individuals. For an explanation see Chapter XII.

[2] Kaŵisa successfully fought the Ŵaluunda, who retreated.

[3] Lesa I successfully fought Chimfumpa (sent by the Yeke chief Mushili), who made a treaty entailing the equal division of tusks when an elephant was killed. Chimfumpa built a walled village at the Musangashi river, where he lived for some time. Lesa I left no heir, and Nyinalufwanshi " came from the west."

41

Katanga, the chief on the Kafulafuta, fled to the Lenje country
with many of his people, while other chiefs submitted to the
despot. Lesa, the Wulima chief, resisted and was undefeated;
he made an agreement with Chimfumpa under which they divided
the ivory equally. Mputu was one of those who submitted to
Chimfumpa, and "drank the potion of submission" to his master
Mushili by surrendering two female slaves and one *impande* shell.[1]

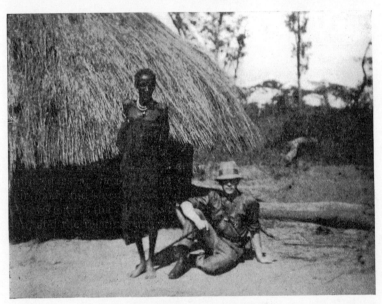

FIG. 19. MUSHILI I AND THE AUTHOR
Photo by the late Rev. J. J. Doke

Mushili of the Garenganze, otherwise known as Mwenda, in
accepting Mputu's submission permitted him to take his name,
which is now the established name of the paramount chief of
British Lambaland.

In February 1893 was published in the *Geographical Journal* a
paper by Joseph Thomson, which he had read before the Royal
Geographical Society in November 1892, entitled "To Lake
Bangweolo and the Unexplored Region of British Central Africa."
With two companions, James A. Grant and Charles Wilson, he had
travelled from Lake Nyasa with a large number of carriers, and
reached the village of "Mshiri" on the Katunga river, near the

---

[1] Though some say he paid fifty elephant tusks.

Lunsenfwa, on November 4, 1890. His carriers had brought with them the smallpox, and of this Thomson wrote:

> On the tenth day I got back to Mshiri's, and not a moment too soon, for the smallpox had spread to the village, and among the victims was the son of the chief. Regretting sincerely that Mshiri's hospitality should have cost him so dear, we hurriedly completed our preparations, and on November 18 commenced the long return journey to Nyasa.

Thomson gives a vivid glimpse of those unsettled slave-raiding days. Of his entrance into Southern Ilamba he says:

> It was more unpleasant to discover that we were once more within the pestiferous sphere of influence of the slave-raiding half-caste Portuguese from Zumbo.[1] We hear much of the ravages of the Arabs on the Congo. I should like, if circumstances permitted, to describe to you the ghastly work carried on by men with European blood in their veins, which has spread death and desolation over many thousand miles of the Zambezi basin. We had soon unpleasant evidence of the reputation the Shakundas, as they are called, had acquired. Invariably we were assumed to be of the same race, and to be engaged on the same bloody mission. Our appearance was the signal for the usual frenzied war-cry, the gathering of excited warriors, and the flight of terror-stricken women and children.

Natives who speak of the visit of these three white men say that they brought a British flag to Mushili's village. In those days the village was near the Lunsenfwa, where the present *imilyashi* (burial-places) of the chiefs are. They remember these men by the names of Mangalaŋanda, Chyochyaŵukala, and Mwenye.

Their arrival was followed by a scourge of smallpox (*ichingwali*), which carried off numbers of people. This again was followed by a failure of the food-crops, and many died of famine. The Lambas called this famine *munshyumfwa-mupopalo*, for whenever they heard a chopping the people would gather to see if there were anything to eat. They ate unripe fruit, and used the famine food *akalembwe-lukasu* as their staple *inshima*.

In 1892 the country was again stricken, this time by locusts (called by the Lenje *ichisoshi*). So bad was the famine that great numbers of the people emigrated into the Lenje country and lived under the chief Chipepo for a considerable time. Of those who remained only a few survived.

In 1895 began the contact of the Lambas with the Swahili slave-

---

[1] That is, the Chikundas.

traders under Chiwala.[1] Chiwala, as he was known to the Lambas, or Majariwa, as he was known on the east coast, was a Yao, born about 1840. He had been a slave, but had scraped together sufficient wealth to purchase his freedom. Possibly the slow process of buying his freedom in accordance with the laws of Islam developed that trait of frugality which ofttimes made him very niggardly. A young Arab, speaking of him, once said, "He is so 'near' that he will save a fowl's feathers to make soup therefrom, and skin a louse to sell its hide." Eventually Chiwala, who had been the skipper of a dhow on the east coast, collected together a quantity of trade goods, and with several native traders set out westward. Chiwala became leader of the expedition, as he possessed most of the carriers and guns. It is estimated that the expedition was some seven hundred guns strong, and each man carried a load of trade goods besides his muzzle-loader. They had with them nine flags, embellished with Koranic texts and other charms.

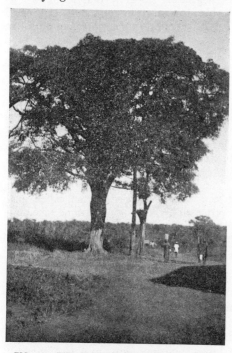

FIG. 20. THE SLAVE TREE AT NDOLA, REMINISCENT OF THE RAIDS
Here slaves were sold.
Photo by Miss O. C. Doke

During the march westward the parties began to separate, going off to various chiefs to trade. After several months' travel Chiwala, at the head of about three hundred and fifty guns, reached the Lamba country. He came to trade for slaves and ivory, and the tariff of exchange was as follows:

---

[1] For my information concerning Chiwala I am indebted to a most interesting article in the *Bulawayo Chronicle*, 1913, written by ' Chirupula '—J. E. Stephenson—entitled " Chiwala, Trader and Raider, a Northern Rhodesia Warrior," which Mr Stephenson has courteously allowed me to quote.

28 yds. of calico, or 1 gun and 1 barrel of powder and caps
$$= 1 \text{ boy or } 1 \text{ woman.}$$

12 to 20 yds. of calico   = 1 man (for he might escape).

200 yds. of calico   = 50 lb. of ivory.

48 yds. of calico, or 2 guns and 2 barrels of powder and caps
$$= 1 \text{ girl.}$$

It is alleged that, on a pretext of obtaining from neighbours a vast store of buried ivory for the traders, the Lambas induced Chiwala to hand over his goods, and then treacherously informed him that they intended to keep the goods and take the lives of the traders.[1] The Lambas had meanwhile built stockades and assembled in great numbers. At this juncture the notorious Chipembere, another of the leaders of the traders, who had been similarly treated by the Lambas, arrived, and at once advised an attack. All the other leaders, similarly duped, came together, and the Lambas were attacked and fled. Chiwala declared that he would not return east until he had got back his goods. 'War' after 'war' was fought, the first against Chilasa, the second against Nkunka, the third against Nkana.[2] The Mohammedan guns executed a great slaughter among the Lambas. The fourth 'war' was against Lilanda, who fled to the top of Chibwe (a huge rock near Chinsenda station), where Chipembere took ample revenge. The fifth 'war' was against Lumina, who sued for peace, and, paying over to the Wanyinasala, as the Lambas called the Swahili slavers, fourteen head of cattle, induced them to make the sixth and seventh 'wars' against Shiwiyungu and Mutofwe. The eighth 'war' was against Mtewa. Two more 'wars' were fought, against Ntututwe and Myele-myele.

The eleventh 'war' was fought in resisting the Belgians, headed by two white officers known to the natives as Kasekele and Kaseya, who were surprised and fled, leaving 200 native soldiers and much booty behind. The twelfth 'war' was against Chinama, Chitumbi, Kalasa, Mushili, Chyongo, Chimese, and others, who built themselves a big stockade on the Luapula river and asked Chipembere (who was now looked upon as Chiwala's fighting general) where he was going. For answer he and his men stormed the stockade, with great slaughter. The thirteenth 'war' was against Kalonga. Saidi bin Abdullah and Mulilo retired from this fight, but Chipembere had a repeating rifle, and himself killed thirty people that day. Then the Lambas broke through their own stockade, fleeing the

---

[1] This is the Swahili version, and is probably exaggerated. The Swahilis saw a quicker way of obtaining slaves and ivory than that of trade.

[2] West of the Kafue.

45

dreadful carnage, but the Mohammedans posted outside put to death 150 of the fugitives. There were other fights, but the preceding thirteen have been designated by the title of 'wars.'

Chipembere acknowledged that at this time "the Lambas were like the leaves of the forest" in number. The fighting spread

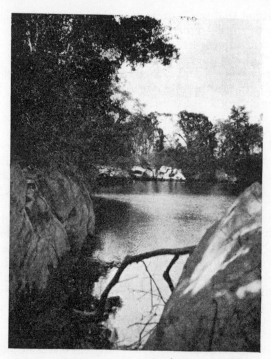

FIG. 21. A CORNER OF THE AKASHIŴA KAŴENA-MOFYA
Photo by C. M. Doke

over several years, and many thousands were slain, and great numbers of youths and girls captured as slaves.

Having subdued a chief, Chiwala's policy was to levy tribute in ivory, and great numbers of tusks passed through his hands every month. Sometimes in one morning as many as twenty tusks would be brought in. Then big parties would set out for Tete, carrying ivory, and return with guns, powder, cloth, and goods. With such wealth, Chiwala's people lived in a most extravagant fashion, until the ivory began to get scarce, the hidden stocks were finished, and Chikunda hunters competed with them.

But the Belgians were not resting beneath the defeat inflicted upon them, and the last war took place at Chiwala's stronghold on the Luapula river, when the Mohammedans were routed and fled from the Congo territory. It was in this fight that Captain Stairs was killed.

After this Chiwala settled down to a more peaceful method of trading, though he could not give up dealing in slaves. The British South Africa Company had sent out Captain Codrington, known as Bwana M'Kubwa, about this time, and Government

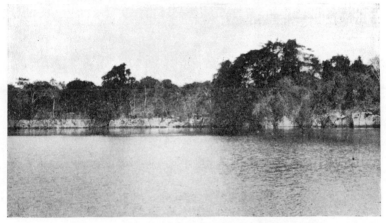

FIG. 22. A GLIMPSE ACROSS " THE JEWEL OF ILAMBA,"
THE AKASHIŴA KAŴENA-MOFYA
Photo by C. M. Doke

officials came to administer the country. Eventually Chiwala was caught red-handed with people tied up in the slave chain, and along with Saidi bin Abdullah, his evil genius, was imprisoned for a period. Thereafter he lived a quiet life, gradually became blind, and died at his village near Ndola in March 1913.

It was just at the close of the century that Bwana M'Kubwa came to the Irume Range with native Ngoni troops. And at that time Mushili removed his village to the confluence of the Myengwe and Mpangamumba rivers. A Government station, or *boma*, had been established at Mwomboshi, on the Lenje-Lamba border. Then in 1900 came the first European trader, Stakes, who traded cloth for rubber.

In 1901 the *boma* was moved to the Manda or Ŵilima river, near the Akashiŵa Kaŵena-mofya. This *boma* was called generally

47

the Kapopo Boma, and was in the Ŵulima country. The Native Commissioner sent was Mr Johnson, who instituted the first taxing in the district; this was in the form of a levy of rubber, or work on the road which was cleared from the Manda to the Mukushi river, *via* Mutofwe and Nkole. At first the natives did not understand what the tax receipts were, and threw them away, complaining that they only received a bit of paper for all their labour. The last rubber tax was levied in 1902.

In 1905 the *boma* was removed, and built by Mr J. E. Stephenson ('Chirupula') at Ndola Yachyani, a site about three miles from the present township of Ndola. The tax was raised from three to five shillings, and in 1910 to ten shillings, at which rate it still stands.

CHAPTER III

TRIBAL ORGANIZATION

Lamba Boundary Disputes

IN Chapter I the territorial divisions of Ilamba were given, showing that the country is divided between the true Lambas of Nselenje and Mushili, the Ŵulimas of Lesa, and the intrusive Kaonde, Lenje, and Lala elements in the territories of Shiŵuchinga, Mukubwe, Nkole, and Chitina. The Lambas and the Ŵulimas are practically one in language, life, and customs, but are under separate headship. There have in the past been numerous boundary disputes, each chief exercising rigorously his rights over his own territory.

The present southern boundary of Mushili's country is the Kafulafuta river, but before the British occupation it lay about fifteen miles farther south, touching on the Nkanga Hills and including the present unoccupied territory from the Nshyaŵala river to the Lwankuni. This territory is now regarded as being Ŵulima, but in the old days it belonged to the group-chief Chiŵombe, whose present representative is Saili. Chiŵombe was a vassal of Mushili, but was also held in renown by the Ŵulima people.

In the past there has been considerable friction over this boundary area, as the following cases will show. The village headman Kalimanama for many years persistently built his village on the south side of the Kafulafuta, cultivating there, and hunting as far as he dared. The Ŵulima people did not themselves inhabit the area, and they feared to assert their claim to it and drive the intruder off. But on the other hand Kalimanama and his sons were also afraid to venture far afield on the Ŵulima side of the river hunting, since the Ŵulimas insisted on their hunting rights.

One day a hunter, Kaluŵe, from one of the Lamba villages on the north side of the river wounded an eland on the south side, followed it up, and eventually killed it not very far from the village of Lumpika, on the Lwankuni river. Lumpika's men confiscated the whole animal, and sent part, as it was royal game, to the chief Malembeka. Kaluŵe took his complaint to his chief, Mushili, who sent an emissary to Lumpika. But Malembeka sent back word to Mushili, "This is our country. You and your people have a large country too. We can give you none of this meat!" And Mushíli had to leave the matter at that.

Chinami, eldest son of Kalimanama, a renowned elephant-hunter, one day killed an eland as far afield as the vicinity of Kalunkumya's village, beyond the Nkanga Hills. Mpupulwa came on the scene and said, "We shall take all the meat to the chief, and you also, to be punished." Chinami said, "No, let me pay you compensation!" So he gave Mpupulwa ten shillings, and was allowed to take away his meat. But Chinami was careful not to hunt again in that direction.

In the old days Nkana's territory extended southward as far as the junction of the Lufwanyama and Kafue (Lufuŵu) rivers, but since the arrival of the white man the triangle south of the Western Kafuŵu river has been given to Lumpuma and his people, who are Ŵulimas from Lesa's country.

Paramounts and Territorial Chiefs

A glance at the map will show that Lambaland proper is cut in two by the international boundary. Nselenje, the present Lamba paramount chief in the Congo, used to be the most influential Lamba chief. At present he is regarded as the chief of his own particular country and that of Chikoloma, his sub-paramount chief. Similarly, in Rhodesian Lambaland Mushili is regarded as para-mount chief over all the Lamba-speaking peoples. In the old days, however, Mushili had less power than Nselenje, and his sub-paramount chief was Nkana. These chiefs used to have no jurisdiction over the people of the Ŵulima, Kaonde, Lenje, or Lala portions of Ilamba. Nkana, however, acknowledged Mushili as his superior, though he was not tribally bound to any service. In case of famine in Mushili's country he would send supplies, as an *umulambu* (offering) and a sign of friendship. Mushili in his turn might act in the same way toward Nselenje.

Group-chiefs of Mushili

We shall now confine our investigations more particularly to Mushili's country. Within this territory there were four group-chiefs of considerable power, Saili, Matipula, Nkambo, and Wasa. Each of these group-chiefs had a number of villages under his immediate jurisdiction.

Saili was the successor to Chiŵombe, who also possessed that portion of disputed land south of the Kafulafuta river. At present Saili's village is situated on the north bank of the river, about eight miles from the Kafulafuta Mission Station. Saili has jurisdiction over a number of villages, which include the following: Katanga, Kacheya, Nkomeshya, Chibweshya, Kalata, Mukungu, and Nsonkomona.

Matipula is situated higher up the Kafulafuta r i v e r, not far to the west of the railway-line.

Nkambo and his villages are grouped about the source of the Kafulafuta river, at the foot of the hills which form the boundary with the Belgian Congo, to the east of the railway-line.

Wasa used to be situated on the Ŵuluŵa river, a tributary of the Upper K a f u e, a b o u t twenty miles north of Kafulafuta Mission Station. Kaŵunda Chiŵele has succeeded W a s a,

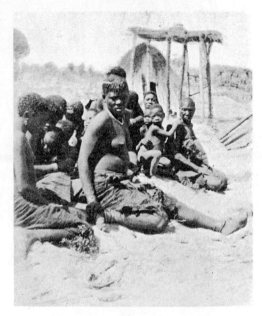

FIG. 23. IN A ŴULIMA VILLAGE
Note the *akapingwe*.
Photo by C. M. Doke

and removed his village southward into the present Ŵulima territory of Malembeka.

Saili, Matipula, Nkambo, and Wasa all acknowledged Mushili's superior chieftainship by sending him meat when animals were killed. Gifts of grain and bark cloth were also sent, but as gifts, never as dues. These group-chiefs were quite independent of any taxation by Mushili.

In case of war, however, Mushili had the right to demand help from them, whereas he could but beg help from Nkana. On the death of one of these group-chiefs, his successor had to send an *umulambu* (offering of servility) of a fowl to Mushili, to announce the death, and later go and present himself to the paramount chief.

51

In law-cases appeal was sometimes made beyond the group-chiefs to the paramount, but Mushili, in order to preserve their dignity, seldom reversed the judgment of the group-chiefs. In

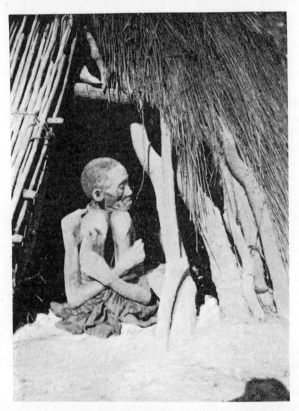

FIG. 24. AN OLD MBWELA WOMAN, A CENTENARIAN,
IN FRONT OF HER INKUNKA
Photo by C. M. Doke

each of these four groups were miniature Mushilis; within their own villages they were paramount. But all villages outside of these four groups, throughout the whole of the Mushili territory, dealt directly with Mushili as their paramount. This was seen, for instance, when an elephant was killed. Both tusks were taken to Saili, Matipula, or one of the others if killed within their immediate territory, otherwise to Mushili himself. The chief chose one tusk, and the hunter took the other and the meat. The chieftainship of the paramount or the group-chief was similarly acknowledged when an eland or a lion was killed. The *akatiŵi* (breast) of the eland belonged to the chief, as did the skin of the lion, though in the latter case the chief compensated the lion-killer with the gift of a slave.

The Dispensing of Justice

These chiefs, the paramount and the four group-chiefs, had power to pass the death-sentence after judging a case. An ordinary village chief or headman, on seeing that a case might involve the death-penalty, would send it on to the group-chief or paramount concerned.

Village chiefs and headmen could settle ordinary cases involving fines, but never pass sentence of death, for the Lambas say *Umwana wambeŵa tatiŵula-chitele*, "A young mouse doesn't pierce the calabash," and a village chief or headman is but a "young mouse" compared to the group and paramount chiefs. The Lambas favour the principle of fines, for they say *Taŵateka-muŵoni sombi umuŵusu*, "One does not enslave a rich man, but a poor!" If, however, the fine cannot be met, the case is sent on to the group-chief, for an ordinary chief cannot impose the penalty of slavery. The group-chief, on hearing the case, might say to the plaintiff, "He is your slave," and the man would be sent to work to pay off his debt, or even sold to the Mbundu traders.

In Ilamba there used to be three main punishments, death, slavery, and fining. Only the third could be imposed by ordinary chiefs. If the accused or the plaintiff were not satisfied with the decision of the ordinary chief, he could appeal to the group-chief, but no further.

Should a man under the jurisdiction of Saili commit murder, and, fearing the consequences, fly to Mushili's village and give himself up there, Mushili would have him thrust into the stocks to await word from Saili. On hearing the evidence Mushili would restore the man to Saili with the advice, "Don't kill him, but fine him heavily!" Should a man of Mushili's similarly escape to Saili or to Nkana, he would immediately be sent back under escort.

Between the Lambas and the Ŵulimas matters were always much more formal. Should a murderer escape from Mushili's country and take refuge in Lesa's, Mushili, on hearing where he was, would send a gun to Lesa, requesting him to seize and restore the man to him. It would be out of the question for Mushili to

53

send armed men into Lesa's country to arrest the man. Should he do so, Lesa would order the arrest of all the men, and Mushili would have to pay heavily for their release. In such a case the murderer would then be protected by Lesa, for "Did not Mushili despise Lesa in sending the men?" Naturally the same procedure would obtain in the case of a murderer escaping from Lesa's country to Mushili's, or between Mushili and Nkole.

In matters of extradition Nselenje would act toward Mushili as Mushili toward Nkana or Saili. In the old days Lamba,

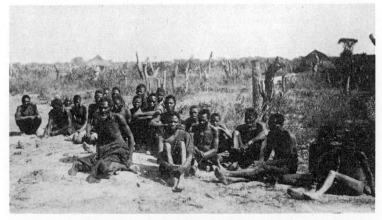

FIG. 25. A GROUP OF LENJE MEN
Photo by C. M. Doke

Ŵulima, and Maswaka territories reciprocated in assisting extradition, but if a man got away to the country of Shiŵuchinga (Aŵenambonshi) or Mukubwe (Aŵenamukuni) he was said to *ililila*, go away for good; his escape was treated as though he had reached Kaonde, Lenje, or Lala country, and there was no chance of procuring his return.

The Origin of Chieftainships

The Lambas say that in the beginning there was only one village in the country. When the chief saw that his village had grown very big he decided to divide it, and, calling one of his principal men (*ichilolo*), who was not of chief's clan, said to him: "Go and build at such and such a stream, and I shall send you people." He acted similarly with other *ifilolo*, forming villages in various places. At first the chief feared to send men of chief's rank, lest

54

they should get sufficient power to rebel against him. When a goodly number of villages under *ifilolo* had been established, he then began to send men of chief's clan to form their villages. First he sent *imfumu ishyamukoka uchye*, chiefs of small rank, not those in his immediate *entourage*. Such inferior chiefs to-day are Katanga, Senkwe, and others. When sending out these chiefs the paramount chief instructed them where to build, and told them not to exploit the people. "For," said he, "they are not your people. All of you belong to me!"

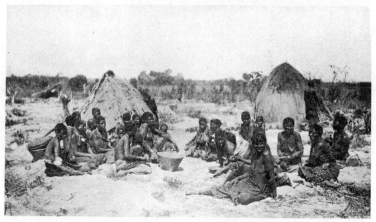

FIG. 26. IN A LENJE VILLAGE—A GROUP OF WOMEN
Photo by C. M. Doke

If the minor chiefs annoyed the *ifilolo* (headmen not of chief's rank), the headmen would complain to the paramount, who would send others of chief's rank to expostulate with them and threaten them.

Later on, when he saw that the inhabited parts of his country were getting thickly populated, the paramount began to send *imfumu shyawuleme*, chiefs of renown, such as Chiŵombe and Wasa, saying to them, "Go and look after those people. Such and such villages are yours. I have given them to you."

Village Distribution

The foregoing account explains the existence of villages of varying standing in the community. There are three main types of villages:

55

THE LAMBAS OF NORTHERN RHODESIA

(1) *Umushi wamfumu*, a chief's village, the headman over which is a man of chief's clan, an *umwinamishishi*. Of these there are three grades, (*a*) the group-chief, such as Saili, (*b*) *imfumu yaŵuleme*, a prominent chief, such as Ntenchye, and (*c*) *imfumu ichye*, a minor chief, such as Katanga.

(2) *Umushi wamuchyete*, a commoner's village, the headman over which is an *ichilolo*, a prominent man, but a commoner. Such villages are Chisachyuni and Kombe.

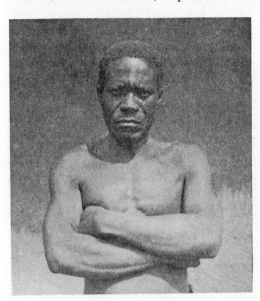

FIG. 27. NSENSENTA, A LAMBA HEADMAN, WHO HAS SUFFERED FROM SMALLPOX
Photo by C. M. Doke

(3) *Ichipembwe*, under the headship of an *umwinamulenda*, a commoner who has succeeded a member of the chief's clan. The Lambas say, *Walya amata amfumu*, "He has eaten [inherited] the weapons of a chief!"

Generally the *imishi yaŵachyete* are larger than the *imishi yamfumu*, because many people prefer the headship of a commoner, who does not 'lord' it over them or oppress them as does a member of the proud *aŵenamishishi*.

The most important *imishi yamfumu* in Mushili's country are the following: Mushili, Ntenchye, Tolo,[1] Muchyenda,[1] Chyembonkonde,[1] Chilenga,[1] Nkambo, Chishiŵanamwansa,[1] Matipula, Kaŵundachiŵele, Kaŵundakasopa,[1] Kampasu,[1] Senkwe,[1] Mukumbi,[1] Katanga,[1] Nsonkomona, Saili, Mutyoka, and Maŵote.[1]

The following are a few representative names of *ifilolo* in Mushili's country: Chisachyuni, Chimbalasepa, Kombe, Masombwe, Kalata,[2] Kachyeya,[2] Kaŵalu,[2] Nsensa, Nsensenta, and Lwembe.

[1] These names are those of minor chiefs ; all the others are *imfumu shyaŵuleme*, and include the paramount and the four group-chiefs.
[2] These are also *aŵenamilenda*.

56

Ifipembwe

The *ifipembwe* are the villages in which are the *imilenda* (shrines with relics) of the paramount and group-chiefs. The *aẁenamilenda*, keepers of the shrines, are *ifilolo* who are headmen of the *ifipembwe*. In Rhodesian Lambaland there are seven *ifipembwe*. The paramount chief Mushili has two, while Nkana, Saili, Wasa, Matipula, and Nkambo each have one. The Ẁulima chiefs do not have *ifipembwe*.

Mushili's *ifipembwe* are Kaẁalu and M̦wema (Lyala), Wasa (Kaẁundachiẁele) has Kachyeya, Saili has Kalata, Nkana has Kampundu, Matipula has Shichyuẁa, while Nkambo has no other *ichipembwe* than his own village.

According to Lamba custom, the *ichipembwe* seems to be a kind of city of refuge. A man who has committed theft, murder, adultery, or some other serious offence, and is pursued by the avenger, will attempt to fly to an *ichipembwe*. The pursuer,

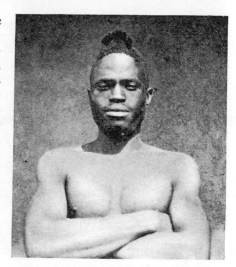

FIG. 28. NDELEMETI, A ẀULIMA
Photo by C. M. Doke

even if he be a chief, will stand without the *ichipembwe*, at some distance. Within the village the fugitive is now caught, secured, and taken before the group-chief for trial. His taking sanctuary has saved him from summary justice at the hand of the avenger. After his trial, "if he is fortunate," they say "he will be fined, for he fled to sanctuary, and we cannot kill him." If the offence is very serious, the fugitive will be bound at the *ichipembwe*, and the chief will come there to try him. Should he sentence him to death, the *umwinamulenda* will carry out the sentence at the *ichipembwe*, and set up the criminal's head outside the village.

Impemba

The paramount chief does not depend upon himself to decide in every case brought before him, nor in every emergency. He

57

has certain councillors, who are called *impemba*. These men, usually four or five, are chosen by the chief himself, and a wise chief chooses men who in his eyes have outstanding ability in counsel. The *impemba* are of varying clan, but always commoners. In 1913 Mushili I had as councillors Nsensa (*-mbushi*), Kachyule (*-ẁesa*), Chimbalasepa (*-ẁesa*), and Masombwe (*-ngo*). Later Shiẁata took the place of Nsensa.

The difference between an *impemba* and an *ichilolo* was given

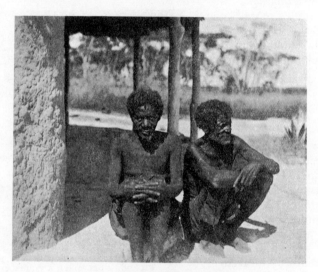

FIG. 29. LUNTANTWE AND AN IMPEMBA
Photo by C. M. Doke

me as this! *Impemba eupembelele'mfumu, ichilolo eupembelele'mishi nechyalo,* "The councillor is one who waits on the chief; the headman is one who waits on the villages and country." The *impemba* always attend the chief as councillors, while the *ifilolo* are his executive officers, to look after the villages and the country.

The present Mushili II has two councillors, Soloshi (*-ẁesa*) and Mukolwe (*-mbushi*), as well as certain other village elders to be called in for advice.

Chiefs have at times resorted to tests in order to prove the ability of their *ifilolo* and *impemba*. For instance, when an eland has been brought to the chief he has been known to call one of his men and say, "*Kalama* [attendant], I want you to cut

58

up this meat ; some take to your house, the rest to mine, and we alone shall eat of it." If he does this there is very soon a chorus of grumbling in the village, and the chief will dismiss him, saying, "He has no sense. Had he sense, he would have said to me, 'No, sir, how shall we eat this meat alone, when the chief's people in this village are many, and all the children too belong to the chief?' Call to me a wise councillor to give me advice!" The chief expects advice, not servile obedience, from his councillors.

Imilambu

In Ilamba there was never any regular tribute paid by the people to the chief. The villagers near the paramount chief would help him with new garden work (*ukukusya'maŵala*), and those who came in to have a case settled or bring a suit would have to do some work for the chief first, and have their cases attended to afterward. , Even Mushili himself, when he gave in to the Yeke despot, did not have to pay regular tribute, but paid a surrender price of two female slaves and one shell.[1]

Nevertheless, in Ilamba is recognized the principle of the *umulambu*, or gift of respect. A village headman will call his people and say, "A long time has now gone by. I want you to thresh out some corn to take *kwipanga* [to the chief's village], that I may go and visit the chief." When the corn is ready three women maybe will carry baskets of corn, and, arriving, set them down in the chief's courtyard. The headman will say to the chief, "We have come to visit you. We have brought food." After greeting him the chief will set a meal before the headman, and when it is time for the headman to return to his village the chief will give him a length of calico as a return gift.

This used to be done occasionally by all headmen, *impemba*, and village chiefs. Foodstuffs such as sorghum, maize, beans, and ground-nuts were taken, but never fowls. Although the paramount chief made a counter-gift of cloth, that was not looked upon as an *umulambu*, for the *umulambu* is an offering made by an inferior out of respect to his superior.

To the native mind there is a tremendous difference between the *umulambu* which they paid to their chief and the *umusonko*, the tax now levied by the European authorities. The *umulambu* was always voluntary, and was made at such times as the headman desired to pay his respects, but the *umusonko* is compulsory, and must be paid at stated times.

[1] The *impande*, which is worn only by big chiefs.

59

War-service

At time of war the paramount chief would summon certain of his outstanding *ifilolo*, of known physical strength and proven courage, to act as captains over his bands of fighting men (*ifita*). These captains were then called *ifilolo fyafita*. The Lambas knew of no such thing as a standing army, nor in time of war was conscription practised. It is said that a chief could not compel one of his men to go to fight, and all who joined the *ifita* did so voluntarily. They were stirred up to go by hatred of the enemy, desire for spoil, the instinct to protect their homes, or maybe by a desire for personal renown.

Inheritance of a Chief

On the death of a chief it is his younger brother who inherits the chieftainship, or, failing him, the chief's *umwipwa*, sister's son —that is, a person of the same clan (*umwinamishishi*) as himself. If there is no *umwipwa*, then some other clan relative, nearest of kin in the village, will inherit. This principle is applied to all chiefs, and even with *ifilolo* the heir to a village headship will be one of the same clan as the deceased headman.

As far as can be ascertained, there has never been any quarrelling over succession, as the relationship system is such that all can see at once who has prior claim among those remaining.

Sometimes it happens that when the chief dies his heir has already a village of his own. Both the villages may then be joined together. If the heir has a younger brother he may leave that brother in the less important village, and himself take the name of the dead chief and succeed him. This is called *ukulye'shina lyamfumu ifwile*, eating the name of the deceased chief.

Installation of a Paramount Chief

At the time of the old chief's death his successor is known, and he immediately apportions the wives of the deceased chief, maybe reserving some for himself. Then directly the burial rites of the deceased chief have been completed corn is threshed and beer brewed in the village. The chiefs and headmen of the nearer villages assemble, and then a greater chief comes. In the case of the death of, say, Mushili it would be Nselenje who would come. On the morrow, with all the people sitting round, the great chief sitting on an *ichipuna mwisasa*, a stool set on a mat, and the heir sitting on another stool set on a second mat, the great chief addresses the heir, saying, *Weŵo waikala pachipuna chyamukwanu*, "You have sat on the stool [throne] of your brother!"

Thereupon all commence the 'beer-drink.' The visiting chief is the first to dip out some beer, and this he gives to the new chief as a sign of his authority, saying, *Nebwalwa wemwine twakupela. Uli mukulu wemwine*, "The beer too we have given to you yourself. You yourself are a great one." He then sits down, and the councillors and people all clap their hands. The councillors then advise the new chief to dispense justice as wisely as his predecessor. All thereafter indulge in beer-drinking. This concludes the simple formalities of installing the new chief.

CHAPTER IV

IMILANDU—LAMBA LAW

Isoŵololo Lyamulandu

THE term *umulandu* is used widely among the Central Bantu tribes with much the significance of the Zulu *indaba* or the commonly used term 'palaver'—a conference, debate, discussion, before an authority. But the term *umulandu* goes a good deal further in being applied more especially to the talking over of a lawsuit before a chief, to the lawsuit itself, and hence to the culpability, blame, and punishment of the party concerned. With the Lambas the idea of judging a case is scarcely conceived. The terms *sololola* and *soŵolola* are used, and these terms indicate rather 'to talk over a case.' This is shown by such a common expression as *Twendeni kubwalo tukasolololo'mulandu,* "Let us go to the chief's village and settle [or talk over] the case." The discussion or settling of a case is called *isoŵololo lyamulandu.*

A Case before a Great Chief

Before the chief hears ordinary cases it is usual for the plaintiff, accused, and witnesses to do a morning's work in the chief's gardens.

Should a very serious case, such as one of murder, come before the paramount chief, the chief will send some of his *ifilolo* who live in his village or near at hand to summon his *impemba* (councillors). When all the *impemba* have come the *ichitenje chyesoŵololo* (court of justice) is arranged. Women take no part in an *umulandu* before a great chief, but all the village elders gather and sit around in an informal way. Children are naturally excluded from participation in court proceedings, but as soon as a young man emerges from boyhood and "shows wisdom, ability, and physical strength" he is called by his elders to quit the play of the boys and to join the older men, take his place in listening to the settling of law-cases, and so qualify to give advice. Neither marriage nor parenthood, as with some Bantu tribes, is a necessary qualification for taking part in the settlement of law-disputes before the chief.

Each witness gives his evidence at length, and is seldom interrupted during his recital. Cross-questioning of witnesses is practically unknown among the Lambas, though the accused may protest at times against evidence brought against him. Neither the accused nor the witnesses are put under any form of oath for ordinary cases, though, as will be seen later, the accused may voluntarily strengthen his denial by oath-taking. Ordeals are imposed only in certain cases of witchcraft, never before a chief at an ordinary trial.

The court is usually the open space before the chief's principal hut, and there is no set arrangement of places for the chief, the councillors, the accused, or the accusers. The accusers are first called upon to state the charge. The accused then gives his explanation or denial, and after him the various witnesses give their evidence.

After hearing the evidence from the witnesses the chief sums up the case. "Listen, my people. This accused man met his companion on the path and killed him; it is my desire to have him put to death!" This he says as a 'feeler' to his councillors. "What do you, my *ifilolo*, think on the matter?" There is silence for a space, and then one of the *ifilolo* may reply, "No, sir, to kill him would be bad. Let the man bring *amaẁoni* [property, wealth, or goods], for it is that which has made him drunk, and give some to the chief, and some let him take to the owner [1] of the man he has killed." For a while the chief sits silent; then again he asks the other *ifilolo* for their advice in the matter. Maybe they too concur in the imposition of a heavy fine. The chief will now say, "No. I intend to have him executed!" Now the *impemba* will join with the *ifilolo* in protesting that they will go and leave the chief to carry out such a sentence by himself if he persists. The chief is, of course, expecting this attitude. It is what he desires. So he sends men to arrest the sisters and mother of the accused. When they are brought, some of the women are handed over to the relatives of the deceased as slaves; others are retained by the chief. The women would be taken whether single or married, and should the husband of one of them desire to retain his wife, he would have to hand over a gun to redeem her, in which case his wife would become his slave.

It is seldom that the *ifilolo* and *impemba* agree at once to killing the accused in such a case. Should they do so, the chief would

---

[1] That is, the relative who has inherited the deceased, or, in the case of a child, the maternal uncle.

63

rightly upbraid them for their lack of wisdom, saying, "Now two of my people are dead!"

Sometimes a man will plead with the chief for his life, offering his mother and sisters. The *impemba* will urge the chief to agree to this; and if the man's father cannot redeem the mother, nor the sisters' husbands redeem them, they will be taken and apportioned. The Lambas have a proverb about an orphan which goes, *Ilamba-nanyina liwule nyina lyamulambula*, "He who pays with his mother, if he have not a mother, is himself the payment."

It has been known for a sister, hearing that her brother is before the chief, to go and hand herself over in his stead. The Lambas say that a man who has two sisters feels perfectly safe, for he always has the means of getting out of a scrape. A Lamba will even call his sisters *imfuti shyanji*, "my guns," because of their value in settling dues.

In minor cases the *impemba* alone give advice to the chief, and generally do so privately. In the more important cases village headmen and other *ifilolo* will also be called, and they may even correct the advice given by the *impemba*.

Punishment

Judgments before the paramount chief generally entail one of the following punishments:

(1) Fining in kind—a gun, a tusk, Mbundu [1] beads, or, for smaller offences, cloth or grain.

(2) Enslavement of the convicted person or of some relations in his place.

(3) Death, though this was comparatively rare, except for witchcraft charges (see Chapter XIX). However, the chief's anger may have been roused, and if the man is not wealthy, and so cannot be heavily fined, the chief may order his execution.

In the old days paramount chiefs have been known, when their anger was roused, to order mutilation, without consulting any of their advisers. This was by no means common in Ilamba, but was a custom taken over from the Lenjes. The hand was cut off for stealing and the ears for informing. The chief would call a strong *ichilolo* to bind the accused and carry out the sentence forthwith. When the ears or fingers had been cut off, the former with a sharp knife, the latter with an adze, a female slave of the chief was sent to foment the wound with hot water in order to stop the bleeding, and to put on healing medicines. Mushili I

---

[1] These beads are described at the beginning of Chapter V.

treated quite a number of people in this way, but Chipepo, the Lenje chief, was especially fond of such punishment.

The Wembas put out the eyes for adultery and cut off hands for thieving.

The Ilas cut off the upper lip for informing and the hands for theft.

The Lenjes severed the fingers at the second joint, cut off ears, and in the case of adulterers removed the Achilles' tendon.

The following are some instances. Masaka, of Chilambe's village, near Kashitu, who was living at Chipepo's in the Lenje country at the time of the locust plague, attempted to escape and return to Ilamba. The chief was notified, and said, "Why has Masaka gone off like this, instead of leaving openly by day?" So Chipepo, annoyed, sent men after him, and Masaka was caught and brought back. Chipepo had his ears cut off and his tendons removed, and said, "Now go!" When his wounds had healed he went back to Ilamba. Similar treatment was meted out to Mwanamusoka, of Chibweshya's village, who lost one ear and had his tendons removed.

Lupiya, of Chishye, near Lesa's village, while a child, stole in the Lamba country, and Mushili had his ears cut off as a warning.

Lyambula, of Mpokota's village, committed adultery with a slave-girl belonging to Chipepo. The chief had his fingers all cut off at the second joint and his ears and tendons removed.

Inkole

In order to secure the restoration of articles borrowed or the payment of some due Lambas used to take the law into their own hands and seize a person as a hostage, or at times property as security. A hostage or property so seized is called *inkole*, or *umukole*. Here is an example of this method of obtaining justice.

A. is plaintiff, belonging to Katanga's village, and B. is defendant, belonging to Mpokota's village. The charge is one of borrowing a gun and failing to return it. A. goes to Mpokota and demands from B. his gun; B., who has used it to settle a debt elsewhere, says he has not yet been able to get a gun to replace it. That evening A. seizes a boy from the village and carries him off to Katanga. As soon as it is found out the father of the lad goes straight to B. and says, "It is you who have caused my child to be carried off!" B. very quickly procures a gun and hands it to the father, who goes with it to Katanga's village to redeem his child. On seeing the gun A. restores the child to his father, and gives

65

the child a gift of calico, saying, *Nakusamfyo'mukole pamuŵili*, "I have washed the stigma of a hostage from your body."

Sometimes, because of the distance they are away, men will put off indefinitely the payment of dues. The exasperated creditor calls his wife to prepare meal for a journey, and then, accompanied by three brawny companions, sets out for the delinquent's village. When still some considerable distance away they prepare an *umutanda* (zareba) in the bush, and put their pots of meal therein. They then proceed to another village, arrive as strangers, and ask for a house to sleep in. They are shown a house, but they carefully watch the village children and the weapons of the villagers. Presently, maybe, some of the children call to their companions to go to the river for a bathe. The visitors watch them closely, and then, emerging one by one, follow the children, and at the river or water-hole seize one of the bigger ones. His companions fly in fright. The captors now throw *amawo* (red millet) meal into their captive's mouth to stifle his cries, and carry him off as quickly as possible. The other children carry the news back to the village, and it is at once known that the boy has been captured as an *inkole*. The captors reach their *umutanda*, eat their food, and sleep. Then in the morning they make for home. News gets to the village as to where the captured boy has been taken, and the relatives arrive to inquire the cause. They are told that the boy was captured because of So-and-so's fault. It is now the business of these villagers to demand satisfaction from the defaulting man in the village near theirs. When they bring the goods to the captor of the child he takes a portion and gives it to the *inkole*, who returns home with his relatives. Should men act incautiously when attempting to secure a hostage, the villagers would kill them if they got an opportunity.

Cases before a Headman

Cases of various types are dealt with by the village headman, whether he be of chief's rank or a commoner.

(1) **Stealing.** If boys have been pilfering in the village the sufferer from these depredations will go to the headman and lay a charge against the children. The headman will summon the parents and children, and order the parents to pay such-and-such an amount to the complainant. The parents will pay over the amount, and then themselves punish the children for the trouble they have brought.

(2) **Immoral Interference.** If during the dancing of an

66

akasela dance [1] some of the young men catch the young married women by their breasts, and if the headman is informed of what is going on, he will summon all the young men who were dancing, and warn them strongly, saying, "When you dance the *akasela*, don't you touch another man's wife, for if adultery is committed by one of you he will be killed before his parents' eyes. Beware. I do not want to hear of this thing again in my village. For if the husbands of the women hear, they will go and beat your parents. You had better stop the dancing, for I do not wish to be called to account at the paramount chief's court!"

If news of such behaviour should get to the ears of a husband, the culprit would make off, and the enraged husband would beat the guilty youth's father and mother. They are held to blame for not having brought up their son properly. When the culprit returns, he keeps to himself for some time, and in all probability would be thrashed by his father. Should he not get away in the first place, the husband would beat him unmercifully. If in addition to his offence of immoral interference he should have suggested adultery to the woman, and she, refusing, had reported the matter to her husband, the husband would still have contented himself with administering a severe beating.

(3) **Quarrelling.** People quarrelling violently in the village are brought before the headman, who will say, "You children of mine are not behaving yourselves here in this village. I do not want quarrelling, as quarrelling induces murder!" Such admonition usually has its effect.

(4) **Reviling.** In the same way the headman will admonish a villager for reviling, *ukutukana'matuka*.

Adultery

In the old days, if a man found his wife and her paramour *in coitu* he immediately killed them both, and then went to the paramount chief and confessed what he had done. In reporting such an affair to the chief the man would approach and hold out his gun to the chief, saying, "I have killed a person, sir, I have killed two, my wife and a man. And I have come to tell the chief!" He would then recount to the chief the whole circumstances. And the chief would say, "You are a man!" In the morning, when the people were all gathered, the man would dance his dance of triumph, surrounded by the advisers and officials of the chief. Thereupon the chief would take some red calico

[1] See Chapter XXII.

and put it on him. In such a case neither the relatives of the woman nor of the paramour could take any action, nor is there any need for the casting of meal (see Chapter XI), as this action resembles that of warfare. But the man would go to an *umulaye* and inform him that he had killed his wife, and make a present to him. The 'doctor' would then bring the medicine necessary for driving off the *ichiẅanda* (attendant demon) of the woman. With the animal's tail which he carries as a switch the *umulaye* would sprinkle the man with the medicine, and with other medicine he would cause smoke to envelop his head. This is done by putting medicinal leaves on the fire and holding the man's head in the smoke; thus he is prevented from dreaming of his dead wife. Similar action is taken on behalf of men who have killed enemies in a war. Dreaming of the dead is believed to be a sign that the *ichiẅanda* is coming to kill the person who dreams.

Lambas believe that for adultery seen by the husband he must kill, or else his heart would never settle down. For adultery which has been reported to him he is satisfied with a trial. This explains the dissatisfaction there is over the administration of English law, which demands a trial in either case.

If a husband, after a long absence from home, returns to find his wife *enceinte*, he will demand of her the name of the culprit. If she tries to hide it, he will bind and beat her. Under this treatment she confesses. The husband goes out, and maybe finds the culprit on his guard. He sends a demand for damages, and the co-respondent sends by the elders goods and a gun. This is generally done before the paramount chief, and if the husband is satisfied with the damages proffered he accepts them, and then says, "Let him also bring *uẅuẅoni bwamankumanya* [goods for meeting]!" The man will then in all probability bring an additional ten shillings, as a sign that the stigma of his action is removed, so that he and the aggrieved husband will be able to meet together as though nothing had happened.

In some cases men divorce their wives if they have committed adultery, as they fear that they can never forget the stigma, but such action is rare.

When a husband has received damages from a co-respondent he never keeps them himself, but hands what he has received over to his wife to give to her mother, who in turn passes it on to her brother, the woman's *mwinshyo*. A man never retains 'adultery money'; it always goes to his mother-in-law, for it has come through her daughter. Should he, however, divorce the woman, he would recover that money.

68

At times, after hearing from his wife the name of her paramour, a man will follow the culprit privily, and kill him with an arrow, without saying anything to put him on his guard. Should he do so, he would follow the procedure of reporting to the chief, triumphing, and then being treated by an *umulaye*.

Another treatment is as follows. A man hears that So-and-so has committed adultery with his wife. He reports it to the chief and demands compensation. Maybe he gets a gun, and *amankumanya* in addition, but still he is not really satisfied in the matter. Later he hears that the man concerned has gone on a journey, so he goes to this man's wife, and, intimidating her, outrages her. On the return of her husband the woman informs him of what has taken place, but since he was the original aggressor he can take no action. Such a man has been known to turn in fury on his wife and kill her, thus incurring a murder charge from her relatives.

In 1925 the chief Lesa-waluluma committed adultery with the wife of a man named Makofi. The case was heard by Mushili II, and Makofi secured a gun and ten shillings for *amankumanya*, but he could not rid himself of the hatred in his heart. When Lesa went on a journey Makofi outraged his wife, and on his return Lesa was told of the affair. Lesa could do nothing except drive away the woman. And now it is said that he and Makofi get on very well together.

There is no 'wife-trade' among the Lambas, and they laugh at the Kaondes for lending out their wives to *awalunda* (blood-brothers).

Seduction

Except in the cases of an *imbuli* (immature girl) or a *moye* (girl who has just passed through initiation), a man is not fined for seducing an *umushichye* (any woman not living in wedlock). He is, however, usually ostracized. If he desires to marry such a woman afterward, the marriage can be arranged if he is considered a suitable husband. There is no *umulandu* for such action.

Rape

As will be seen later, rape, carried out in the bush, is a most serious anti-social crime, one to which a man is prompted by an *ichiwanda* (demon). The penalty for such is the death of the man and the enslavement of his sister.

Incest

Incest of every type is with the Lambas a most serious anti-social crime. A man committing such must have been incited thereto by an *ichiŵanda*. The committing of incest entails the breaking of strong exogamic taboo, and it must be remembered that many cases which in Ilamba are regarded as incest would not be so regarded under European systems of kinship. In Lamba incest is called *ishiku*.

(1) *Ishiku lyamuntu nenkashi*, of a man with his sister or a woman in his age-grade bearing his sister's clan name. In such a case the man is driven from the community by the woman's brother, and can never return to it. The woman, if she reports the matter, is not in any way blamed. If both, however, were consenting parties, and the truth came out, as in resulting pregnancy, in the old days they would have been burnt as *imfwiti*, witch and wizard.

The Lambas have peculiar beliefs concerning the result of the marriage of a man who has committed incest. If a man, driven away for such a crime, goeś elsewhere and marries, when the time comes for his wife to give birth the labour is prolonged. At this an *umulaye* is sent for. The doctor questions the husband concerning the reason for his having left his home, and warns him that unless he speaks the truth his wife will die. In fear the man confesses: "It was *ishiku* I committed with my sister!" At this confession the *umulaye* goes for special *umusamu* (medicine); some he gives to the woman in labour and some to the husband. The woman now gives birth. More medicine is procured for the husband to bathe himself in it completely; afterward he gives his wife certain goods as compensation. It is said that some *aŵalaye* agree to hush up the matter, perform the ceremonies secretly, and receive the compensation goods themselves. It is part of the work of an *umulaye* to find out the breaking of taboo. Breaking of taboo is always shown in the sickness of friends or relatives of the culprit. Similar results come when a man has relations with a widow before the death-dues have been paid and she is released for marriage. This breaking of taboo, however, is not termed *ishiku*.

In certain cases when a man has committed incest the fear of the consequences drives him to take his sister and go straight to an *umulaye* to be cleansed and freed from the *ichiŵanda*. After this, though the man will be driven away from his home village, he will be able to marry elsewhere, without fearing any evil consequences.

(2) *Ishiku lyamuntu nawanyina*, of a man with his mother. This is treated as a case of witchcraft. It is not caused by the evil influence of an *ichiŵanda*, for that would have driven him to his sister, a crime less heinous, as the *ichiŵanda* is said to have some *inkumbu*, or pity. In the case of a man committing incest with his mother both man and woman would be burnt.

(3) *Ishiku lyamuntu nemwana umwanakashi*, of a man with his daughter. Here it must be remembered that the clan totems differ, as the girl takes her mother's clan. Nevertheless, she has her father's blood in her. Generally both would be treated as *imfwiti* and burnt, but if the girl were very young she might be spared and taken to the *umulaye* for cleansing.

(4) *Ishiku lyamuntu nemulamu wakwe*, of a man with his wife's sister or one in similar relationship. This used to be no uncommon occurrence, as instanced by the proverb, *Umulamu mulamu pamenso, kafishyoloko'lukolo mukashi*, "A sister-in-law is a sister-in-law in public; when they go behind the house she's a wife!" As soon as such an occurrence, however, is known a hue and cry is raised, and the man hides himself. When he is caught he is made to pay to his injured sister-in-law a gun, and he has then to go to the *umulaye* for cleansing from the baneful consequences. The girl would in such a case hand the gun to her mother.

If the matter were not discovered at the time, both parties, fearing lest the consequences should be shown in sickness, would agree to go privately to an *umulaye* for cleansing, and the affair would be hushed up.

(5) *Ishiku lyamuntu nemwipwa*, of a man with his niece of the same clan as himself. This would be treated as (3), and the man would be put to death in any case as an *imfwiti*.

(6) *Ishiku lyamuntu namukamwinshyo*, of a man with the wife of his maternal uncle. A man is, as a rule, on peculiarly friendly terms with this aunt, and misbehaviour would be treated as witchcraft, and the man killed. A man capable of such behaviour, say the Lambas, is capable of anything. The elder brother of Lifwa, a one-time pupil at Kafulafuta Mission School, was guilty of this, and it was only fear of the white administration that saved him. As it was, he had to give his maternal uncle a gun.

Procedure between Group-chiefs

The following hypothetical case will illustrate the procedure followed when two group-chiefs are affected. A. of Nkambo steals or burns the property of B. of Saili. B. catches and binds

A., and takes him before Saili. Saili asks A. where he comes from, and A. replies, "From Nkambo." Saili instructs B. to go with A. to Nkambo, fifty miles away, and to put a rope round the prisoner's waist. The prisoner, they say, would not attempt to escape, and the shame he would feel in the villages is such that he would refuse food. Nkambo, when he sees one of his people brought in in this ignominious fashion, roundly abuses B. for treating A. "like a dog" instead of merely accompanying him. If Nkambo loses his temper B. will be thrashed. After passions have subsided, and Nkambo has heard the case, he will give B. compensation, and later on A. will have to restore to Nkambo the goods he has handed over. Should the man have been caught redhanded burning the grain-house or other property belonging to B., he would have been killed immediately.

War-challenge

Should a chief, A., think his renown is such that he can make demands upon a distant chief, B., he sends word to B., "If you do not send me an *inkombe* [a present as a sign of submission] we shall fight!" Chief B. calls together all his people, councillors, headmen, and youths to consider the case. He informs them that A. has sent him a demand for submission, and then, in order to test whether his people are courageous or not, he says, "My headmen, I want you to send to him an *inkombe* with slaves male and female!" But his headmen and councillors refuse, saying, "No, sir, that means servile submission. Send him word saying, 'Let him come and let us fight!' and revile [*tuka*] him too!" The chief replies, "My children, it is not well to kill one another." But they reply, "No, sir, but he is the aggressor." The chief, having tested the feeling, says, "It is well. Prepare your arrows throughout the villages! Those who have guns, let them come here and get powder!"

A haughty message is sent back. It is now A.'s turn to consult his advisers, and if he really does not want to fight he himself sets out with three of his *impemba*, and, reaching a near-by village, sends on word announcing his arrival to the chief. Chief B. inquires of the messenger as to the number of men with the visiting chief. On hearing that he has only the three *impemba*, B. knows that the other does not desire to fight. In the morning, when chief A. arrives, they talk the matter over, and, to settle it, A. gives B. a slave.

Sometimes when a haughty reply is to be returned to a challenge a youngster is sent, if the distance is not too great. The youngster on arrival says, "My chief says that to-morrow he will meet you at such-and-such a stream and fight. *Teete teete napankashi yenu!* [1] ['Come and fight, if you don't want to marry your sister!']" On hearing this abuse the chief, disregarding the youngster, calls together his people, and says, "Tighten your bowstrings, for to-morrow we fight." And he sends back the youngster, saying, "If he does not set out quickly, *paliŵanyina* [2] ['It is on his mother']. Go and tell him that!" On getting this reply the chief is roused, and the two parties meet and fight on the morrow.

Hired Assassins

Even as the youngster who carries the insulting challenge is not held in any way blameworthy, so in Lamba law with hired assassins. The Lambas have a proverb *Kamunkomene taŵona mulandu*, "The little one who wounds does not carry the blame." If certain people are sent to kill a man, and when they have done the deed they are brought before the chief, they will say, "O chief, we were sent!" The chief, quoting the proverb, will order the arrest of the man who sent them, and have him put to death. The assassins whom he employed may be lightly fined.

Sundry Cases

(1) **Accidental Homicide.** The unfortunate culprit will, if he can do so, go straight to his paramount chief and tell him that he has killed a man. The paramount will call the relatives of the deceased, tell them that the killing was not intentional, and ask them whether they desire a gun or the sister of the culprit as compensation, warning them not to persecute the man. The culprit would fear to go to the deceased's relations to tell them, lest they should kill him in anger.

(2) **Disrespect to an Elder.** At a 'beer-drink,' if A. tries to start a quarrel with B., one younger or feebler than himself, B., afraid, will go and sit near one of the elders. A. will now fear to touch B. But if he should go and strike him the elder would consider himself affronted, and deal drastically with A., because B. had taken refuge beneath his reputation.

(3) **Harmful Frightening.** If an armed man, for fun, pretends to stalk youngsters while they are playing, and the youngsters scatter in fright, he is held guilty if one of the youngsters hurts

---

[1] This is provocative abuse, telling the chief to commit incest with his sister.
[2] Abuse telling him to commit incest with his mother.

himself in his eagerness to get away. If the child is not badly hurt the elders content themselves with scolding and reviling the causer of the trouble. If an arm is broken, he might be fined two lengths of large beads; if the child is totally disabled, blinded, etc., a fine of a gun or two guns might be imposed; if the child is killed, a fine of a gun or a sister as a slave might be demanded. Blinding was always reckoned by the Lambas as being a terrible calamity, the eye being reckoned presumably of greater value than life, for invariably two guns would be demanded for the loss of an eye.

(4) **Wrongful Arrest or Charging.** If a man is wrongfully arrested through a mistake in identity, and an innocent man is charged before the chief, the accuser will, on proof of innocence being produced, have to pay the accused two strings of large beads.

(5) **Cause of Suicide.** A. is wrongly accused by the wife of B. as co-respondent, and sentenced. He goes into his house on the pretence of smoking and blows out his brains. The relatives of A. now make a case against the wife of B. They go to the *umulaye* for him to divine, as is done in witchcraft cases, for A. is dead. The *umulaye* demands of the woman the name of the real adulterer. She tells. The person responsible for the spirit of A., probably his younger brother, now takes the woman and enslaves her. The man whom she had shielded will have to pay a gun, but the husband, B., gets no compensation at all.

(6) **Suicide.** Suicide was by no means uncommon in Ilamba, not only because of fear or worry preying on the mind, but also because of the deliberate intention of bringing trouble upon the one who was causing the fear or worry. The person whose action has caused another to commit suicide is held responsible for the death.

A. continually pesters B. for the settlement of some debt, and threatens him with enslavement, or otherwise makes his life miserable. B., in exasperation, takes a length of bark rope (*ulushishi*), tells some of the youngsters in the village what he is going to do, and goes and hangs himself from a tree at the side of the path, some distance from the village. People passing find him, cut the body down, bury it, and then gather to wail. As they seek for the cause of his death, the youngsters will tell them that B. said his life was made miserable by A., and that that is why he has killed himself. The relatives now charge A. with his death, and if A. is wise he will procure a gun and pay it over at once; otherwise the case will be taken before the paramount chief.

(7) **Borrowing.** Many of the continual lawsuits of the Lambas
are due to their habit of borrowing. If a man has a death-due to
pay in order to free himself to marry again, he usually borrows a
gun for the purpose, and then lightly puts off the day when he
will procure the means to get another gun to repay his debt.
Suits are continually being made for the restitution of articles
borrowed or for their equivalents. Should a man die before
making such restitution, his *impyani*, or heir, would be held
responsible.

The Lambas have a proverb *Mwapu usekaseka napakuluŵula
usekaseka*, "A smiling loan, and a smiling when redeemed."
A man must not be angry when the creditor comes to claim back
what he has lent.

With the Lambas, an article borrowed is returned and no
addition is demanded. They do not know of interest or usury
charges. In buying, however, they have a custom which seems
peculiar. A. agrees to buy an article from B. for, say, nine
shillings. When the article is brought and the money passed
over B. will say, *Nundileni-po*, "Add on for me!" and A. will
perhaps give him an extra shilling. It is the one who brings the
article to sell who asks for the addition, "because of the distance
I have come to bring your goods," he says. Possibly because of
this, the store principle of the *imbansela* (the Lamba equivalent
term) has caught on in Ilamba. The people have a saying,
"*Nundile-po*" *tabwelelwa-makweŵo*, "Saying 'Add on for me' does
not mean the returning of the articles!"

(8) **Trespass on Garden Rights.** If a man hoes beyond his
recognized patch, and encroaches upon a portion belonging to his
neighbour, the case may go before the headman. Such cases are
usually settled without much wrangling, for the headman will
quote *Mushili-mfumu tekumulwila*, "Don't fight over the soil,
our chief!" and will add, "One of you can fell timber in another
direction!"

(9) **Responsibility for Messengers.** A. sends B. on a message
to the village where C. lives. B. meets C., quarrels with him,
and kills him. A. is held to a certain extent responsible.

In such a case B. is arrested. B. says, "But it was A. who sent
me here!" A., when called, protests, "I merely sent him to
take some cloth to my mother-in-law!" Possibly B. will then be
killed, but the relatives of B. will go to A. and demand certain
compensation from him as having been the cause of B.'s coming
to the village and dying while in his employ.

Should B. be the slave of A., A. would have to face the full penalty of the death of C. and pay the necessary full compensation to C.'s relatives.

The Lambas say, *Chiŵasa-munko walimuloŵele,* "The carver of the porridge-stick bewitched him!" A charge of witchcraft poisoning can go farther back than to the one who cooked the food; it may implicate the one who made the utensils.[1]

(10) **Life-saving.** If a person, in trying to get honey, or some small animal, such as a galago,[2] from the cleft of a tree, should get his hand caught, so that he cannot free himself, he will shout and shout for help. If some one hears him and comes to his aid he will have a life-debt to pay to his rescuer. In order to secure his own freedom from slavery he may have to pay over a sister as a slave.

(11) **Denial of Guilt.** *Mukana-lweŵo alakana nefyakwe* is a Lamba saying—"He who denies the charge denies his all as well." A man denying guilt must deny ownership of all the goods brought as evidence of his guilt. This principle is carried further. If villagers condemn a certain man as unworthy of their society, and drive him away, they dare not keep any of his belongings; all must be counted as unworthy, and he must be allowed to take them with him.

(12) **False Evidence.** A man who desires vengeance on another may call assistance from another village. These helpers, on arrival, will talk over the case, and if the man has brought them on a trumped-up charge they will revenge themselves on him. So the Lambas say, *Muloŵafita alaliloŵela,* "He who betrays to assassins betrays himself."

(13) **Enforcement of Payment.** It is a Lamba custom that a man, if he cannot get payment of a debt, will at evening fetch a long log of firewood and put it through the door of the debtor's house, reaching to the fireplace within and protruding outside. The creditor will light a fire at the outside end of the log, intimating that he is going to remain until the case is settled. The door cannot be shut, nor can the debtor go to sleep. Sometimes a mat is brought and laid in the doorway with the same intent.

(14) **Accidental Burning of a Grain-house.** If the parties concerned cannot agree upon the amount of restitution to be made, the case is brought before the paramount chief. If A. demands

[1] See the Lamba story of " Mr Wild Dog and Mr Duiker " (Doke, *Lamba Folk-lore,* p. 233), where the guilt for the chief's wife's poking a needle in her eye is traced back from the cock to the hornbill, lark, night-jar, elephant, monkeys, shrew, snake, duiker, wild dog, and eventually to the women of the village.

[2] Kind of small lemur or large night-ape.

exorbitant restitution, say, ten *ututundu* (large baskets) of grain at a time of food shortage, B. will bring the headman as witness to the shortage, and the chief may award, say, three *ututundu*.

(15) **Death of a Stranger.** Lamba hospitality demands that if a stranger comes to the village he must be given a hut to sleep in. There is more than mere hospitality in this, for should he sleep outside and be caught by a lion the villagers would be held responsible to the paramount chief. If such a thing were to happen, and the stranger were a visitor from another tribe at a great distance, the headman of the village would report to the paramount chief, who would await news from the man's relatives. In the event of no news coming there would be no further action taken.

Cursing

In Lamba *ukufinga* or *amafinje*, cursing, is believed to have its effect. Should death come upon a person cursed, even after a lapse of years, the curser would be reckoned as an *imfwiti* (witch). The following are typical curses:

(1) *Neli ninkalamu ikwikate, neli ninsoka kekulya, neli kufwa ufwe lelo!* "May a lion catch you, or a snake bite you, or may you die to-day!"

(2) *Wafwa walowa!* "You are dead, you are bewitched!"

(3) *Neli manata kolwala, kawichyele lukoso muŋanda!* "May you suffer from leprosy and have to sit in your hut!"

Filthy Reviling

Ukutukana or *amatuka*, filthy reviling, is a very common cause of fighting in Lamba communities. If a person repeatedly indulges in it he may be taken before the chief. *Umuchyobwe*, abuse in word or action, is a term which includes *amatuka*.[1]

Oath-taking

Ukulapa or *ichilapo*, an oath, is taken in order to strengthen a statement, generally when a man is denying his guilt. The Lambas used to believe thoroughly in this method of establishing a man's innocence, and would say, "Leave him alone, he is innocent, for he has named a powerful name!"

---

[1] The following are typical examples of *amatuka*:
(1) *Kakala kanoko!* " Little penis of your mother!"
(2) *Kanyo kanoko!* " Little anus of your mother!"
(3) *Kakala kowe!* " Your little penis!"
(4) *Kawóloko!* " Your little testicle!"

77

The following are examples of oaths:

(1) *Newo kani nshikesa-po'ko Lesa uyu akandye!* "As for me, if I do not come there, let God eat me!"

(2) *Kani nachita-po ichichintu Shyakapanga andye wopelo'yu!* "If I did this thing, may God himself eat me!"

(3) *Kani newo napepa-po fwaka wenu yalile umukwasu!* "If I smoked your tobacco, a lion has eaten my brother [*i.e.*, it will therefore come and eat me too!]!"

(4) *Kani nalya-po amatawa enu mulwanshya umulela'wakwasu!* "If I ate your maize, it is at the Lwanshya river, where my brethren lie [*i.e.*, you can take me there to the cemetery!]!"

(5) *Nalesa!* "And God!" (A recently imported oath, said to have come from Nyasaland.)

(6) *Kani nachita-po ifyo ulusengo lwambowo ululele-ko umukwasu!* "If I did that, the horn of the buffalo at which my brother lay!" (The brother killed by the buffalo is invoked, and therefore "I can go the same way!")

(7) *Chingwali*[1] *kani nachita-po ifyo!* "It is smallpox, if I did that!" ("Let it kill me!")

(8) *Ichipumpula!* "Famine!" (Old Lambas used to swear by the great famine.)

Divorce

See Chapter X, on "Marriage."

Trial by Ordeal

See Chapter XIX, on "*Uwufwiti*—Witchcraft," in connexion with which it is used.

---

[1] *Mwalo!* and *Chilwashi!* are other similar expressions, the latter borrowed from the Lenje.

CHAPTER V

SLAVERY

Slave-trading

ACCORDING to Lamba accounts, Ilamba was for many years the happy hunting-ground of the slave-traders. Lamba women are generally very comely, and were greatly prized by slave-traders. The first regular slave-traders were the Mbundus from Angola. The Lambas say they were peaceful traders who brought calico, guns, and beads to trade for ivory and slaves. Mbundu beads are but rarely to be seen in Ilamba to-day. Those used in buying slaves were of two kinds; the first, called *imikoshi yamabwe* (stone necks), had a diameter of about two inches, and a necklace of these reaching as far as the diaphragm would purchase a female slave; the second, called *utunkolomwena*, were smaller, with a diameter of about two-thirds of an inch, and were red in colour; five strings of these, measuring from the small toe to the hip, would purchase a female slave, while three similar strings would purchase a male slave. A female slave (*umushya*) was thus of more value to the trader than a male slave (*kalume*).

The Mbundu traders were often treated treacherously by both the Lambas and the Lenjes. In some cases they were robbed by the Lamba chiefs. It is said that the Lenjes used to bring their own children to the Mbundu traders in order to buy calico, powder, and tins of dynamite. After conveying their purchases to their houses they would arm themselves with the guns and powder just acquired and in the evening attack the Mbundu camp, scatter the traders, and recover their children. This is said to have happened at Chipepo and on the present site of Broken Hill.

Later the Chikundas from the Lower Zambesi came trading for slaves and ivory. But perhaps it is the Swahili traders who have left the strongest impression of this nefarious traffic in the country. Many of these very traders are still to be found living in the villages not far from Ndola. Old Nkana, of Nkana's country, to the west of Mushili's country, a few years before his death, which took place about 1924, gave me a most realistic account of

THE LAMBAS OF NORTHERN RHODESIA

how the Swahili slave-raiders—for they were not peaceful slave-traders—depopulated that vast stretch of country to the west of the Kafue river. I had travelled from Chipulali's village, on the Lufwanyama, to Nkana's, on the Kafue, a distance of over fifty miles, and had found only one village between, although we passed stream after stream and fertile valleys all the way. Nkana told me that some years ago that whole country was thickly populated, but the Swahilis came, working up the streams systematically, burning the villages, shooting the men, and taking the women and children captive. They said that the men gave them too much trouble on the long march to Zanzibar!

Domestic Slavery

The Lambas, in common with the surrounding tribes, practised a type of domestic slavery from which the horrors of the slave-raiding and slave-trading were to a great extent absent. As we have seen already, men and women were enslaved as a punishment for some misdeed or in settlement of some debt. So in many cases the slaves were deserving of their state. In European communities they would have been convicts, and in fact many of them were guilty of murder and other serious crimes. But the hardness of this system was that accidental damage or accidental homicide often resulted in enslavement; and to hold a man responsible for an injury whether he has committed it of intent or by misfortune is not an equal dispensing of justice. The domestic slave in Lambaland, however, enjoyed freedom of movement, and, as we shall see, was often at liberty to go in search of employment to redeem himself. Men became slaves in various ways—in settlement of debt, by misdeed, by capture in war, and by self-enslavement.

Self-enslavement

In the old days *ukuliteka* or self-enslavement was quite a common thing.

(1) **Of a Male.** A man finds that he cannot get on with his relatives and others in his village, and so, having heard of some distant village headman of repute, he leaves his home, goes to the village, enters the house of that headman, and sits down on the hearth. The headman asks him, "Where have you come from?" "I have come from yonder, sir. I have come to eat here with you." The headman now asks him, "Have you no relatives?" "I have!" "Why, then," he asks, "have you left your relatives to come and enslave yourself?" And the man

80

explains that he cannot get on with his relatives. At this the headman gives him a hut and food, and thereafter sets him to do such work as he desires, hoeing, felling timber, cutting firewood, or building. The slave dare not now run away. In time the headman will give him a wife. If he behaves well, after many years such a slave may become an *impemba* (advisor) in the village. He would not be treated as an ordinary *kalume*, for he could not be sold by his master. He might, however, be temporarily handed over as a hostage, should the headman get into serious trouble, and then be redeemed later on.

Self-enslavement has generally been the result of *insala* (hunger) through inability to manage one's own garden, or inability to get on with one's relatives, or inability to face the payment of a large due.

(2) **Of a Female.** If a woman enslaves herself she may be married by the chief if she is prepossessing, but even then she would be called *umushya*. Such a woman, when enslaving herself, would not stay outside when she reached the chief's house, but would go straight in and sit by the fire. Should the chief not desire to marry her, she may be married to some one else; in this case the calico of the marriage pledge would be given to the chief to whom she had enslaved herself, and she would no longer be accounted *umushya*, but *umukashi*, or wife. In case of the death of such a self-enslaved woman her husband would have to go to her relatives to clear himself of the death-dues; so would the chief have had to do had he married her, but in his case he would pay over only a small amount of his own choosing in order to satisfy and allay the *ichiŵanda* (attendant demon) of the deceased woman. Should such a female slave not get married, she would have her own house, and do certain work for the chief, water-drawing, hoeing, weeding, sweeping, grinding, and so on. Such a woman is called *umushyakashi*, or *chipishyamenda*, the latter term meaning 'water-warmer,' because she takes the early morning warm water to her master.

(3) A man's father has died without settling a debt, and at his death his creditors come to his son and say, "Give us a gun!" When the son finds he cannot procure a gun he makes up his mind to enslave himself. Going to some chief, he says, "I have come to enslave myself, sir. Give me a gun to settle my debt. If I cannot procure another to repay you I am your slave." And the chief gives him a gun, which he hands over to his creditors. If he does not procure a gun to pay back the chief, the latter will either keep him as his slave or sell him for a gun to some one else.

If, however, the man desires to go away to work, and the chief sees that he is honestly trying to get the necessary money, he will not trouble him. The Lambas say, *Ufwayafwaya taluŵa*, "He who is looking for money to redeem himself is not lost." For even if he should go far away he will come back; are not his relatives present who can be enslaved? A further proverb in Lamba gives wise instruction in these matters—*Talipula muɲombe kalikala mumuntu*, "The [spear] does not pass through the ox and rest in the man!" For if a person desires to kill another for some misdeed or debt, and he meets the other bringing an ox as payment, let him be satisfied with the ox and not pursue his vengeance on the man!

Slaves Acquired

Says the Lamba slave-owner, *Uyu nikalume nemwine wakunonka wakapini kamulombe*, "This is my slave, whom I have acquired like an axe-handle of *lombe* wood! He is my own."

A man may demand a slave in settlement of a debt. If his debtor has no slave to give he may give a gun, with which the creditor is able to buy a slave.

If a man has committed adultery, and then made his escape to a neighbouring territory, the aggrieved husband may seize the delinquent's sister and enslave her. He may marry her if he cares to, or he may sell her. Should she die, her relatives must *pooso' ŵunga*, throw on him the meal as a sign of his liberation from the consequence of her death, without demanding any payment at all from him. No one else would marry such a slave as this.

Marriage of Slaves

If two slaves of one master marry, their children are also his slaves.

A. owns a male slave, B. a female slave. Should they marry, A. will come to B. and say, "Give me a gun, because your *umushya* has married my *kalume*, and I shall see him no more at my house; he will be as though he were your son-in-law!" B. will do so, thus buying A.'s slave. Any children will naturally belong to B.

Slaves Captured

In inter-tribal fighting, and even in faction fighting within the tribe, when an enemy village was raided, the men were slaughtered, but the women and children were carried off as slaves. When the fighting was over the captives were all brought before the chief.

SLAVERY

If a man had caught, say, three persons the chief took one and handed two over to their captor. Such slaves were treated as those enslaved for debt or misdeed, the master in reality having absolute power over them. In such fighting the men were speared lest they should organize the women to escape back to their country.

Redemption of Slaves

Strong-hearted relatives of slaves captured in fighting have been known to come to the conquering chief and tell him that they are looking for captured relatives in order to ransom them. The chief would summon the man who captured the slaves, together with the captives themselves, and instruct him to hand over his captives and take in their place the slaves brought by the relatives as ransom.

There is a Lamba saying regarding an industrious slave, *Kalume aliluŵuchile mumbono shyakwe*, "The slave ransomed himself with his own castor-oil." An industrious slave can do little odd jobs and continually bring things to his master. After several years of this he may demand his release, on the plea that he has brought to his master more than the amount of his debt, and may thus be released. No stigma attaches to a one-time slave in Ilamba. As soon as he has gained his freedom he becomes once more an *umwana waŵene* (free man).

Should a slave kill an elephant, or, when alone, find one dead, one tusk will go to the paramount chief, and with the other he will redeem himself and go free. But should he be out hunting with his master, any elephant he found would belong to his master.

Responsibility for the Misconduct of Slaves

If a slave is the cause of the burning of a grain-store it will be the responsibility of his master to make reparation. If this was an accident, nothing would be done to the slave. Should a dwelling have been burnt, the slave may be sent to build another.

Should a male slave commit adultery, he would be killed by the aggrieved husband and his master beaten for not looking after his slave properly.

If a slave steals, his master must make restoration; and the master will probably beat his slave to warn him against doing it again. A master may beat his slave for lying or for insolence.

For continued thieving a master may kill his slave. If this is done, the person or persons who last laid a charge of stealing against the slave are brought before the paramount chief and sued by the owner as being the cause of his slave's death. The chief will confirm upon them the blame of being the cause of his death, and will say that the master of the slave acted as a *kamunkomene*,[1] one sent to kill by those complaining of the thefts. They will have to bring a slave or a gun to the dead slave's master, and pay the chief two strings of Mbundu beads, practically the value of a slave.

If anyone injures a slave, compensation has to be paid to the owner of the slave. Suppose the slave loses an eye, a compensation of two guns would be paid to the master, who would give his slave one and send him home free.

Should a slave belonging to one man injure the slave of another, the settlement of the case would be between the owners.

[1] See Chapter IV.

CHAPTER VI

VILLAGE LIFE AND CUSTOM

WE now come to consider more closely the village life and the customs and habits of the people in the villages of Ilamba.

A New Village

When the soil in the vicinity of a village has become worked out —a thing which happens after a few years, inasmuch as hoe cultivation does not go very deep—or when the environs of the village have become insanitary owing to long residence on one spot, the village headman will call together his *impemba* (advisors) and inform them that it is time to search for better soil. His advisors will assent, and in all probability tell him that they have been waiting for him to broach the subject, as the first approaches in this matter cannot come from the *impemba*. Should the *impemba* desire to remain longer on the old site, the headman would not force his desire to move, but would wait for a more opportune occasion. The subject of village moving would only be raised *pamwela*, during the dry season.

For moving a village in the old days no permission from the paramount was necessary as long as the site chosen was still within that chief's territory; for instance, Saili's villages could not move from the territory belonging to Saili. Established villages welcomed newcomers to their vicinity, for these provided an added protection in time of war; and since game was plentiful, there was never any jealousy.

The chief generally chooses the direction of the move. He will say, "Let us go to such-and-such a river. There is good soil there." When this has been decided, maybe four young men are sent out *ukwendelo'mushili*, to go over the soil in order to choose the best spot, keeping in mind the proximity of good drinking-water. On their return these men make their report. If it is satisfactory, the women are now sent to grind corn for the pioneers of the new settlement. In the morning the men of the village fill bark bags with meal, tie up their cooking-pots, and set off *mukwikato'mushili*, in order to 'catch the soil.' All the women

85

remain at the village. The last of the men to leave the village and go to the new site is the headman.

When the men reach the proposed site they erect one big *umutanda*, or stockade, which they share. That very evening the village headman takes a small quantity of meal (*uŵunga*), and addresses the spirits of the people who used to inhabit the country round that stream: *Twamupeleni mwemulele muno, twamupeleni uŵungo'ŵu, tulukufwayo'kwenda nenu. Kani tamulukutufwaya, uŵungo'ŵu tusangane mwapalaya*, "Ye who sleep here, we have given to you, we have given to you this meal; we want to live with you. If you do not want us, let us find that you have scattered this meal!" This he says in order to propitiate them for the intrusion and to gain their good wishes. And he adds, *Kani mulukutufwaya, tusangane ŵonse ŵulikumene*, "If you do want us, let us find it all intact!" After this he pours the meal in a heap outside the stockade, behind it to the eastward. Then, with more meal, he goes to another spot, and says, *Kani pali ŵambi aŵachikani aŵataŵenda naŵantu, naŵo uŵunga bwaŵo mbu!* "If there are others, evilly minded, who do not get on with people, this meal is theirs!" Thereupon the old man goes into the stockade, and they all sleep.

At dawn the headman emerges, and goes to inspect the various heaps of meal. If he finds the heaps intact, he goes back to the *umutanda*, and says to his people, "They have accepted us!" And all are relieved.

If he should find the meal scattered about, perhaps by mice, the headman reports, "They have not greeted us here; they have driven us away!" Perhaps some will protest, "Let us stay here. The soil is so good!" And they will stay, but not without some misgivings. Should a man die, the headman would immediately say, "Did I not tell you that they have driven us away, and you would not listen?"

When the men come out in the morning, should one find a dead genet or a dead hare, intact with head, it would be considered an ill-omen. All would gather together to consult with the chief. In all probability they would decide to move to another stream, as such an occurrence is considered an indication of approaching death or disaster.

Should, however, all the omens be favourable, the men leave the *umutanda* that morning to choose their various garden sites, and each chooses his own plot and marks the trees. The next day they all go to commence the timber-felling, which takes several weeks of labour. At a new village site (*umusokolwe*), as each tree is felled the branches are lopped and piled about the tree to dry for burning; the *ifiteme*, as these piles of branches are called, are not packed regularly, as is the case with already established gardens.

Meanwhile, if the distance is not too great, the women will bring regular supplies of meal. They do not do the cooking—the men cook for themselves—for the women have the bird-scaring to do at the village, and can be away from it only during the heat of the day. If the distance is great, the men will go from time to time to fetch their food. Sometimes, though rarely, men will return for spells to their wives at the village.

At the end of about a month the men will all return to the village to assist in reaping the harvest of sorghum (*amasaka*). The corn-stalks are first cut down (*teŵula*); then, when they have lain thus a day or two, the heads are cut off (*chyesa*) and gathered into stacks (*ififufu*) on stands raising them just off the ground away from termites. Next, grain-houses (*amatala*) are erected in a secret place in the bush, in which the corn is stored (*longela*).

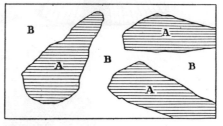

FIG. 30. PLAN OF A NEW GARDEN

A, ash-covered soil where trees have been felled and burnt ; B, *inkuule*, roughly hoed soil.

When this is done, all, men and women alike, go to the new site to commence the hoeing.

On their arrival they erect each man his own *umutanda* around the site of the big stockade, and an embryo village springs up. Bamboo doors are made for each *umutanda*, which is generally bushed over the top as well. Now men and women set about the first rough hoeing (*ukukuula*), turning up the great clods. Sometimes the woman does this while her husband is extending his *ifiteme* by felling more timber. Should the *ifiteme* be large enough, the man does the rough hoeing and his wife comes after him, breaking up the clods (*ukupume'nkuule*). Hoeing thus consumes many days, and from time to time visits have to be made to the old village to fetch food.

When the timber is dry the time for burning it comes, and when this is done the women commence to sow the *amasaka*, some in the ash-covered soil, some in the hoed ground as they smash the sods. The ground beneath the ash is not hoed, as it is held that

87

as the tree burns it softens the soil, so the hoe is merely struck in to make a hole for the seed. In these new gardens maize and sorghum are sown long before the first rains.

As soon as the sowing is complete *inkunka* huts are built, the men cutting the poles and bringing the bark rope, while the women bring the grass. The *inkunka* is a lean-to hut. Heavy poles are planted in the ground in a circular trench, the tops of the poles being brought together to form a cone. This is thatched

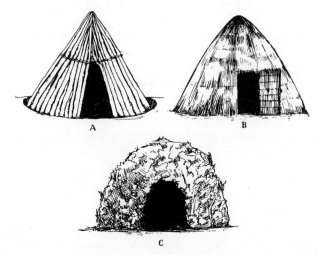

FIG. 31. INKUNKA AND UMUTANDA
A, *inkunka*—poles assembled ; B, *inkunka*—thatched, with door ; C, *umutanda*.
Bamboo doors are made for each *umutanda*.

over, the grass reaching right to the ground, where sods cover the ends and make the whole secure.

By the time that the settlers have moved into the *inkunka* the first rains are upon them. Pumpkins are planted, and very soon the weeding of the gardens commences. As soon as the sorghum has grown to a certain height the women thin it out and transplant. The first crop they get is that of pumpkins, and as these are ripening the people have to erect shelters (*ututungu*) in the gardens themselves, into which they move temporarily to protect the pumpkins and maize from bush-pigs and monkeys. The next crop to ripen is maize, and after that the sorghum (*amasaka*), which necessitates the bird-scaring.

The *inkunka* village has been built *ichiŵakeŵake*, without plan or order, but when the sorghum has been harvested grain-stores are built on the outskirts of the site chosen for the permanent village.

The Village

One day the headman will summon his people to go with him and choose the site for the *amaŋanda antanda*, the permanent houses of upright walls and conical roofs. When they reach the site the chief selects the spot for his own house, and says, "I shall build here; my brothers-in-law will build there; and my

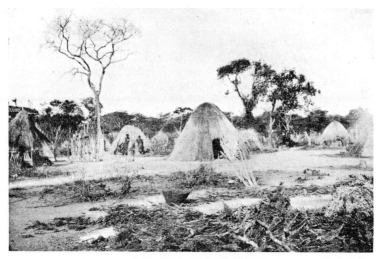

FIG. 32. INKUNKA VILLAGE OF KAPOPO, 1913
Photo by C. M. Doke

sons-in-law yonder!" Under his direction each man marks out the spot for his own permanent dwelling.

Key to Plan of Village (Fig. 33):

The village lies east to west, with the chief's huts at the eastern end and grain-stores outside to the east.

    (1) and (2) are the chief's huts, and unless this is the village of a commoner he will be an *umwinamishishi*. (1) is the hut of the principal wife, *mukolo*, of clan perhaps *umwinambwa*, (2) the hut of the younger wife, *mutepa*, say, *umwinachyulu*.

    (3)–(7) are occupied by the brothers-in-law of the chief who have married his clan sisters, *aŵenamishishi*. Of these the clans of the men may be as follows: (3) *umwinambushi*, (4) *umwinamaila*, (5) *umulembo*, (6) *umwinambushi*, (7) *umwinanswi*. The men of (3) and (6) are *aŵanaŵankashi*, brethren, and they regard those of (4), (5), and (7) as *aŵofi ŵaŵyaŵo*.

(8)–(19) are occupied by both men and women, commoners not related in any particular way to the chief. Some may be relatives of the men of (3)–(7). (18) is a hunter, *umupalu*, and behind his hut is the *uluŵansa*, court, where the *ichinsengwe* dance is performed before the hunting shrine, *ichipanda*.

(20)–(23), huts of *aŵenshikulu aŵachyete*, grandchildren of commoner's clan. If some of them are young women, they may be married to *aŵenamishishi*. If they are young men married to *aŵenamishishi* they would be termed *aŵako*, sons-in-law.

(24)–(28), huts of *aŵako* who have married *aŵenamishishi*. (26) is a blacksmith, *umufushi*, and behind his hut stands the *ichintengwa*, or smithy.

(29), *ichyambawilo*, or meeting-house for talk and discussions.

(30)–(34) and (37), huts occupied by boys, both of chief's rank and commoner's.

(35) is the communal grinding-house, called *ichimabwe*. Each house has in addition its own grindstones under the eaves.

(36) is the goat-house, *ichimpata chyambushi*.

Small circles indicate the positions of various fowl-houses.

On the *uluŵansa lwamfumu*, the chief's court, are held *imilandu*, courts of justice, and the majority of the dances. Here the *ŵamoŵa* and the *aŵayambo* dance.

On the *uluŵansa lwaŵanichye* the children play their games and the women dance the *ifilaila* dances.

There are no ceremonies when building the new permanent *intanda* village. Some lazy people remain permanently in *inkunka*, but unless they are aged folk they are despised by the others, who say, "Why do you like to live in *inkunka* like *aŵatwa* [Twa people], who have no trees with which to build proper houses?"

The Building of the House

The building of the permanent *intanda* is carried out as follows:

First the ground shape of the house is marked out (*ukutala*). A peg is driven into the ground; a piece of bark rope is tied to this, and with another stick at the end of the rope a circle is described, with the peg as centre. A shallow trench (*umufolwa*) is dug where the circle was marked out. Upright poles are

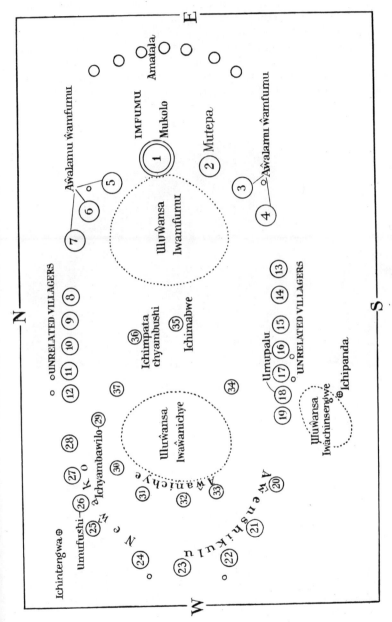

FIG. 33. PLAN OF A LAMBA VILLAGE

91

planted in this trench, a gap being left for the doorway; the poles are bound together with long pliable bonds made of split bamboo and bark rope, or withies of the *umusamba*-tree with bark rope twined round them, or reeds. The bark rope used is stripped from within the hard outer bark of the *umusamba*- or *akasabwa*-trees, and is not plaited. The topmost bond, called *kankasa*, is of exceptional strength, and completely encircles the

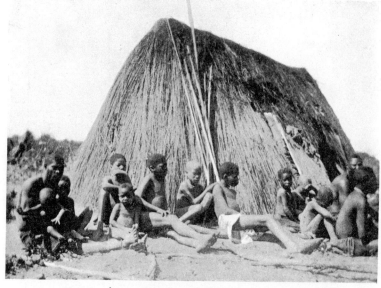

FIG. 34. WULIMAS OF AN INFERIOR TYPE IN FRONT OF A
PERMANENT INKUNKA
Photo by C. M. Doke

hut, going over the top of the doorway. In large buildings the next thing done is the erection of the *ulupumpu*, a temporary supporting pole in the centre of the hut. Four *impanda shya-mutenje*, forked roofing poles called *insonta*, are now brought together above the top of the *ulupumpu* and tied with bark rope, the forked ends resting at equal distances apart on the *kankasa*. An *ichiŵango*, a circle of withies, is now prepared below, forced up into the apex within the roof, and secured to the outside by *ulushishi* (bark rope). Many more *insonta* are added to strengthen the roof and close up the large interstices. Encircling bonds are now fixed without and within, and when all is tight the *ulupumpu* is removed.

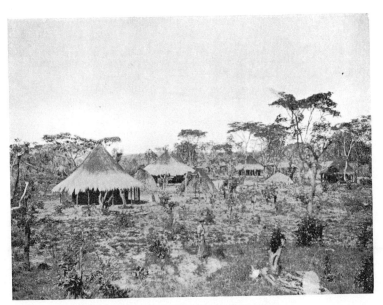

FIG. 35. A VILLAGE OF INTANDA
Photo by C. M. Doke

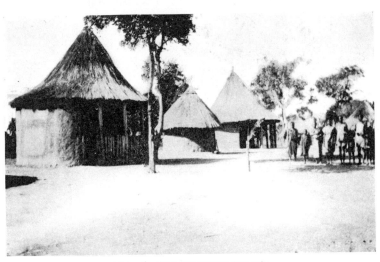

FIG. 36. IN A CHRISTIAN VILLAGE
Note the tidiness.
Photo by Miss O. C. Doke

The next operation is that of thatching the roof. From the first layer round the bottom edge of the roof each bundle of grass is placed with the head of grass hanging downward. The bundles are thrown up to the thatcher on the roof; he loosens them out and secures them with *ulushishi* to the roof-bonds. The uppermost capping of the thatch, the *sunsa*, is prepared on the ground. On the roof it is opened out; a long peg (*ulupopo*) is placed in the centre and driven in between the *insonta*, thus making it rigid. The next thing done to the house is the plastering (*masa*); usually the inside of the walls is plastered first, well-worked, heavy mud being placed in all the interstices between the wall poles; then the same is done from the outside.

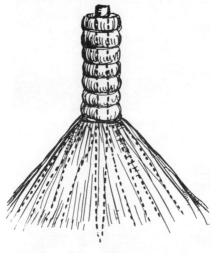

FIG. 37. SUNSA

When enemy attacks were feared, the outside was often plastered first. When the rough plastering is complete, the whole is smeared over with thinner mud by the hands: this is called *ukushingula*. The floor is next attended to, earth being brought in and well trodden down. Water is poured on to it, and it is smeared over (*ukushingula*) and left to dry and harden. In these days the floors are beaten (*pamantila*) with short pieces of flattened wood, but this method of dealing with them has been learnt from the Europeans. Lastly, the door (*ichiŵi*) has to be made, and for this bamboo, bound together with cross-pieces and *ulushishi*, is generally used, or sticks of *umusuku* or *umusamba* if no bamboo is available.

The Calendar of Work

To the superficial observer the life of the average African native often seems to entail very little real work and an enormous amount of leisure time. Other equally superficial observers are apt to say that the women do all the hard work and the men practically nothing. To get a complete survey of the activities of men and women in Ilamba throughout the year it is well to classify (1) the calendar of work according to the thirteen Lamba lunar months and (2) the division of labour between the sexes.

The Lamba year (*umwaka*) commences with the month of the first rains.

(1) *Ntenkentenke* or *lukundula-fiŵunsa*, late October to November. This is a month of food-shortage. There is no special work apart from the daily rounds during this month.

(2) *Ŵangashye*, November to December. During this month the *ifiteme* are burnt and the *inkuule* broken up, maize, sorghum, and pumpkins being planted. Honey, extracted by the bees from the flowers of the *imisamba*-trees, is collected, and fish-spearing is possible as the water begins to rise.

(3) *Umwenye* or *umwenye-masuku*, December to January, is reckoned the height of the *umuŵundo* or rainy season. During this month ground-nuts are planted, gardens weeded, fruits such as *impundu*, *imfungo*, *amasuku*, and *amasafwa*, honey, and mushrooms collected. The small red millet called *amawo* is sown during this month.

(4) *Akakuŵo*, January to February. The weeding of gardens continues; the first pumpkins, melons, and cucumbers are gathered; the raised mounds (*imilala*) for sweet potatoes and cassava are prepared; wild fruits such as *amakonkola*, *imfungo*, and *inkomfwa* are collected, as well as such caterpillars as the *ififumbe* and the *ifisukuŵya*. Bridges are constructed (*ukusanshike' fyaŵu*).

(5) *Inkuŵo* or *inkuŵonkulu*, February to March. Green maize is eaten, also such caterpillars as the *ulumombwe*. Garden work is suspended, except that upon sweet potatoes and cassava. The women make *amasasa ampoolo*, soft grass mats. This season is called *imintimpa*, the end of the rains.

(6) *Akaŵengele-ntanga* or *iŵengele linini* or *akalusafya-manika*, March to April. During this month fresh *inkuule* are rough-hoed to enlarge the gardens. If a move to a new village site has to be made, it is during this month that the men set out.

(7) *Iŵengele* or *iŵengele likulu* or *seŵa-pachyulu*, April to May. Bird-scaring (*ukwamina*) is commenced, anthill shelters (*utupingwe*) are made in the gardens, and *amankuŵala* (sounding boats) carved to scare the birds. Sweet potatoes are dug, *amawo* harvested, and weirs (*ifipanda*) constructed across the receding streams to catch fish.

(8) *Ichishika*, May to June. Bird-scaring and *amawo*-harvesting continued, beans picked, *imyumbu* marsh roots dug, and ground-nuts, *uŵuleya*, and *umuninga* dug up (*tula*). This is the middle of the dry season, called *umwela*. Tree-felling (*ukutema*) is commenced during this month.

(9) *Akapyantoto*, June to July. The main staple crop of sorghum (*amasaka*) is harvested, entailing *ukuteŵula* (cutting down), *ukuchyesa* (lopping of heads), building of stands (*ififufu*), and erection of grain-stores (*amatala*). The women convey the crop to the *amatala* and store (*ukulongela*) it. During this month there is building of *inkunka* if a new village site has been chosen.

(10) *Nkumbinkumbi*, July to August. With the commencement of grass-burning cane-rats (*insenshi*) are hunted. *Umuninga* is scratched out (*ukufuka*). Tree-felling continues at the new village.

(11) *Kasabwa* or *akasako-kanduŵa* or *ichibwela-mushi*, August to commencement of September. The garden workers return to the village. Clods are smashed in the new gardens. This is a time of rest at an established village. The first maize and sorghum are planted. Timber for building is cut. Bundles of grass are fetched and stacked in the village.

(12) *Ikungulu* or *ikungulu lyamitondo* or *injelekela* or *akapalala*, September. During this month the permanent *intanda* houses are built, and the women have considerable work bringing in thatching grass.

(13) *Akasuŵa-kachye* or *temangume* or *kamalekano-nalesa*, October. This is the hottest month, just before the rains, and is reckoned the middle of *ulusuŵa*, the hot season. House-thatching is the principal work of this month.

Division of Labour between the Sexes

The Lambas say that the sign of the man is "the axe and the spear" and the sign of the woman "the hoe." This to a great extent determines the division of labour between the sexes. Hoe-work is primarily women's work, though men may take a hoe to assist them. Axe-work is primarily men's work, though here again women may use an axe on occasion. A woman would not use a spear. A tabulation of the work of men and that of women will help the better realization of the fundamental principles underlying this social division.

VILLAGE LIFE AND CUSTOM

	MEN	WOMEN
(1) Daily Duties.	(a) ——	(a) Draw water.
	(b) Inkuni (heavy firewood).	(b) Insamfu (kindling wood).
	(c) [May help sweep courtyard.]	(c) Sweep house and courtyard.
	(d) ——	(d) Ukwanshika (make bed).
(2) Gardens and Food-preparation.	(a) Ifiteme (tree-felling).	(a) ——
	(b) Ukukuula (first hoeing in clods).	(b) Ukulima (ordinary hoeing).
	(c) Ukochya (burning ifiteme).	(c) ——
	(d) ——	(d) Ukupume'nkuule (smashing the clods).
	(e) [Help in sowing and weeding.]	(e) Sow and weed.
	(f) Ukusema (scare pigs, monkeys).	(f) Ukwamina (scare birds).
	(g) Ukuchyesa (cut cornheads).	(g) Ukutewula (break down corn).
	(h) Make stands and grainhouses.	(h) Carry corn to stand (ukutunta); put corn in grain-house (ukulongela).
	(i) ——	(i) Ukuwansa, take out daily corn supply.
	(j) ——	(j) Ukupuma (thresh).
	(k) ——	(k) Ukwela (winnow).
	(l) ——	(l) Ukupela (grind).
	(m) ——	(m) Ukutwa (pound).
	(n) [On journeys, etc.]	(n) Ukunanya (make porridge).
	(o) Search for mushrooms, caterpillars, fish, meat, etc.	(o) Search for edible leaves for relish (uwuchisa), caterpillars, mushrooms, etc.
	(p) Gather wild fruits and roots (ukusepa).	(p) Ukusepa.
	(q) ——	(q) Extract salt.
	(r) ——	(r) Brew beer of all kinds.
(3) Other Preparations.	(a) Akapofwe for soap.	(a) Akapofwe for soap.
	(b) Tobacco.	(b) [Tobacco, old women.]
(4) Hunting, etc.	(a) Hunting proper (uwupalu).	(a) ——
	(b) Trapping: game, birds, mice, etc.	(b) ——
	(c) Honey.	(c) ——
	(d) Fishing: nets, weir-traps, spearing, hooking.	(d) Fishing: treading, bailing, string with worm-bait (no hook).
(5) Domestic Animals.	(a) Attention to goats.	(a) ——
	(b) Attention to fowls.	(b) Attention to fowls.
(6) Building.	Ukutala (marking out), ifiti (bringing poles), ulushishi (bark rope), ukufimba (thatching), ukwiwaka (erecting), ukuwanga (placing bonds), treading mud for plastering, ukumasa (rough plastering), ichiwi (door).	Ichyani (grass for thatching), water for mud, [ukumasa], ukushingula (smearing walls), preparation of floor, beating of floor, making of interior screen (ichipembe).

97

THE LAMBAS OF NORTHERN RHODESIA

	MEN	WOMEN
(7) *Clay-moulding.*	(a) [A few men mould pots.] (b) Pipe-bowls.	(a) Cooking and other pots. (b) ——
(8) *Baskets and Mats.*	(a) *Ututundu* (large baskets of bamboo). (b) *Ifisele* (shallow baskets of split bamboo). (c) —— (d) *Imichyeka* (palm - leaf mats). (e) *Imisengelo* (reed and split bamboo mats), *impasa* (of split reeds). (f) [*Amasasa* by few old men.]	(a) *Ututundu* (large baskets of reeds). (b) *Ifilukwa* (grass meal baskets). (c) *Imfuma* (grass beer basket), *ichisumiko* (beer strainer), *uluwanga* (rush fish basket). (d) [A few *imichyeka*.] (e) [*Imisengelo* by few unmarried women.] (f) *Amasasa* (of marsh grass).
(9) *Wooden Utensils, etc.*	(a) Eating bowls, ladles, stamp-blocks (*ifinu*), stools (*ifipuna* and *amatewe*), stirring-sticks, dug-out canoes, drums, axe, hoe, and spear handles, sticks, door-fasteners, etc. (b) *Inkombo*, drinking calabashes.	(a) —— (b) *Ifyeso* (calabashes halved).
(10) *Musical Instruments.*	*Ingoma, akalimba, akankoto, ubwesela, isese, umusembe, ilinkuwala.*	*Insai* (wild-orange rattle), *umutungu* (gourd drum), *insangwa* (seed rattles).
(11) *Weapons and Instruments.*	Spear, axe, bow, arrows, knife, hoe (*ise* and *ubweya*), adze, dancing axe, *akaweshi* (type of small knife carried in the hair), wire, brass bracelets, rings, combs.	*Uwuyombo* (grass dancing waist fringe), *amabwe* (stones for grinding picked up).
(12) *Bark and Skin Preparations.*	(a) *Ukusale'nguwo*, the preparation of bark cloth (*umusompo*). (b) *Ukupashila* (sewing). (c) *Ukunyuke'fisewa*, the preparation of skins as sleeping mats. [N.B. The Lenje and Ila wore skins, the Lamba bark cloth.]	(a) —— (b) —— (c) ——
(13) *Personal Adornment.*	(a) *Ichingalangala*, the feather headdress. (b) Tattooing.	(a) *Inkuku*, bead headdress woven in girls' hair. (b) Tattooing.

All wood-work (9) and metal-work (11), without exception, is the province of the man. Tree-felling, the procuring of heavy firewood, the essential parts of house-building, the use of bamboo in baskets and mats, and bark preparation all entail the use of the

98

axe, and therefore are done by the man. Hoeing, garden-work,
clay-work, and food-preparation are the province of the woman,
though when it comes to the heavier, or maybe more dangerous,
parts of this the man is required; he may do the hard initial
breaking of the ground in the new gardens, and while the woman
scares the birds, the man is needed to watch at night for the wild
pigs. Men must fetch the bamboo—it needs the *axe* to cut it
down and to split it for use afterward; but the women must
fetch the thatching grass, for, having no sickle, the Lambas use
the *hoe* to cut it through just above the roots. The divisions of
the types of fishing are equally suggestive; [1] the men fish with
the aid of metal and traps which require the use of the axe in their
preparation, while the women use the basket and similar means.
Again, that the 'heavy' work is given to the men is shown in the
fact that the heavy plastering (*ukumasa*) is done by men, while
the women put the finishing touches by smearing (*ukushingula*).
In basket- and mat-making men work predominantly in bamboo,
which requires the axe, while women work in grass and in reeds,
which require at most a knife to treat them. Not only is the
making of musical instruments of every kind practically confined
to the men, but the playing of them is similarly so restricted.
One never sees a woman playing any of the instruments made by
men, and, *vice versa*, the rattles and the gourd-drum which the
women prepare are never used by men. It is a significant thing
that since the preparation of clothing (bark cloth) used always to
be done by the men, with the substitution of calico in these days
the preparation of this into garments has also devolved upon the
men, and any sewing-machines that there are in the country are
used by the men. To a slight extent this tradition is being
countered by the teaching of girls by the missionaries.

Food and its Preparation

With the Lambas the three important things have always been
food, shelter, and clothing, in that order of importance. The
months or moons are regarded principally in reference to the food
there is to be had, to planting, garden preparation, and the
ripening of crops.

The staple food is *inshima*, thick porridge made from sorghum
meal. Sorghum or Kafir corn is called by the Lambas *amasaka*.
The preparation of *inshima* is called *ukunanya*. A large cooking-
pot is three-quarters filled with water and brought to the boil.

[1] See Chapter XX.

When the water boils handfuls of meal are added and the whole vigorously stirred. Meal is continuously added until the *inshima* is stiff. The last meal is naturally not fully cooked. The pot is now taken from the fire, held firmly by the feet, and the stirring continued for some time, when the steaming mass is turned out into a dish, a wooden bowl, or eating basket.

Accompanying the *inshima* there must be a bowl of *ifyakutoŵela*, relish. Generally the men eat together, and the women and children together, but at times the family—father, mother, and children—will eat from the one bowl. The participants in a meal are scrupulously careful to wash their hands before eating, for they use no spoon or suchlike implement to help them. They all squat round the common eating-bowl, and, breaking off with finger and thumb a morsel of the porridge, roll it round in the hand, dip it into the pot of relish, and eat it.

All Lamba foodstuffs are thus divided into those which comprise the main part of the meal and those which are used as relish. Here is a brief survey of the main commodities which they use under these two headings.

(1) **Food.** *Inshima* is made from *amasaka* (sorghum), *amataŵa* (maize), or *amawo* (a very small millet, of which there are several kinds—*kaŋonde*, *kapepele*, *mutuŵila*, and *chiŵungwe*). Maize and sorghum, when fresh and young, are also used boiled; this is called *umusaku*.

The following are boiled (*ukwipika*): *chipushi* and *mwanamusungu* (pumpkins); *ichilungu* and *akalungwa* (yams); *umumbu* (a marsh cultivated root, of which there are several kinds—*kafukwa*, *chyumbumapondo*, *ikumwa*, *chikata*, *kasununu*); *inyangu*, *utunyanguŵulamba*, and *nyinamatoŵomatoŵo* (beans); *umungu* (marrow); *ichitungusa* and *katende* (cucumbers); *kandolo* and *chilolwe* (sweet potatoes, both red and white); *tute* (cassava); *umuninga* and *uŵuleya* (ground-nuts).

Certain of these are also baked on the coals (*ukochya*)—for instance, *umuninga*, *tute*, *kandolo*, *chilolwe*, and sometimes *chipushi*—while a number may be eaten raw, *ichiŵimbi*, *ichitungusa*, *katende* and *ichikowa* (cucumbers), *kandolo*, *chilolwe*, *tute*, also the marsh roots *umumbu*, *mukuŵa*, and *kasununu*.

(2) **Relish.** The general term for relish is *ifyakutoŵela*. One of the principal types of relish is, as we shall see, *uŵuchisa*, and this latter term used to be applied to all types of relish, even meat, in order to hide what delicacy it might be. Using the terms strictly, the Lambas have the following types of relish:

(a) *Uŵuchisa*, cooked leaves.

(b) *Umulembwe*, greens pounded and cooked to a soft mash.

(c) *Ifishimu*, caterpillars squeezed out, skins thrown away, and interior juices boiled.

(d) *Ifinani*, meat (i) of *inama*, animals large and small, (ii) of *imbeŵa*, types of mice.

(e) *Ifyuni*, birds.

(f) *Isaŵi*, fish.

(g) Foodstuffs used as relish.

(h) Miscellancous.

(i) *Ifyakulunga*, condiments.

(a) *Uŵuchisa*. The following are the commonest leaves used in this way: *umusampala* (pumpkin leaves), *impumpule, umushikalilo, umunemena, chimboyi, kaliilwanse, ichimbulumutumba, iŵondwe* (wild spinach), *sosa, saasa* (cassava leaves), *ichitashi, umusaasa, ubwakaka, tandaŵala, funte, mwaŵo* (species of grass), *ichisosola* (eaten raw), *amakasa anchyenchye, akapulula, kalembula wamuchinika*, and *indulwe*.

(b) *Umulembwe*. These include the following: *mukona, pupwe, insanchi, umukungu, kalembwelukasu, ichilembwelembwe*, and *akafunda*.

(c) *Ifishimu* constitute a great delicacy with the Lambas. There are many kinds, which they collect from the trees at regular seasons. In many cases the caterpillar bears the name of the tree on which it feeds. In the following list the name of the tree is in parentheses after the name of the caterpillar: *ichinkuŵala (umutondo), umushila* or *umwandakoso (umutondo* and *umwandakoso), ichifumbe (ichifumbe), umukoso (umukoso), ulumombwe (ulumombwe), akaŵambe (umutondo), umusalya (umusalya), akakoto (umutoŵo), ichisukuŵya (umusuku), mwenje (umwenje), munshisondwa (ichimpampa)*—very few eat these last two—*akampakamwa (umusalya), umupetu (umupetu)*—eaten only by a few old people—*mumpa (umutondo), umushyankoko* (eats sorghum and grass), *ichiŵalatende* (eats grass), *chimamba (chimamba), ichilengwa* (a white grub 6 inches long, 2 inches in diameter, which lives inside *umunga*, the thorn-tree).

(d) *Ifinani*, meat, is treated in several ways by the Lambas. Fresh meat is either boiled or grilled on the coals. If a quantity of meat has been obtained, a portion is dried on a stand with a slow fire beneath—this means smoking as well as drying. Meat dried like this lasts for a long while, unless the *ifyundu* (zabrus, meat-eating grubs which become beetles) get to it. Dried meat is generally boiled to make a relish. Salt is greatly prized to boil with meat.

Following are lists of the more common animals (*inama*) and members of the mouse family (*imbewa*) eaten by the Lambas. It will be noticed that certain of them demand special treatment, owing to ill-omen which is associated with them.

(I) INAMA. *Insofu* (elephant). Lambas do not bake the trunk in the orthodox Bantu fashion in a heated trench. Pieces of the elephant are cut off and grilled on the embers. The tasty pieces are the trunk, the feet, and the flesh above the eyes.

Imfuwu (hippopotamus). The tasty pieces are the entrails, the head, and the feet. The feet are chopped up and pieces put into a large pot and boiled.

Kakwele (rhinoceros). Only a few people eat this.

Imbishi (zebra). It is taboo to bring the hoofs of a zebra into the village lest a death should occur; they are always cut off and thrown away.

Inkulo (black waterbuck).

Impelembe (both roan and sable antelopes).

Inkonshi (hartebeeste). The front feet are not eaten; between the hoofs is a deep cleft, and it is said that the *uwungwa* ('roguishness') of the animal is there. Natives fear that they may become 'rogues' if they eat it. The hartebeeste is credited with *uwungwa* because of its method of running and the way in which it eats, away in the middle of the plain.

Inshya (duiker).

Senya (oribi).

Insewula (puku).

Ichikokamabwe (klip-springer).

Inja (lechwe).

Impoyo (reed-buck).

Insowe (sitatunga).

Impala (gazelle).

Timba (grysbok).

Imbowo (buffalo).

Ichikwindi (yellow-backed duiker). This animal is not eaten by women, as it has quantities of blood. Women fear lest at childbirth they should lose a great deal of blood.

Shiwolwe (bush buck). One must never beg the neck of this buck, for it has a white hairless patch. It is feared lest a child born should have a similar spot on the neck. With this the evil seems to be in the begging; if offered, it can be eaten with impunity.

Insongo (eland). This animal is prized above all others for its fat. The tasty bits are the shins and feet.

Inguluŵe (bush pig) and *injili* (wart hog) are highly esteemed. When killed, these animals are held over a fire to burn off the bristles, and eventually eaten skin and all.

Inunji (porcupine). The meat is fat and greatly relished. The intestines are thrown away, as they are bitter, and it is said that dogs die if they eat them.

Impendwa (ant-bear). It is taboo to bring an ant-bear's head to the village, and it is always cut off and left in the bush.

Akampalanga (steinbuck).

Imbushi (goat). Not eaten by some natives.

Kolwe and *musemeni* (monkey and baboon). Eaten only by old people and little children.

Inshimba (genet). The *ichifungo* (scent-excreting gland) is first cut out, and then the animal is boiled, never grilled.

Inchyema, ŵumbe, akasakanenga, and *akapolobwe* are small animals boiled, not grilled.

Fulwe (tortoise). The old people eat this; they first put it on the fire to take off the shell, and then boil it.

Katumpa (civet). The scent-gland at the tail is first cut out, then the animal is grilled and afterward boiled, when it is said that the meat is good.

Akalulu and *ichilulu* (hares). It is taboo to bring the head to the village; it is cut off and left.

Chyanga and *akaŵundi* (galagos).

Ulupale (squirrel).

Shiŵembele (flying squirrel).

Kambole (ratel), always boiled.

Ipulu, akakwiso, chikankati, and *kandende* are small animals like mungooses and weasels.

Unborn animals are never eaten, but are thrown away. Meat *pakusasa*, when 'high,' but not yet putrid, is greatly prized. The natives say of it, *Fyaito'muto*, "It is calling the soup!"

(II) IMBEŴA. Under this heading the following are eaten, generally boiled: *insenshi* (cane-rat), *imfuko* (large mole), *akakoko* (small mole), *imfumbe, tunga* (by children and very old people only), *polongwe, ipanga, chishye, iŵende, mwansakala, pena, imfulwe, ingali,* etc. (all species of mice).

(*e*) *Ifyuni*, birds.

(i) Those eaten whether boiled or grilled:

Insumbi (domestic fowl). The eating of this is often connected with ceremonial.

THE LAMBAS OF NORTHERN RHODESIA

Inkulimba (pigeon), *chiŵa* (dove), *musokoshi* (pheasant), *ikanga* (guinea-fowl), *chintalantala* (partridge), *pwele* (thrush), *shimutengu* (lark).

Akatutwa, a small bird which is never eaten by anyone who still has his own mother and father living. It is believed that if this taboo is broken the bird can curse the eater.

Iŋanga yashiŵakota, chintole, impolcŵe, mukwe, ifukulansyama, ichisokosoko, akaundu (quail), *chyandwe* and *chyelemfu* (parakeets), *muŵangwa* (woodpecker).

(ii) Those only eaten boiled: *ichyoso* (duck), *ishipi* (goose), *ichipampamanshi* (a water-fowl), *mulondwe* (cormorant), *akaseŵe* (buzzard), *akaseŵa* (sparrow), *induŵa* (lurie), *umukuta, fumfunkanana, mulongwe* (hornbill), *mutongola, inkonje* (egret), *imbuŵute* (hoopoe).

(iii) Only eaten grilled: *akatinga* (type of tomtit).

(*f*) *Isaŵi*, fish. Fresh fish are usually boiled, but the larger ones may be grilled on the coals. Generally, however, fish when caught in quantities are cut open, dried over slow fires, and then when used are either boiled or grilled. The commonest fish in the rivers is the barbel called *umuta*, of which there are several kinds—e.g., *kambale, akatanaŋanya, sampa*, and *ichiŵoŵe*. Other edible fish include the following: *isuŵula, ikamba, chikuwamawo, sampa, chipuŵamulomo, akafumbe, umusenga, ilemba, umupofwe, shimwenje, ulukomo, ulupumbu, chinimba*. In addition the crab (*inyanje*) and a certain species of water-beetle (*imbushi yapamenda*) are eaten.

(*g*) The following foodstuffs are also used as relish:

Inyangu (small beans). These are crushed on the grindstone, winnowed clear of husks, boiled, and stirred into a kind of gruel. It is called *kwela wanyangu*.

Umuninga (pea-nuts). Roasted with salt.

Intetele (pips of pumpkin and marrow). These are used either roasted with salt or stamped, boiled, and made into gruel called *umusanta*.

Uŵuleya (a species of ground-nut). Broken up in the stamp-block, winnowed, boiled, and made into gruel, called *kwela waŵuleya*.

(*h*) Miscellaneous relish:

Londwa (flying termite). Roasted.

Umutende (small flying termite). Roasted.

Ulushye (locust). Used when they appear, and treated in one of three ways: (i) boiled, (ii) roasted, (iii) dried by old people and stamped to a meal.

Ichipembya (countess beetle). Roasted.

Amaluko (young of bees). Boiled or roasted.

(*i*) *Ifyakulunga*, condiments, are used when they can be obtained, and are principally of three kinds: (i) salt (*umuchyele*), (ii) chilies (*impilipili*), and (iii) onions (*ifitungulu*). Natives often make up a type of pickle of all three mixed with water.

(3) **Supplementary and Famine Foods.** In the various seasons the people supplement their menu with gleanings from the forest; these, called *ifisepo*, consist of fruits and roots. They also avail themselves of the various types of honey and the many kinds of edible fungi. In famine time certain of these wild roots become their mainstay of life. As will be seen, some of them have to be treated in a special way.

(*a*) *U ŵ u c h i*, honey. Bee-honey is to be found at different seasons

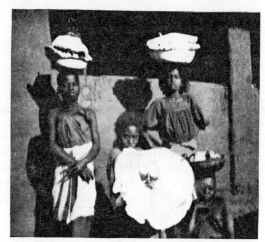

FIG. 38. MISSION SCHOOLCHILDREN WITH TELYA MUSHROOMS

Photo by Miss O. C. Doke

according to the type of nectar procurable by the bees; and the natives recognize the following: *kasabwa, kumba, akankobwe, umusamba,* and *umutendefu.* But apart from the ordinary bees there are several kinds of small honey-making insects which the natives call *utushimu* (the ordinary bee being *ulushimu*). Most of these place their honey deep down in the ground or in anthills. They include *uŵungulwe, ichipashi, umwande, insolwe, uŵunyanta, ichiŵonga,* and *chintimba,* the last of which makes a strong intoxicating honey if it has used the nectar of the *kasabwa*-tree.

(*b*) *Uŵowa*, fungi or mushrooms. It is wonderful to see how well the people, young and old, are able to pick out the edible from the poisonous types, and I have not heard of a case of mushroom poisoning among the Lambas. Edible mushrooms are of many kinds, and during the rainy season are generally

105

plentiful. The following is not a complete list: *winyanta, ulumbulula, chimpape, akatyotyo, tande, uŵukwesenje, sukwa, ichisamfu, akatulukwa, nsanda, telya, uŵunkungwa, akankolenkole, munya, uŵusepa, kaŵansa, musefwe, kakonso, imfuti, ubwitondwe, ichilomonamuŋomba, ichiŵengele, ilimfwemfwe, ikaŵakaŵa, akapolo, mushinje.* As a rule these are eaten boiled, but the *kaŵansa* is also eaten raw, while the *munya* may also be grilled.

(c) *Fruit.* The following are some of the commonest fruits eaten by the natives in Ilamba: *ulupundu, ikonkola, ulukomfwa, imfinsa, ifufuma, ikole, iŵungo, ikukwe, mukolamfula, impo, ichikundunkuluŵyu, ilinkulimba, uluchyenja, ichichyenjeshilu, ilolo, isuku, akakonko, ichisombo, akalunji, chyangwemuleya, akatonga, akaŵungombalala, akampamapebwe, muŋomba, ulukulungufya, ulufungo.* The last named is also eaten when boiled and stirred into a kind of gruel.

(d) *Roots.* The following provide substitute food in times of scarcity of the crops planted:

Uŵusala. This resembles a sweet potato when it is cooked.

Umupama. Boiled.

Kasaŵo. This root, on account of its poisonous properties, has to be treated in a special way. The root is white, and is cooked in large pots. After it has been thoroughly cooked, the next day the skin is scraped off and the roots sliced up. They are then placed in an *umusantu*, a grass bundle, and put to soak in running water, where they are left for two days. On the third day they are taken out and put in water boiling over a fire, stirred up, and treated like *inshima*.

Natives say that if hyenas are troublesome about the village they take bones with a little meat on them, soak them in water with raw *kasaŵo*, and then place a pot of this at a crossing of the paths. A hyena will come and eat the meat and bones and drink the water. He will then be rendered so helpless by the poison that he will be found there by the villagers in the morning and killed. Sometimes villagers in famine time have been poisoned through not waiting to soak the roots for the full time required.

Ulukolongo. This is a red root which is treated in the same way as the *kasaŵo*, except that it has to be soaked in swiftly running water for four days. After that it may be eaten straight away or made into *inshima*. If not treated in this way it is said to cause 'drunkenness' and even death.

Ulufumfutu. This root is not dangerous, but on account of its bitterness and slimy nature it too has a lengthy treatment.

It is cooked, taken out, scraped, and cut up; then it is soaked for two days, after which it is eaten.

Ulusasa. A root eaten raw.

Mukwilwa. Eaten raw or cooked.

Ilintabwa. Dug up, brought to the village, and sliced up after being scraped clean of rind. Certain bitter leaves called *ŵufunde* are placed in a pot, the *amantabwa* is placed on them, and more *ŵufunde* on top. With water this is set on the fire and boiled for a long time, until the whole settles to the bottom. It is then dished up and divided out; all use ladles and drink it as gruel. The *ŵufunde* in the mixture is said to have become sweet and the whole to taste like honey.

Ilumbwe. A root resembling sweet potato, eaten raw or boiled.

Umunkombwa. Eaten boiled.

Isafwa. Eaten raw.

Ulupalwa. The roots of the water-lily (*ichikwiŵu*) eaten grilled or boiled. This is the main food of the Twa people of the swamps, and is said to taste like *amawo* millet.

From this list it will be seen that the bush of Lambaland provides very many kinds of famine foodstuffs. Such is the improvidence of the people that, despite the number of kinds of cultivated food grown, they very often have to depend upon *ifisepo*, veld food, in the period before their crops ripen, and when it is realized that *kasaŵo* and *amantabwa* have frequently to be relied upon it can be seen how hard-pressed they sometimes are.

(4) **Drink.** There are two principal kinds of beer made by the Lambas, *ifisunga*, which is non-intoxicating, and *ubwalwa*, which is very intoxicating. The only other intoxicating beverage which they make is *imbote*, honey-beer, which may be intoxicating or not, according to the method of brewing. But there are several other kinds of non-intoxicating drinks which the people are able to make only at special seasons. From sorghum, in addition to *ifisunga*, they make *intongo*, *akatete*, and *funku*; from maize, *ichisekele*; and from various fruits, such as the *impundu* and the *amasuku*, they make *timbwa*.

To brew (*ukukumba*) the intoxicating *ubwalwa* the Lambas soak (*aŵika*) sorghum in water for two days, until it begins to sprout, when it is called *amamena*. This they spread out to dry (*anika*). When dry, it is ground, and the flour is then boiled for a long time. Meanwhile a portion of the *amamena* is taken when dry, mixed with ordinary sorghum, ground, cooked, cooled in a large pot (*umutondo*), and set aside to ferment (*ŵila*). This is called *umusunga*. This 'leaven' is then mixed in small quantities with the boiled *ubwalwa*.

Beer-drinks take place after working-bees or working-parties (*imbile*), when the one whose garden is hoed supplies his helpers with the beverage, also during the dancing in connexion with mourning and other types of spirit-worship. Women brew the beer, but they do not gather at the beer-drinks as the men do. They often wait on the men, handing the beer round, and may drink moderately by themselves, though I have never known of a Lamba woman getting drunk.

Honey-beer (*imbote*) is of two kinds, an intoxicating and a non-intoxicating.

(*a*) INTOXICATING. The young of bees (*amaluko*) are taken and put into a calabash with a little maize flour; the calabash is closed up and the preparation set for one day to ferment. In the morning a mixture of honey and water is poured in and stirred up, the calabash being filled, and then set out in the sun for a day. In the evening it is set near to the fire and kept warm during the night. After another day in the sun it will be ready for drinking by night. This beer is violently intoxicating, and is indulged in only by small parties. The drinking of honey-beer is not connected with any of the social or religious gatherings.

(*b*) NON-INTOXICATING. Water and honey are mixed in a calabash and set in the sun for a day. That same evening it is drunk. This beer is called *umumfundwa*.

Tobacco

Tobacco, *fwaka*, is grown in every Lamba village, principally on the sides of the enormous anthills, where the soil is very rich. Sometimes the leaves are plucked, quickly dried before the fire, crushed, and then smoked. But when large quantities are dealt with the leaves are picked and packed in a large drum of bark called *imfuulu*, which is mudded up to render it airtight. This bark drum is then put into the fire, baked carefully, and put aside for four or five days. After this it is broken and the tobacco taken out and pounded in a mortar (*ichinu*). The tobacco is then put out to dry slightly, pounded again, made into little cakes (*ifimpwampwa*), and again put out to dry. These cakes are then put into a basket (*ichilukwa*) and pressed and kneaded together (*ukukatika*) with the pounded leaves or bark of a shrub called *umulolo* to make the mass bind. It is then taken from the basket, polished, and put out to dry. This result is called *umwambwa*.

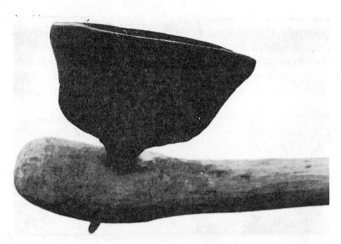

FIG. 39. ICHIPAMBA
See p. 121.
Photo by W. Paff

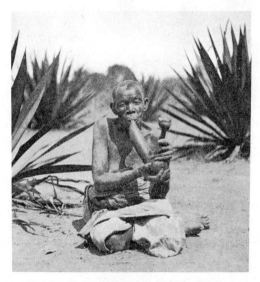

FIG. 40. OLD CHYALWE AND HER IMBOKOMA
Photo by C. M. Doke

THE LAMBAS OF NORTHERN RHODESIA

There is another type of prepared tobacco, called *kansai*. Green leaves of tobacco are bound together in a bundle of grass (*umusantu*) and left for five to ten days, until the tobacco rots, when it is treated as above. *Kansai* is extremely strong.

The common Lamba pipes are of two kinds, the *impoli*, a small clay bowl at the end of a long reed, and the *imbokoma*, or calabash pipe. The *impoli* holds but little at a time, and is often used for

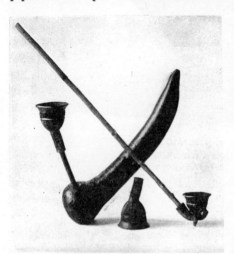

FIG. 41. IMBOKOMA AND IMPOLI WITH CLAY PIPE-BOWL
Photo by W. Paff

uluŵangula or h e m p. The *imbokoma* is composed of three parts. A large clay bowl (*intuntu*) with a neck, into which is fixed a reed stem (*itete*) connecting it with a long-shaped calabash water-container (*umuchinda*). Tobacco is placed in the *intuntu*, live coals put on top, and the smoke drawn through the water in the calabash with a gurgling noise.

In the old days hemp was grown in most villages. When it is full size the people cut it down and dry it; they then tie it up in bundles, and use it after crushing it in the hands. When smoked to any extent this *uluŵangula* has a maddening effect, far worse than that of intoxicating beer. In Rhodesia and the Belgian Congo it is now illegal to grow hemp.

Salt-making

Before European salt was imported the Lambas used salt of three kinds: (1) a brown salt imported from the Kasempa district, (2) a black salt, called *nyinalochya*, imported from the Congo, and (3) their own, obtained from the burning of certain grasses.

Nyinalochya is prepared by the Congo Lambas, who dig a species of black mud, put it into *imfuulu* (bark covers), and then cause water to percolate through it (*ukusumika*). The dry mud which is left over is then burnt by turning the container over a

110

fire as on a spit, the bark cover not being allowed to burn. It is then put aside to cool. When cool, the bark is broken off, and the mud is found black and hard. This is used for salting food.

Various types of salt grass are used for salt extraction—e.g., *umunyanja, chikukulu, chikankati, chiŵangalume, nteŵe*—as well as the plant *ulwisonga* and the leaves of the *ichitashi*-tree. When preparing this salt, women who are not menstruating go to the

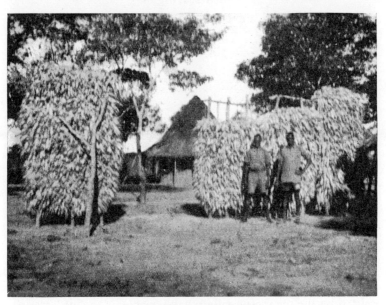

FIG. 42. HOW MAIZE IS STACKED
Photo by Miss O. C. Doke

river, gather the grass, maybe *nteŵe*, and spread it out there to dry. In the morning they come and gather more. When dry the grass is burnt and the ashes gathered and carried to the village in baskets (*ututundu*). Salt percolators (*ifyeso* or *ifisumiko*) made of finely woven palm leaf are brought and the ashes placed therein. Water is poured on, and this trickles through into a pot below. This salty water is used to season meat. At times salt-ash is stored in bags and treated as above when required. Salt made from the *ichitashi*-tree is not greatly relished on account of its smell, as also that from the chickweed, *ulwisonga*.

At places a salty incrustation is found on rocks, ground, and *chyembe* grass. This looks like hoar frost, is called *chyembe*, and

III

is merely gathered together and used in that state for salting relish.

The soil of certain of the large anthills is decidedly salty, and this has been discovered by the large game, who resort to such places to lick. Some of these salt-licks have been used for many years, great cavities being made in the anthills. These the natives call *imbu*.

Bird-scaring

One of the regular annual duties, which takes up considerable time and the attention of all the women and children, often

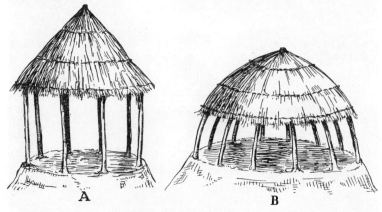

FIG. 43. TWO TYPES OF INSAMA
A, with upright poles and thatched roof ; B, with poles bent to meet
at top and upper part thatched.

assisted by the men, especially the old people, is the bird-scaring, *ukwamina*. This generally commences at the end of April, and lasts some seven weeks, until the harvest of sorghum is gathered in. Small shelters, *insama*, are erected on the anthills to shelter the scarers from the sun, though the work is confined mostly to the morning and the evening, the birds not being active at midday. If there are insufficient ant-heaps, *utupingwe*, platforms on poles, are erected to elevate the scarers. The birds which cause most damage are the *utuseŵa* (sparrows), *uŵuchyonko* (finches), *ŵachiŵa* (doves), *ŵachyandwe* (parakeets), and *ubwilangwe* (mecklings). In these days tins of all sorts, in addition to the *amankuŵala* (hollowed boat-shaped logs of wood), are beaten to make a noise and scare off the birds. The little boys make miniature bows with grass-stalk arrows (*intende*) and shoot at the birds to keep them on the move.

Threshing and Winnowing

When the sorghum is harvested the cut heads are stacked on low stands (*ififufu*) to keep them off the ground, away from termites. In front of the stand the hard ground is swept clean. A certain amount of the gathered heads is put down on this

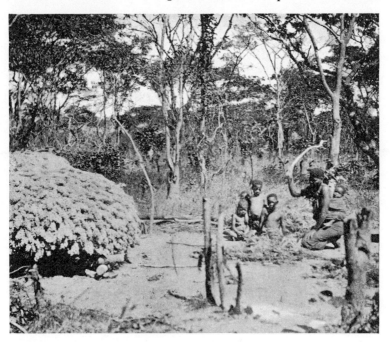

FIG. 44. THRESHING SORGHUM, AND AN ICHIFUFU OF SORGHUM
Photo by C. M. Doke

threshing-floor. A woman will break off any serviceable stick, and, kneeling down, often with her baby asleep upon her back, will beat (*ukupuma*) the corn, continually turning it over. The empty heads are thrown aside and the threshed corn gathered into baskets. She will now proceed to winnow (*ukwela*). Taking a quantity of corn in a small basket called *ulupe*, standing at full height, she pours it out in a stream into a large *akatundu* basket standing on the ground. If the wind is blowing this process is repeated only a few times to clean the grain of all refuse.

Grinding (Ukupela)

After the corn-heads are harvested into the permanent grain-houses, the people prefer to thresh and winnow small quantities from time to time, as the unthreshed corn is less susceptible to the ravages of the weevil (*uŵusumfi*). Sorghum and the small

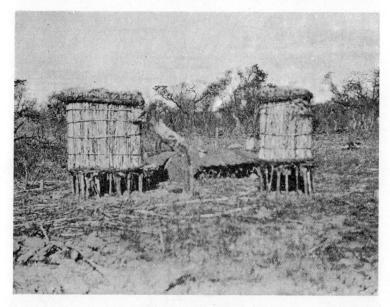

FIG. 45. GRAIN-BINS
Photo by C. M. Doke

millet are ground on the grindstones. Each woman has her stone beneath the eaves outside her house. A hole is dug, in which the stone is set; mud is pressed down all round the stone and moulded carefully round its edge. The nether grindstone is called *ibwe* (the stone). The upper stone is called *impelo* (the grinder). The women use a third stone, called *insono*, for chipping and roughening the lower stone when it becomes too smooth. In front of the *ibwe* and below it is a scooped-out hole, well plastered, into which the flour falls as the corn is ground. The woman kneels behind the stone, takes a handful of corn from her basket, places it on the stone, and works the *impelo* over it with the motion of a washerwoman using a washboard; the ground meal goes into the hollow below, and more corn is added to the

114

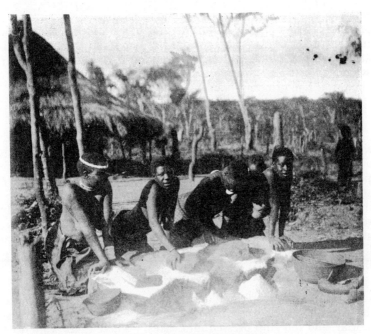

FIG. 46. A COMMUNAL GRINDSTONE
Photo by C. M. Doke

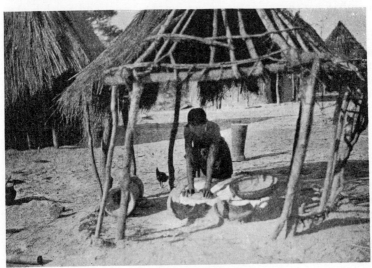

FIG. 47. AN ICHIMABWE
Photo by C. M. Doke

stone as required. The Lamba method of grinding while kneeling is in marked contrast to that of the Ila, who stand at raised grind-stones. Most villages have a communal grinding-house, in which as many as five stones may be seen together beneath a shelter. The grinding-house is called *ichimabwe*.

Stamping (Ukutwa)

Maize is generally treated in the stamp-block or mortar [1] called *ichinu*. This is a partly hollowed log of wood which stands about 2½ feet in height, the lower part being of solid wood. The pestle (*umunshi*) is a heavy smoothed piece of wood. Women sometimes stamp singly, but more often in pairs, alternate stamping crushing the foodstuffs very quickly; and I have frequently seen three working in rotation at the same mortar. The maize, after being stamped, is generally husked by sifting or shaking up. Cassava, various leaves for relish, and tobacco are all treated in the *ichinu*.

Soap Substitute

In the place of soap the Lambas used to use the *akapofwe* bush, the roots of which were dug up, scraped clean, pounded in the mortar, and the pulp pressed into cakes. These cakes were used as is a cake of soap, and much froth was produced. Usually a small portion was pinched off and rubbed over the body. The Lambas say that this was known to the Ngoni and Swahili also.

For cleaning the teeth they have a substitute for the tooth-brush. They take a thick twig of *umusuku* or *umupundu*, scrape it free of bark, beat the one end with an axe-handle on a stone, and use this fibrous end for rubbing their teeth. It is called *umuswachi wameno*. Sometimes ash is used as a tooth-powder.

Fire-making

The Lambas used regularly to make fire by friction, though this method is seldom seen nowadays. The lower stick, called *ichipantu*, is in the rainy season always made of *indale* wood, but in the dry season any stick is chosen for the purpose. The upper stick, called *ulushiko*, is made of the bush *umushikalilo*. The upper stick is twirled between the opposed palms of the hands until a small pile of powder is ground off from the lower stick and commences to smoulder. A bit of cloth is put to this, and when it has caught alight grass is lit by pressing it against the smoulder-ing cloth and blowing upon it. The lower stick is always notched,

[1] Note the two mortars in Fig. 47.

to give the upper stick a grip. The Lambas have always vener-
ated the *ulushiko*; they say, "It is our father, for it makes fire
for us."

Clay-moulding and Pottery

Apart from the moulding of pipe-bowls from clay, all clay-
moulding and the making of pots is the province of the women.
It is not every Lamba woman who can do it, but certain *aŵamano*,
clever ones, regularly do this work and barter what they make.
In the plain or near the river they dig up suitable clay, called
iŵumba, which they bring to the village and pound on a stone.
Old potsherds are now brought, broken up, and mixed with the
clay, the resulting mixture being called *inshiŵo*. A little water is

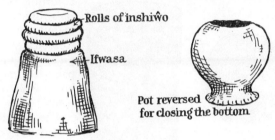

Rolls of inshiŵo

Ifwasa

Pot reversed
for closing the bottom.

FIG. 48. STAGES IN THE MAKING OF A POT

now added. When this mixture is ready a large *ifwasa* (nodule
ant-heap) is brought, the top cut off level and smeared with mud,
and the ant-holes all stopped with mud. All this is done within
the house. The *inshiŵo* is now kneaded up, and a long roll of
the damp clay prepared and placed encircling the top of the
ifwasa. On top of this another roll is placed, and so on, gradually
building up the pot. When one layer is set on the other an
oyster shell is taken and used to smear the two together. When
the mouth of the pot is finished decorative markings are made all
along the lip. The pot, with the hole in the bottom, is then
taken off the *ifwasa* and stood inverted in order to dry. The
moulder then takes an *ichipyolo*, a type of wooden knife, which
has been used for marking the lip, and with it works over the
outside, bringing the superfluous clay forward to fill up the hole
left. When this is closed up the pot is put aside to dry hard.

When a number of pots have been moulded and dried firewood
is brought; some is put on the ground, with the pots upon it,
while the rest covers the pots completely. The pile is then
burnt and the pots thoroughly baked.

Lamba pots are of various sizes and types. The general term by which they are indicated is *inongo*. Others are *ichimfwembe* (a large pot with a large mouth, used for cooking and washing purposes); *ichisanshilo* (a large pot for brewing beer); *umutondo* (water-pot); *ichisanji* or *uluŵya* (a small pot with a wide mouth, used for relish); *intalo* (the regular medium pot for cooking *inshima*); and *insukuso* (a warm-water finger-bowl).

Mat- and Basket-making

It has already been observed that the making of mats and baskets is carefully divided between the men and the women

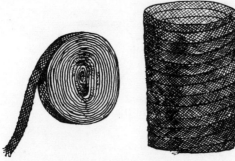

according to the materials used in their manufacture. The women use grass and rushes, the men palm-leaf and bamboo, while both use reeds.

The finest type of mat made by the Lambas is the *umuchyeka*, the manufacture of which is almost en-

FIG. 49. MAKING OF UMUCHYEKA

tirely confined to the men. Sometimes there are women found who plait and weave this type of mat, but they do this after the men have procured and prepared the materials. Branches of the *ulunchindu* palm are cut down and put out to dry. When dry they are dipped into water to soften them. In order to obtain dark leaves for weaving the pattern some are left in the water for a whole day. When the leaves are ready they are cut and torn down into strips. The weaving is done by hand, great lengths of woven material, each 2 to 3 inches in width, being produced and wound into a coil like a roll of ribbon. When the weaving is finished the length is worked together in spiral fashion to make a huge mat cylinder, which is cut through and laid out flat.

Working in Wood

Men only make implements and instruments of wood, using the axe and the adze. Drums (*ingoma*) are hollowed from logs of the *umuchinka-*, *umusase-*, and *akalunguti-*trees, stools (*ifipuna*)

118

from the *umuchinka*, and *amankuŵala* (used in bird-scaring) from the *akalunguti* and *ichiŵoŵo*, on account of their resonance.

Makers of boats, dug-outs, are called *aŵaŵashishi ŵamato*, and they command considerable respect in the community. As much as fifty shillings is paid for a good dug-out canoe, and in the old days the price was a gun or a female slave. The trees used are the *umupundu*, *umupapa*, *umululu*, and *umuchyenja*. The tree selected is felled; the next day the top is cut off; the next day the bark is beaten and removed; on the next notches are cut across the log (*ukuŵange'mango*) and the hollowing commenced. When the log is hollowed out the outside shaping is done. Usually two men work together, and the work is completed in about a month.

A bark canoe (*ichikondo*) may be made in a very short time. I once watched one being made for the purpose of retrieving a hippo which I had killed in the Upper Kafue, and it took just two and a half hours from the choosing of the tree to the launching in the river. My guides quickly picked out a large *umuputu* - tree

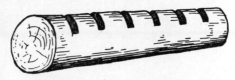

FIG. 50. LOG NOTCHED PREPARATORY TO BEING HOLLOWED OUT FOR MAKING A CANOE

growing near the river, ringed it round near the base with an axe, leant against it a pole, up which one climbed and ringed the tree round again at a height of about twelve feet. A vertical incision was then made in the bark from one ring to the other, poles being inserted into this incision and used to lever the bark from the tree. As soon as it was loose the whole strip of bark slid to the ground and was pulled away. A fire was kindled, and into this the ends of the cylinder of bark were placed. They soon became pliable, and were doubled up and secured with cross skewers of wood. Other cross-pieces were placed at intervals along the length of the canoe to keep the bark open. The canoe was now ready. A couple of cracks, where hasty work had penetrated the bark, were plugged with clay, and the boat was launched, two men paddling it quickly to the other side of the river, to secure a long bark rope to the hippo.

Bark-cloth Making

Until the introduction of calico, first by the Mbundu and Chikunda traders and later by Europeans, the Lambas depended entirely upon bark cloth for their supply of clothing, both to satisfy the demands of modesty and for warmth during the winter nights. The Lenje and Ila peoples as regularly used skins, and to a very slight degree this custom was followed by some of the Lamba-speaking people, especially the Southern Wulimas. The preparation of bark cloth was no small undertaking. Usually a

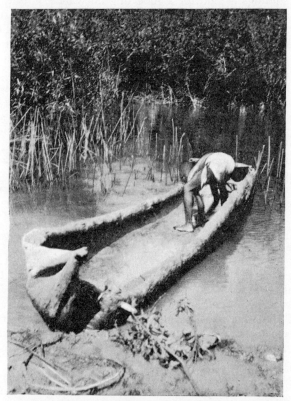

FIG. 51. BAILING OUT A BARK CANOE
Photo by C. M. Doke

party of men went together to sleep in the bush at a place where there was a supply of suitable *lwenshi*-trees. Food for the journey and the stay there would be prepared by the women beforehand. The trees have to be tested; small chips of bark are cut out and broken to examine the fibre. Satisfactory trees are cut down, and the branches cut up to make a pile of logs, each about 4 feet long, with a diameter of about 6 inches. Each log is then taken and the hard, rough bark carefully removed with an axe. After

120

this an incision is made down the length of the log, and the soft inside bark, *ulukwa*, is taken off whole. This complete process is called *ukukombole'nkwa*. The stripped logs are thrown away. When they have stripped all the logs the men carry their *inkwa* to the *umutanda* where they have slept. In the morning they clean from the *inkwa* all remnants of the outer bark (*ifipapwa*) which had escaped the work of the axe. This is called *ukupale' nkwa*. Each man will do from fifteen to twenty strips at a time, and then put them in the sun to dry. The next morning these strips are tied into a bundle and taken to the village. Several more days are taken to dry the pieces of bark completely, and then they are soaked in *ichilambe* (muddy water) for a whole day and night.

At the village flat boards (*imikunko*) are prepared, about 4 feet by 1½ feet by 4 inches, carefully cut and smoothed with adzes so as to lie flat and steady on the ground and present a flat surface for the work. *Umuchinka-* and *umuchyenja*-trees are used for this purpose. These boards are taken to the marsh where the bark is soaking. The bark strips are taken out of

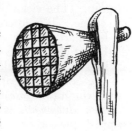

FIG. 52.   ICHINKUW̊U

the water one at a time, carefully washed clear of mud, and laid on the *imikunko*. The hammering (*ukusala*) of the cloth then commences. It is done with an *ichipamba*.[1] One kind of *ichipamba* is of metal, shaped like an ordinary axe-head, but with the cutting edge split open. It has a short wooden handle, and is but rarely to be seen in these days, except in spirit huts. Another is made of wood, and called *ichinkuẘu*. The *pupwe*-tree is used for the head, which is set in a handle, as is the other. Sometimes rhinoceros horn is used for the purpose. With the *ichipamba* the *ulukwa* is hammered thoroughly all over, water being sprinkled on to keep it wet. When one side is done the bark is turned over and the process repeated. When the second side is finished the cloth is folded over, and two men together wring out the water (*ukupota*). The finished cloth is much wider than the bark was when it was first stripped from the tree. When complete it is called *umusompo*, or, more generally, *inguŵo*. *Umusompo* is a necessity to the young men, who sell it in order to get the necessary *ichyupo*, or pledge for marrying. Unmarried women will supply food to them when at this work so as to get a piece of cloth in return.

When the cloth-beating is complete, the edges of the pieces are

[1] See Fig. 39.

trimmed and the strips sewn together with twine made from hemp (*uluŵangula*) into four-yard pieces (*ifilundo*). As an *ichyupo* two *ifilundo* are given to the mother-in-law, one to the bride, and one to the bride's maternal uncle.

Rope-making

Rope and fine twine are made from the *umukusa* (sanseviera plant), the soft inside bark of the *umusamba*- and *lwenshi*-trees, and in the old days from *uluŵangula* (hemp).

The *umukusa* strips are beaten with a stick on a log of wood, and then squeezed or scraped with a piece of bamboo to extract all pulp. The clean fibre left is rolled on the thigh and twisted into twine. It is interesting to note that the Qhung Bushmen of the Kalahari use the same plant, but do not beat it; they finish off the article by polishing it with kapok.

The soft inside bark (*ulushishi*) of such trees as the *umusamba* and the *lwenshi* is stripped off, soaked in water, and then rolled on the thigh (*ukuposa*) and rolled in reverse (*ukupyata*).

When *uluŵangula* is used, the stalks are broken, and the bark stripped down them; from that the string is twined.

It is perhaps not out of place to note here some of the customs of the Lambas concerning their personal adornment in hair-dressing, teeth-filing, and tattooing.

Hairdressing

Ordinarily, hair that has been cut off is thrown away on the ash-heap. Men, women, and children make no distinction in their hairdressing; they all usually keep it cut short. In the old days it was cut with a knife (*akaŵeshi*), a tedious business, but in these days scissors are used. At the time of death the relatives of the deceased *shave* their heads clean as a sign of mourning.

With the Lambas hairdressing is not significant, but merely ornamental. It is indulged in by the men as a rule, though the women at times let their hair grow long, and then weave (*ukuposa*) it in little plaits all over, some of which are worked together. The men have various eccentric ways of cutting their hair, dividing it into sections and patterns. Sometimes huge ears of hair are left—the chief Nkomeshya favoured this style—and sometimes *umwala wambishi* (a zebra's mane) is left down the centre. Others have an *ichipachilo*, like a raised vizor above the forehead, the back and top of the head being shaved clean. Sometimes *ifipupu*, combs or horns of hair, are left, one in front and one at the back, shaved round and between.

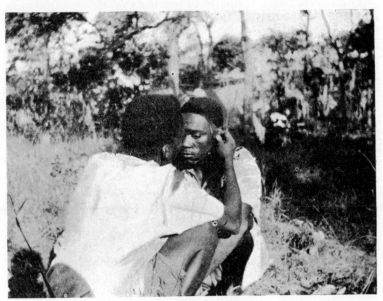

FIG. 53. SHAVING THE CHIEF KAWUNDA CHIWELE
Photo by Miss O. C. Doke

Many men shave back regularly from the forehead so as to increase the size of the forehead, and thus gain more respect. This custom they say they derived from the Wembas.

An *ichisungu* girl does not cut her hair during the period of her confinement; at the end of her time the special adornment of the head with beads is carried out.

A *mukamwami* also does not cut his hair, but lets it hang in plaited tassels all round his head, adorned with castor-oil and red ochre.

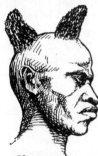

Ichipachilo   Ifipupu

FIG. 54. TWO METHODS OF DRESSING THE HAIR

123

Teeth

The Lambas used regularly to practise the custom of filing or chipping the teeth (*ukuŵasa'masonje*). A man with his whole teeth (*amankamba*) was laughed at by his companions. They used to say that when such a man went to sleep "his teeth came out, ate dung, and when replete went back to him in the morning," but that the *amasonje* went out at night and ate meal. This ridicule was effective in driving the young people to have their teeth chipped. On the day that a child is to have his teeth treated his father, mother, and maternal uncle each make him a present of a fowl, as a sign of honour. The Lambas have special *aŵaŵashishi ŵameno* (teeth-chippers), among whom are Makwati and Chilyobwe, of Nsonkomona's village. The chipping is done

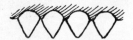 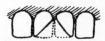

FIGS. 55, 56. TWO METHODS OF FILING THE TEETH

with a small, sharp adze. Friends of the patient hold him by the head during the operation. All the single teeth are done, on the first day all the top ones and on the next day the lower ones. The result is 'crocodile teeth.' This is, of course, conducive to early decay, as the enamel is destroyed, and in these days very few indulge in the practice.

Another practice, which is stated to be of Kaonde origin, is to chip the two upper front teeth so as to part them. A further practice borrowed from the Kaonde is that of extracting the two centre lower teeth. These are knocked out, sometimes by a piece of iron, sometimes by a specially shaped piece of stick hammered in between them. These practices are purely for personal adornment.

Tattooing

With the Lambas tattooing is never a tribal mark as it is with the Ŵemba people, who make tribal incisions between the eye and the ear. There are three significances of tattooing, that in the initiation of hunters, that for curative medicinal purposes, and that for personal adornment.

(1) *Ubwanga bwanama*, the hunting charm, consisting of incisions in the hand, is described in Chapter XX.

(2) As curative medicine. If a person suffers from continued headaches a friend, or maybe his wife, will cut small incisions

lengthwise across his forehead, and rub into them *umusamu* (medicine) prepared from *chilangalume* roots, pounded into a wet paste. This burns violently, and no doubt acts as a counter-irritant. When these *inembo* (incisions) heal up no mark is left. Similar incisions are made on the back for pain in that region. A professional 'doctor' (*umulaye*) is not called in to do this.

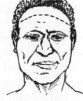

FIG. 57. CURATIVE INCISIONS

(3) For personal adornment incisions are made on the chest, upper arms, and back. On the arms the marks are cut in short dashes lengthwise from the shoulder toward the elbow. Men tattoo the chest, while women tattoo from below the breasts to the navel.

Recently the women have begun to imitate from the Kaonde the tattooing of two long incisions above each breast, also of six

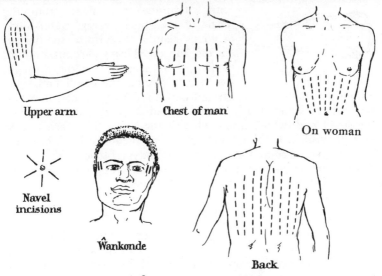

Upper arm.   Chest of man.   On woman

Navel incisions   Ŵankonde   Back

FIG. 58. EXAMPLES OF TATTOOING

radiating from the navel. Both men and women have begun to copy incisions between eyes and ears, which are called *ŵankonde*. The Kaonde people, both men and women, make six incisions on the pubes, but these the Lambas fear to copy.

Tattooing on the back is also of downward incisions, reaching as far as the waist.

All this tattooing is carried out by a professional *umulembeshi* (cutter). He is paid with small quantities of beads. This art is considered a great accomplishment, and not many have it. At Nsonkomona's village is Muka-Maŵutau. In tattooing the skin is cut with a sharp razor, and much blood is let out. Ground charcoal is then rubbed into the incisions. The operation is described as very painful. On the next day the places are washed, and castor-oil is rubbed on until the sores heal up. The operation is generally carried out beneath the hut eaves, and usually a crowd of interested spectators gathers round, though nervous 'patients' would be operated on in private.

Cupping

This is an operation not confined to the *aŵalaye*; anyone may cup (*ukusumika*) a sick person. Supposing a man is suffering in his legs and unable to walk, a friend will suggest cupping. The

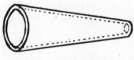

'cups' (*imisuku*) are made from the horns of reed-buck, young water-buck, or young eland. The tip of the horn is cut off, and the thicker part cut straight, so that there is a hole right through. Beeswax is put on the small end. In-

FIG. 59. UMUSUKU

cisions are made on the affected part, the 'cups' dipped in water, set over the wounds, and the air sucked out with the mouth from the small end, which is closed with the wax. They are left on until they fill with blood and fall off of themselves. They may be put on a second time when emptied of blood. The blood thrown out is by this time clotted and hard. The Lambas believe that the sickness comes out with the blood.

Hospitality

The hospitality of the Lamba villagers is almost proverbial. It is with them a law that no stranger shall be allowed to sleep hungry. It must be conceded, however, that villages on main routes of travel are becoming very lax in this regard, on account of the constant calls they have from passing strangers. Ordinarily the traveller in Lambaland can go from one end of the country to the other with no provision for the journey. He will have shelter and food provided gratis wherever he needs to spend the night. This is so taken for granted that should a stranger happen to be treated inhospitably he would loudly voice his grievance in the morning, saying, "Do you not know that I am a person? How is it I have to sleep like an animal in your village?" This will bring the headman quickly to make his excuses or apologies—maybe that his wife did not return from her fish-bailing until late at night—and to offer a bowl of *ifisunga* to mollify the aggrieved stranger. Nevertheless, a visitor must be careful not to overstay his welcome, and if he accepts repeated hospitality something is expected in return from him. The pot of beer, the dish of *inshima*, and the common pipe are all cheerfully shared with a complete stranger. The Lambas are brought up on such proverbs as these: *Umweni tapinta ŋanda*, "A visitor does not carry a house" ("You must provide him with shelter!"), or *Umwensu woŵe kakulya*, "Your visitor means food!"

The Paramount Chief's Village

In the olden days the village of the paramount chief was always greater than any other. In these days Mushili's village is one of the smallest and most insignificant. Many are the Lamba sayings concerning the wonders of "the Court of the great chief." Approach to it must be with the greatest respect, the body sagging, the spear, bow, and axe held hanging low in the hands, never over the shoulders. One must approach as though one were bound, and when the village is entered weapons must be laid on the ground and further advance made unarmed. The chief's Court, *kubwalo*, is called *mwilole*, the place where people stare. To the country villager it was a place of wonderment, full of objects of magnificence. The place was known for the generosity of the chief, who always treated his visitors well. "It is at the chief's residence," they say, "that one eats sumptuously." It is called *mwitumbatumba* also, the place of many lawsuits, for all the important cases are settled here by the great chief. The awe in which the great chief's village is held is well shown by a proverbial saying: *Twafika muno mwityatya, muchiminine, ichilele chifwile, muchifunshya-mwana, ukufunshyo'mukashi tekumuŵona*, "We have arrived here in the swish-swish [of grass when one walks through a place overgrown—even as one fears long grass because of wild beasts, so one fears the chief's abode], in the standing-up [the place where the chief exercises authority, where the people are so busy that they find no time to sit about], where what is lying down is dead; where one can inquire after one's child, to inquire after one's wife one won't find her [the place is so big and busy that one's wife, who is able to walk by herself, would speedily get lost]."

Hermit Life

The Lambas have a very independent trait in their characters. If a man cannot get on with his village headman or his companions he, with his wife and family, may select a fertile spot by some stream several miles away, and go and build his house and have his gardens and set up for himself there. Sometimes such a family lives almost a hermit life, out of contact with everybody else. At other times other villagers, sharing the man's grievance, go with him, and he sets up his own village, with himself as headman. A village headman can have no constraining control over such a person—it is only the group or paramount chief who has power of life and death over the individual—and, provided the man does not remove outside the territory of his group chief, he is free to live by himself if he so desires it.

It is no uncommon thing for villages to split up. The young people of the large village of Chimbalasepa some years ago wanted a school and mission church in their village. After considerable opposition from the chief and elders the school was obtained, but the old people continued to do all they could to harass and obstruct the young people, many of whom had professed Christianity. Eventually things became so intolerable that Soloshi, one of the most prominent of the young men, left and established a village of his own at some distance. More than half of Chimbalasepa's people went with him, and now Soloshi's village is larger than Chimbalasepa's.

Uŵulunda

On the other hand, lasting personal friendships between Lambas are common. Many a Lamba has his *umulunda* or 'half-section.' Such friendship is always initiated with reciprocal gifts, and kept up by a constant interchange of gifts, cloth, food, fish, meat, etc. Lambas say, *Ichiŵusa chitanshi kuula*, "Friendship begins by barter." Among the Kaonde this principle is carried to an extreme, and the Lambas ridicule the *uŵulunda* of the Ŵakaonde, who go so far as to share their wives, lending them out when a friend comes on a visit. Nothing of that is found among the Lambas.

Height by Gesture

The Lambas differentiate between animals, people, material objects, etc., in the way in which they indicate height. The accompanying diagrams of the hand position indicate these

128

differences. The position of the hand generally signifies the position of the head—for an animal horizontally on edge, for a person vertically, for a baby at an angle, etc. It is significant

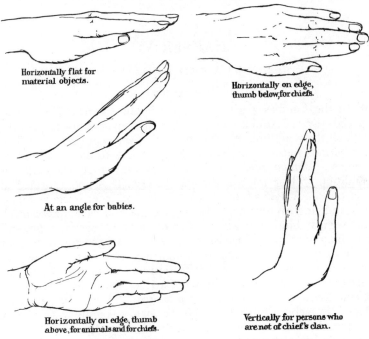

Horizontally flat for
material objects.

Horizontally on edge,
thumb below, for chiefs.

At an angle for babies.

Horizontally on edge, thumb
above, for animals and for chiefs.

Vertically for persons who
are not of chief's clan.

FIG. 60. HOW THE HAND IS USED TO INDICATE HEIGHT

that a chief is indicated in the same (or the reverse) way as a lion. This parallelism is further indicated when it is remembered that the word for chief, *imfumu*, belongs to the 'animal class' of nouns, in which also is found *inkalamu*, the lion.

CHAPTER VII

BIRTH AND INFANCY

Pregnancy

With the Lambas a first pregnancy is always treated in a very special way. A young recently married woman is not acquainted with all the symptoms which indicate that she is pregnant. When her periods become interrupted she will say to one of the elder women, *Nshilukuseesa*, "I do not have my periods," and her condition will be known, though she herself is not informed of it at once. A *nyinachimbela*, a midwife, will inform the woman's husband, and say to him, "Get a small piece of calico [*ichipande*], that we may bind your wife with an *inyemba*, for she is pregnant." The man goes to tell his sister, and says, "To-morrow you must come early in the morning to announce to your sister-in-law, for she is pregnant." Man and wife retire as usual that night, but very early in the morning the sister arrives, and calls at the door, *Weŵo, weŵo, isuleni-ko, ŵanangwa ŵafwa!* "You, you, open the door. Somebody's dead!" The woman wakes up with a start to open the door and hear who has died. Directly she pulls back the door her sister-in-law squirts *umufuŵa* from her mouth on to the young woman's chest and back, and says to her, *Tiina'ŵantu wakula!* "Fear people, for you are mature!" The *umufuŵa* is mixed meal and water, and is used on this occasion as a sign of distinction.

The meaning of this procedure is clear to the young wife, and she goes back into the hut and gives way to a fit of tears. Her husband now brings the *inyemba* and fastens it about her abdomen; she continues to carry it about her person during the period of her pregnancy.

After this the older women of the village instruct her how to look after herself. She must not bathe in cold water. She must lie on her side, not flat on her back (*akampabwa*), *amala engaya peulu*, "lest the intestines should move upward." She must not run quickly.

To the woman who has already had children the symptoms of pregnancy are clear. She notices that the periods have ceased, and that as the womb enlarges dark rings are formed around the nipples on the already swelling breasts. Then, too, the nausea appears, *kumutima alukufwayo'kuluka*, "in her heart she feels like vomiting," and she begins to refuse one and another kind of food —maybe she turns against *inshima* porridge. She gets longings (*ukutinamina*) for meat, honey, or some other rare commodity, and the people say, *Ipafu lyamupoosa ukulye'nama*, "Her pregnancy has caused her to long to eat meat." This whole state is called *ichipoosela*, a state which covers the feeling of nausea, the longings, and the revulsion that often comes toward her husband. Sometimes the revulsion is so strong against her husband that she quarrels violently with him, and the village elders advise him to go away for a time on a journey, *pakuti chipoosela ichi, uka-bwele pakukule'pafu, epakuchileka*, "for this is a 'longing,' and you can come back when the pregnancy is advanced and it ceases."

As a rule the expectant mother continues her work of hoeing, grinding, etc., in the usual way. At times some women lie up, and are reckoned by their neighbours as lazy. All kinds of work are continued right up to the time of giving birth.

Birth

Women who have had several babies before take little notice of the first pains of labour, but a fearful woman will send at once for the midwife, and then it is believed that the labour will be long. Her friends will say, "How is it that the birth is so long delayed?" The midwife's reply is, "She was in too much of a hurry to send for me!" As soon as labour commences all guns, axes, spears, and hoes are removed from the hut, for it is believed that these weapons of war will bring ill-fortune to the child. The child must be born into peace. During the whole of the labour no food or drink is allowed to the mother, but from time to time water is sprinkled on her face to give her relief.

Older women, *ifimbela*, or, as they are more commonly called, *wanyinafimbela*, assist the mother in giving birth (*fyashya*). They often call in younger women who are already mothers to watch them and so to learn the art of midwifery. These midwives have considerable skill, and are able to turn the child if it is not presented correctly.

Birth generally takes place in the hut, but if there is too much noise and disturbance in the village the mother and her attendants go into the forest to the secluded shade of some bush, where the child is born. No idle onlookers are allowed, but the husband is permitted to stay in order to see that there is no foul play. If he has a midwife whom he can trust he will sometimes absent himself at such a time. All small girls and young women who have not yet given birth are driven out and not permitted to see what is going on. Whether the woman cries or endures the pain without crying is without significance in a Lamba birth.

As soon as the child is born the navel cord is cut from the *ifinsangwe* (afterbirth), after being tied by a bit of cloth (*akasansa*). The child is then washed in warm water. The midwife takes the afterbirth and buries it just behind the house, but never away in the bush. Great care is taken lest birds or dogs should touch it. A strip of cloth (*umukopo*) is tied round the abdomen of the mother in order to steady her breathing, and hot gruel (*uŵusunga*) is given to her to drink. The baby is put to the breast as soon as it is washed. If the baby does not cry at birth it is said to *fiso' ŵulishi*, to hide its crying.

In some cases as soon as the child has been successfully delivered the midwife goes out and dances in the courtyard (*uluŵansa*) before the house. This is called *ukuchindilo'mwanichye*, dancing to the child.

On the day of birth the midwife takes charge of the child, but that same evening hands it over to the mother and returns to her home, leaving the mother to have complete charge. The father of the child will kill a fowl in honour of the midwife (or midwives), make a present of *umusompo* (bark cloth), and have some *amasaka* (sorghum) threshed for her to take with her. Nowadays cash to the value of about two shillings is given in place of the sewn piece of bark cloth. Should the mother need subsequent attention or medicine, it is usually her mother who attends to her.

There are several special cases of birth which must be noticed.

Ulunyena. If the child excretes (*pambuka*) immediately on birth he is called *ulunyena* or *ulumbashi*. The midwife fetches the leaves of the *intelele* plant, and makes medicine with which to anoint the eyes and feet of all the people in the village, lest they should suffer from the disease called *akapoopo*.

Mwika. If the child is born with a leg presentation it is called *mwika*.

Chikuto. If the membranous covering is on a child when born he is called *chikuto*. These names often cling to a person all his life.

Akafunga. A still-born baby, like a miscarriage, is called *akafunga*. When this occurs the midwife finds *ulupaapi* leaves, and makes medicine for all in the village, men, women, and children, to drink in order to ward off the evil consequences, which may mean illness or even death. Another medicine is prepared from the *ichinchyeŵa* bush, for smearing over the body and the feet. The midwife and a companion will carry the body with the afterbirth in a large cracked pot (*ichiyinga*) into the veld and bury it secretly. For a month after this the woman may not touch another's fire. This regulation is the same for a woman who has given birth to a live baby.

On the day, however, when the woman and her husband are about to resume marital relations the husband goes into the veld and builds an *umutanda* (zareba) at a distance from the village. He then obtains from an *umulaye* certain medicine, which he puts into a large bark trough (*umukwa*) with water. With this medicated water both husband and wife bathe their bodies ; they then take up their abode in the *umutanda*. This is done when the moon has waned (*lombo'mwenshi waya mumfinshi*). When some one wants to go and talk to the couple he first goes to where the bark trough of medicated water is and washes ; then he is permitted to enter the *umutanda*. At the time of the new moon the couple may move back again to the village and resume their ordinary life.

Umuŵishi. A baby born prematurely is termed *umuŵishi*, an unripe one, and is cared for indoors until it is strong. There are no special ceremonies connected with premature birth.

Akasenshimbeŵa. Occasionally a baby is born with teeth. This is looked upon as very lucky, especially as there is no apprehensive waiting to see that the lower teeth are cut first. A baby born with teeth is called *akasenshimbeŵa*, a name also applied to a species of mouse.

Twins

There are two terms in Lamba which are used to indicate twins. *Wampundu* is used when both are boys or both girls, and *amapasa* is used when the twins are a boy and a girl. The birth of *ŵampundu* is treated exactly as an ordinary birth, but that of *amapasa* is looked upon as *ishyamo*, ill-luck, and the father immediately goes to a doctor (*umulaye*) in order to obtain the necessary medicine (*umusamu*). A certain medicine is given to him, with which he smears (*suŵa*) himself, his wife, and the twins; another medicine is placed in water and drunk ; while yet another is thrown upon the fire, so that the smoke fills (*puuta*) the hut. It is feared that if the *umusamu* is not obtained the children will die. The parents too need the medicine, because *chyeeŵo chyaŵo*, "it is their fault."

While they are small twins must be dressed alike and given clothing at the same time, provided they are *ŵampundu*. They must not be parted. These regulations apply until they are about twelve years of age. The Lambas profess to know nothing of triplets.

A child born with a hare-lip or any other deformity, such as a shortage of fingers, is believed to have been bewitched, but in such cases no action is taken to try to identify the witch.

Confinement

After giving birth the mother remains in the house for one day, and if strong enough goes to the river on the next day and bathes herself completely. She is then permitted to grind, draw water, etc. The child, however, is left in the house for five or six days, until the navel cord drops. Meanwhile he is in the charge of his maternal grandmother. The mother is not, however, permitted to *nanye'nshima*, prepare the stiff porridge, until the passage of a whole month. The moon is used for this calculation. Often this period is longer, sometimes even until the succeeding moon is finished, a period of maybe five weeks.

Until this period is completed the father is not permitted to touch the child in any way; he may not touch the child while he or she is still *koti menda*, like water—*tanje akose aŵe neŵuntunshi*, "first let him harden and get his humanity." A new-born babe is not considered an *umuntunshi*, a human being, until this period has been passed.

When the confinement period is over the husband may resume marital relations with his wife. On the day on which this takes place neither husband nor wife is permitted to leave the hut. This restriction is said to be in honour of the child. Every one knows that *ŵalukuchindiko'mwana lelo, ŵapoko'mwana waŵo*, "they are honouring their child to-day, they are receiving their child." Friends will come in to visit and compliment the parents. On this day the father presents the child with an *akeshiŵilo kakumuchindika*, a token of praise. This used to be a present of beads, but in these days is usually two shillings for calico.

Meanwhile, about five or six days after birth, the umbilical cord has dropped off. Charcoal mixed with castor-oil is rubbed on the navel for about four days in order to strengthen and harden the place. As soon as the cord has come off the child may be brought outside the hut. He will be carried by his mother, brothers and sisters, or friends, but not by his father, who may not touch him until after he has again had intercourse with his wife. This restriction is confined to the father himself; the father's brothers are not so restricted.

Naming the Child

If the labour is long and the birth difficult a doctor (*umulaye*) is sent for. When he comes he divines and says, "It is So-and-so, who died long ago, who wants to be reborn." Then the child is born, and the name of that ancestor is given to the child.

If the birth is normal it is the maternal grandmother who decides upon the name of the child. This will be the name of a dead relation or ancestor, whose spirit (*umupashi*) is believed to be reincarnated in the newly born babe. Should the child fall sick after a day or two, or even after a week, the people say, "He has refused the name!" An *umulaye* will have to be summoned, and he will say, "He has refused this name, because it is So-and-so [naming some other dead relative] who is this child who is born." This new name is the one by which the child will be known.

The spirit of the same ancestor may be reincarnated in more than one child at one and the same time. This is discussed in the chapter on "Spiritism," but the following case of which I know is a good illustration:

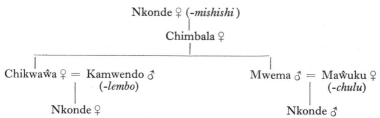

The two Nkondes, who were named after their great-grandmother, were cousins of about the same age, the girl being born in 1912 and the boy in 1913. These spirit names given at birth are afterward abandoned by the children when they are old enough to select one for themselves.

The Lambas use a peculiar phrase when indicating the order of birth. They say, *Liŵe waito'mwanichye wakwe*, "So-and-so has called his younger brother," or "Chinemu called Nkonkola, Nkonkola called Ŵombwe, Ŵombwe called Shiŵata, and Shiŵata called Nsensa." Chinemu was the eldest of the family and Nsensa the youngest.

135

Illegitimacy

Illegitimate children suffer no disability: they are treated as orphans who have no father, and are accepted as clan members by the members of the mother's clan, to which they naturally belong. The mother also, if an unmarried woman, is shown no disrespect. Her state before giving birth is called *ipafu lyaku-pumba*, a begged or borrowed pregnancy. The onus is upon the father, though no case is made against him unless the woman dies in childbirth. There is no hindrance to her securing a regular marriage afterward. An illegitimate child is called *umwana waŵushichye*, a child of an unmarried state.

If a married woman has had illicit intercourse with another man, it is firmly believed that when it comes to the time for her to give birth labour will be long and difficult. An *umulaye* is called, and after divining he will say, "You had another man while your husband was away at work." If the woman confesses the doctor will give her medicine to facilitate the birth. The procedure against the man involved will afterward be commenced in accordance with Lamba law (see Chapter IV).

Ichipaapo

Like the Ŵembas, the Lamba mothers carry their babies on their backs in a carrying cloth (*ichipaapo*) made of softened bark (*umusompo*), never of skins, as among the Lenje, Ila, and Soli peoples. The Lambas and Ŵulimas use the bark of the *umu-samba*-tree, the Ŵembas use that of the *umutaŵa*-tree, while the Lala people use both. This discrimination is due to the prevalence of a particular tree in any district. The father prepares the *ichipaapo* for the baby to be carried in.

Nursing

There is no special restriction of diet for the mother during the nursing period, though *uŵusunga* (gruel) is taken to induce a plentiful supply of milk.

If the milk becomes insufficient while the child is still very small *umuninga* (pea-nuts) is pounded up, mixed with water, and strained through an *ulusanso*. The milk-like fluid strained off is given to the child. At times *uŵusunga* is given to the child. No stated periods for suckling are observed. The child drinks whenever he wants to, and if satisfied or sleepy he leaves off. Whenever he cries he is given the breast to soothe him. Should the mother die while the child is still at the breast, it seldom survives in a country where the fly prevents the keeping of cattle, unless there happens to be a younger sister of the mother who is in a position to suckle the orphan.

Clothing and Ornamentation

No clothing is given to the newly born baby. As soon as he becomes ' intelligent ' (*chyenjela*) and is able to sit up a string of beads is put round his waist. Before this, however, after the drop-
ping of the navel cord, an *ichiponje*
is placed round his neck in order to
strengthen it. The *ichiponje* used to
be a piece of bark cloth shaped like
a collar, on the ends of which strips
of bark are left for tying round the
neck. Beads are threaded, and lines

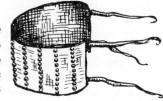

FIG. 61. ICHIPONJE

of them fastened to the collar in vertical rows. Nowadays the *ichiponje* is made of cloth.

At the time of the ripening of the maize (*pamatawa*) a small horn of *umusamu* is given to the child to prevent him from getting convulsions (*umusamfu*). Little babies may also wear wristlets (*amakoosa*) of cloth and beads.

Haircutting

Long before teething time, when the child's hair is somewhat grown, it is shaved off with an *ichimo*, a small metal razor which is often carried by adults secreted in the hair. Before the shaving is begun the head is well washed in order to soften the hair. The shaved hair is buried in the *ishyala*, the midden. Hair is never burnt, for the natives say the smell of burning hair is offensive.

When the nails begin to get long they are cut with a sharp *ichimo*, and the parings are thrown away.

Cutting of Teeth

The cutting of the first teeth of any child is a most important occasion, and one which is awaited by the parents with extreme anxiety. Normally the lower front teeth come through first, and when this takes place the relief of the parents is tremendous.

If the teething worries the child the mother foments the in-
flamed gums (*ukuchine'fishili*). A piece of medicinal bark is warmed in hot water and rubbed gently on them. Sometimes medicinal leaves are similarly used.

THE LAMBAS OF NORTHERN RHODESIA

When a tooth is discovered in the early morning the maternal grandmother brings the child outside the hut and utters the shrill lululu-ing indicative of joy (*ukulishyo'lumpundu*), in order that everybody may know that the child has successfully passed this critical stage. She addresses the child, saying, *Wakula wamena'meno*, "You are grown up. You have grown your teeth." After this he is able to begin to eat *inshima* and soft vegetables.

Amankunamwa. If, however, the upper teeth show signs of coming first a doctor of repute is summoned. He brings medicine for drinking and for smearing on the gums, and is believed to be able to prevent the upper teeth from coming out and to induce the lower ones to come first.

But if the upper teeth come first the people say, *Tekwelelwo' kushyo'mwano' wamankunamwa, mumupoose*, "It is wrong to leave a child who has cut the upper teeth first. You must throw him away!" In the olden days such a child was thrown into a pool. An *ichimbela* (midwife) wraps the child in calico, binds it, and carries it on her back to the pool. She then stands with her back to the pool and throws off the child without looking round (*amamfutenuma*), to be drowned or devoured by the crocodiles. The state of cutting the upper teeth first is called *amankunamwa*, and such a child is thus termed *uwamankunamwa*. It is popularly believed that should one of these children be spared, many people would die as a result of the influence from the child, who is considered to be an *imfwiti* (wizard) embodying an *ichiŵanda* (demon). In fact, it is believed that as each milk tooth of an *uwamankunamwa* comes out some relative dies. The mother and father of such a child must not mourn when he is thrown away. They fear also that should they spare the child all their children to be born will be *aŵamankunamwa*.

Talking

When the child begins to speak (*taata*), to say "Father," his father makes him a present of a fowl, and when he says *kapa* ("Grannie") his maternal grandmother also presents her grandchild with a fowl to greet him. Natives say that the order of the first words which a child learns is (1) *tata* (father), (2) *kapa* (grandmother), (3) *mama* (mother). Despite the fact that the third is the more likely beginning, they say that the mother constantly tries to get the child to say *tata*, and that he hears her using that term more than any other.

138

BIRTH AND INFANCY

Walking

The child usually crawls first and then gradually begins to walk. No special notice is taken of the child when he achieves this, but a child who does not walk at the usual period is called *ichite*.

Weaning

Weaning (*ukusumuna*) is not carried out until the child has his teeth and is able to run about, often between two and three years of age. Should another baby come along, however, weaning will take place at the birth of this next child. The child is said to fear the new one who sucks, though very often the mother does not refuse to let both children drink. At times, in order to expedite weaning, chilies (*impilipili*) are rubbed on the nipples, or the child is sent away to spend some time with the grandmother. No ceremony is performed at weaning or after.

The Losing of the Milk Teeth

When the first tooth comes out the child takes it and a piece of cinder (*umushyangalala*). The tooth he throws to the east and the cinder to the west, saying, *Welino kawise'fisa'kasuŵa! Wemushyangalala kauye'fiwa'kasuŵa!* "Tooth come back in the way the sun comes back! Cinder go in the way the sun sets!" This is done in order to ensure the proper growing of the new teeth—the sun comes up again in the east. A gift is necessary to satisfy the west, and the cinder or a piece of charred wood signifies the darkness which is the quality of the west.

CHAPTER VIII

CHILDHOOD

The Grandmother

THE child sleeps in his parents' hut until he reaches an age sufficient to allow of his going to live in the hut of his maternal grandmother. If the grandmother lives in the same village the child may go to live with her as soon as the next baby is born. If she lives in another village the child may be five years of age before going to live with her. Sometimes, if the maternal grandmother has other grandchildren to look after, the child will go to the paternal grandmother. The duty of the grandmother in the community is to provide the grandchild with food (*teŵeta*), protection (*lama*), and shelter (*ukulala muŋanda*). Generally the children spend their time in play, though at times they will be sent to draw water or to gather kindling wood (*utusamfu*). When they are big enough the girls are required to grind, stamp, cook, bail fish, and sweep out their grandmother's hut. They will be taught how to make baskets (*ukupose'filukwa*) and screen-mats (*amasasa*). The little boys will be required to cut firewood, hunt for honey, and kill birds and mice for their grandmother. Later they learn to make sleeping mats (*imisengelo*) and doors as they are needed.

Games

There are many games which native children play to while away the leisure hours, besides the various dances, which for the most part take place at night.

Ukusamba. Lamba children are very fond of bathing (*ukusamba*), generally in the more or less shallow fords of the rivers, where there is no danger from crocodiles, or in the *ifisapa*, the draining-off channels of water from the plains, when they are flooded in the rainy season. Little boys and girls bathe together until they reach the age of about seven or eight years, when the little boys are able to accompany their elders on their hunting and foraging expeditions into the bush. The little ones splash about in the shallow water and play at diving, putting their faces

140

under the water, while their backs are still exposed. When they get older their diving becomes more serious. One will sink

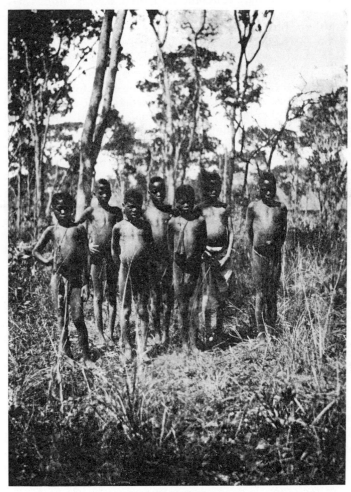

FIG. 62. TWA CHILDREN
Photo by C. M. Doke

out of sight, and his companions will guess where he is going to come up. In their frolics the children chase one another, running through the shallow water, and when one stumbles they all throw themselves down in the same place.

THE LAMBAS OF NORTHERN RHODESIA

Intafu. Playing ball is a favourite pastime, and one indulged in even by grown-ups, from one side of Africa to the other. It is called *ukwante'ntafu* (catching the ball) or *ukutane'ntafu* (playing ball). The *intafu* is made of solid rubber. Boys go into the bush where the rubber-creeper (*umuŵungo*) is growing and collect the juice on their arms, where it quickly hardens; it is then peeled off and worked, with continual additions, into a ball the size of a golf-ball. Two teams play, and each tries to keep the ball among its own members. The ball may not be kept for a moment in the hand, but as soon as it is received it has to be bounced on the ground to another member of the holder's team. Boastful expressions are freely indulged in as the play goes on, and the excitement of the game is enhanced by the wit of these expressions. When one side captures the ball from the other the victory is announced by a loud Lamba cheer (*ingwele*), which incites the others to strive for its recapture.

Ichisolo. Another game which is found right through Africa is *ichisolo*, or African 'draughts.' Four rows of holes are made in the ground, and small stones are used for 'men.' Each player distributes his men along the rows of holes on his side. Then he begins to move the stones along, capturing those of his opponent according to certain definite rules.[1] The one who clears the 'board' of his opponent's men wins the game. Much cheating, through very rapid moving of the pieces, often takes place in this game. Quite small children become most proficient in playing *ichisolo*, but it is a game which has a strong fascination for the older folk also.

Inshingwa. The children have whip-tops (*inshingwa*), which they spin. The top is made of a cone of wood, bark string is wound round it, and the top is then thrown down and kept spinning by whipping. The whip (*ubwembya*) consists of a stick to which is attached a bark-string lash.

Inondo. Lamba children have a game which closely resembles that of ninepins. A number of shelled mealie-cobs, called *aŵantu* (men), are set up in two opposing lines about 12 feet apart, and behind these are ranged the players. The *inondo*, a kind of teetotum, is spun across the intervening space, in order to knock over the opponent's men. This *inondo* is made of a convex circular piece of calabash, with a stick inserted in the

---

[1] For careful descriptions of this game see Smith and Dale, *The Ila-speaking Peoples of Northern Rhodesia*, vol. ii, pp. 232–237, and Junod, *The Life of a South African Tribe*, second edition, vol. i, pp. 345–349, where the game is called *tshuba*.

centre to act as a spindle. If one of the men is knocked over it may be restored if its owner can knock over an enemy cob. If all the cobs of one side are down their owners may throw until the teetotums are exhausted; then, if they do not succeed in raising any of their men, the game is over and they have lost.

Other Games. There are many other ways which the children have of amusing themselves. The boys indulge in wrestling (*ukusunkana*), in which the winner has merely to throw his opponent. Wrestling is often used as a means of settling quarrels, though in this case the under man is usually severely mauled when he falls. Lambas do not know how to use their fists in fighting, and wrestling takes the place of this. Boys also go in for tug-of-war (*ichyandaŋombe*). The two centre players catch one another's hands, the others holding on in a row, each with his arms round the next boy's waist, much as is done in our Oranges and Lemons. No rope is used, and the Lambas say of this, *Ulushinga lwaŋombe taluputuka*, "The ox-thong does not break."

Others play at walking on stilts (*ukuchito'tukonkola*), and others at a hopping game, in which many children, holding one leg, hop about, calling out *Shimunkonkoli! Shimunkonkoli!* anyone falling causing great merriment. Little children are fond of swinging (*ukuchita'kampelwa*). Two long bark ropes are suspended from a tall tree, and a short stick is used as a seat. Then they have games resembling our Hide and Seek, and indoor games like Hunt the Thimble, one of which is called *ichipyolopyolo chyaŵana ŵankanga*, "the Guinea-fowl Chick."

Amansanshi

Most of the children's play, however, centres in the *amansanshi*, miniature huts, which they build outside the village and where they reign supreme. There are three types of these *amansanshi*: the *amansanshi atwanıchye*, play huts of the little children, the *amansanshi ambuli*, the play huts of the girls, and the *amansanshi aŵalalume*, the play huts of the boys.

(1) *Amansanshi atwanichye.* Little children will club together to go and build a miniature village of their own. They steal some axes belonging to their elders, go to the outskirts of the village (*ifitumbo*), cut down bushes and branches, and build their miniature huts. These *amansanshi* are lean-to huts (*inkunka*), and look like *imilenda* (spirit huts). When the huts are built the children appoint one of their number as village headman (*umwine wamushi*), and go off to steal monkey-nuts (*umuninga*) and other

143

foodstuffs from their elders in the village. Sometimes they even go and dig up *umumbu* (certain succulent roots cultivated in the marshes), but if they are caught at this they can be certain of a sound thrashing. Some of the children will play the part of strangers visiting: this is usually done by the boys. They come to visit the *amansanshi*, and the girls prepare food for them. When they have eaten, obscene language is often indulged in by the girls, who will say to their boy visitors, *Pano ukulya walya fungulule'ŵolo lyoŵe ulale-mo!* "Eating you have eaten. Now unfold your scrotum and sleep in it!" On saying this the girls slip quickly into the *amansanshi* and shut the doors. Meanwhile others of the girls have hidden themselves in the shrubbery, pretending to be hyenas (*ifimbolo*). They now spring out, howling like hyenas, and the boys run off in pretended fear. The girls in the *amansanshi* now in their turn rush out to drive off the hyenas. If one of the visitors is caught by the hyenas all the others will gather together to wail. Some will be sent to the village for food for the time of mourning (*amalilo*), pretending that their companion has been killed by a wild beast. The one who has been caught they cover over with calico, as though he were a corpse, until the food is brought, when the dead one is restored to life. They all now shout, *Pano mweŵame ninkondo!* "Now, mates, it is war!" They divide themselves into two parties, and attack the food to see who can eat the most and the most quickly. The one who gets the least in this contest usually finishes up in tears.

Sometimes the children go down to the river-bank and make toy pots with the moulding clay there. In the evening they troop back to the village and leave their play for the next day.

(2) *Amansanshi ambuli.* Older girls, not yet initiated (*imbuli*), together with some already initiated (*ŵamoye*), build their own secluded *amansanshi*. One of their number they appoint head of the village, and the rest are looked upon as wives and children. When they have been there for a little while they say (in play), "Now the sun has gone. Let us go in and shut the door." This they do. Later one of them acts the part of the cock (*kombolwe*), and crows that they may know that the dawn has come. So they open the door and come out. In the *amansanshi* the girls boil *umusaku* (fresh, unground corn) ; one of their number waits on the others as though they were visitors, and they eat. Girls will go from one hut to another where their companions are and tell folk-tales. In this way they play until it is time for them to return to the village for their evening duties. Many of

144

the practices indulged in by growing girls are carried out by these unmarried girls in the *amansanshi*. Here the *ẁamoye* practise vagina-distension, which, as we shall see, is believed to assist in child-bearing.

(3) *Amansanshi aẁalalume.* In some cases boys at the age of puberty erect *amansanshi* in which to practise the *ukukuya*, but generally this takes place in their own huts in the village and no bush-huts are erected at all. As we shall see, there is no initiation or puberty rite for boys among the Lambas, as there is with the girls, but the boys have certain practices which they carry out among themselves at this time. The boys choose certain roots which grow across the path, such as those of the *umukole-, umu-ẁanga-, kaẁumbu-,* or *umusaalya-* trees. Such roots are con- sidered to be strong, because people tread

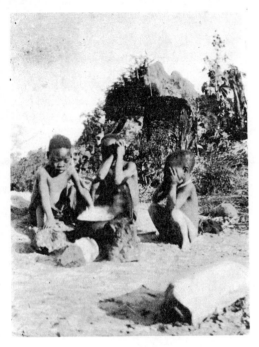

FIG. 63. SHYNESS AROUND THE POT
Photo by C. M. Doke

over and on them and yet they remain across the path. They therefore are believed to have the virtue of passing on strength. From the root a medicine is prepared for the boys to drink, but the chief preparation is for external application. A section of the root, about eight inches in length, is cut out, shaved down, and shaped. At night the wood is heated before the fire, turned round and round until thoroughly hot, and then pressed on to the penis (*ukukando'ẁukala*) all round, in order to enlarge and harden the organ. The stick is hidden in the thatch, and the operation repeated each night. In addition to this, similar roots are pounded and rubbed on to the

145

testicles (*amakandi*). This is done in the belief that unless the organs are thus enlarged the young men will not beget children. It is a parallel practice to that of vaginal distension among the girls. Every young man carries out this practice—fear of the scorn (*ukutongala*) of his companions is sufficient to make him do it. Christian influence naturally is beginning to have a deterrent effect on these customs.

Names

Each child at birth, or soon thereafter, as we have seen, receives what is called his spirit name, the name of that deceased relative whose spirit is believed to be reincarnated—a relative of the same clan as the child. A child may even be named in honour of a relative though the clan may be different, but in this case reincarnation is not possible, nor is it believed to have taken place.

When a child has reached years of discretion in such matters—from ten to twelve years of age—he chooses a new name. The old spirit name is despised, and should it be used by a companion after another has been chosen a quarrel would in all probability be the result.

The new name may be given to the child by an elder or by relatives, and a gift of beads is added to confirm the naming. But usually the child himself assumes the name he has chosen. The name may be one of self-praise, such as Nsandaŵunga, "Scatterer of Gunpowder"; Ntambika, "Offerer of Food"; Kanyakula, "Killer at one Shot"; Kalimanama, "Cultivator of Animals"; Chinami, "Bluffer." It may be one of self-commiseration, such as Kanamakampanga, "Little Buck of the Veld"; Chipeso, "Sleeping-mat"; Chyoŵola, "Blasphemy"; Chilupulamatipa, "Mud-treader"; Chyendanaŵulwani, "Traveller with Ferocity." Names of objects to be desired are often used, such as Nsalamo, "Ring"; Nsapato, "Shoe"; Malupenga, "Trumpet." In these days the vogue is to adopt the names of common English objects; *e.g.*, "Soap," "Table," "Five," "Sixpence."

The adoption of new names is less followed by girls than by boys, and among the Lambas there seems to be very little sex distinction in names. A name may equally apply to a boy or a girl. There are a few exceptions. I have not heard the name of Chilyelye ever applied to a boy, while such names as those taken from English common nouns are practically confined to boys. Naturally Biblical names and English proper names are applied now with sex distinction.

CHILDHOOD

Grown men, later in life, at times supplant their youthful names by praise-names, either chosen by themselves or given to them by others. Such are Konibwile, "Little Bird with Darkness here"—*i.e.*, "I've no fear of night"; Fumfunkanana Uwakwenda Kachyeneme, "Hornbill who flies with Open Mouth"; Bwashinganya-milyango Uŵushiku Bwamanyinsa, "Rainy Season Night has darkened the Doorways."

CHAPTER IX

ICHISUNGU—INITIATION

The Main Crises of Life

AMONG the Lambas there are no rites or ceremonies initiating boys into manhood. The elders, on noticing that a youth shows wisdom, ability, and physical strength, tell him that it is time he quitted playing and talking with the youngsters and joined the *amaŵumba aŵakulu* (the groups of grown men) and took his part in listening to the settling of law-cases (*imilandu*). Marriage, even, is not necessarily a sign of manhood, as many youths marry while they are still looked upon as boys. Circumcision is not practised by the Lambas, and the change from boyhood to manhood is gradual and imperceptible. Not so the change from girlhood to womanhood. Here, in the first menstrual appearance, is to the Lamba the sign of a definite and sudden change, one which demands some special rite. In the life of the individual there are four of these main crises, of which three only apply to males. At each of these crises, or, as they are sometimes called, "marginal periods," [1] rites of spiritistic or dynamistic significance have to be observed. The four main crises are birth, teething, initial menstruation, and death. There are other crises, such as the falling of the umbilical cord, the first talking of a child, the marriage of a *moye*, but these are not treated as of such importance as the main four. Additional crises happen in the lives of individuals, such as illness (brought on by the action of spirits, demons, or witches), and to meet these special spiritual, dynamistic, or other occult powers are necessary. Again, the spirit-possession which affects certain individuals, causing them to become *ŵamukamwami*, *ŵamoŵa*, or *aŵayambo*, constitutes a period of grave crisis for those individuals. In this chapter we are to consider that tremendous crisis which takes place in the life of every Lamba girl—her first menstruation, her initiation into womanhood, with all its possibilities of marriage and motherhood.

[1] *Cf*. H. A. Junod.

148

ICHISUNGU—INITIATION

Ichisungu

Of all the marginal ceremonies of the Lambas this one, *ichisungu*, is the most prominent. It is spread over a considerable time, and most of the members of the community take some part in its various sections at one time or another.

At the first signs of the first menstruation (*ukuseesa*) the older women say to the girl (*imbuli*), *Pano wakula, ukwelelwa'ti uwe' chisungu*, "Now you are mature. You must pass through the initiation!" Some girls do not wait to be told, but act at once on their own initiative. The girl steals away by herself, usually in the early morning, though it may be during the day or even in the afternoon, and goes and lies down beneath an *umwenje*-tree. Occasionally an *umusamba* or an *umuŵundikwa* is chosen for the occasion, but generally it is an *umwenje*. This action on the part of the girl is called *ukuwe'chisungu*, falling as an initiate. The place chosen by the girl is called *kuchiŵuula*, at the place of instruction, for it is here that the *nyinachimbela*, an old dame who also acts as midwife, commences the instruction of the initiate.

The girl is soon missed from the village; the cause of her disappearance is either known already or immediately suspected, and a number of her companions set out to hunt for her. Usually they have not very far to go in their search before they find her, and then they immediately *lishyo'lumpundu*, utter the shrill cries of joy and excitement, at the spot under the *umwenje*-tree where they have found her. Now her companions cover the girl completely over with a piece of calico, for she must not be seen. Leaving her thus covered beneath the tree, they return to the village and announce, *Lelo awe'chisungu'yo mwalukufwaya, twamuŵona*, "To-day the one whom you were wanting has fallen an initiate. We have found her!" On hearing this the women set out for the near-by villages (*imitala*), to call their companions to come and help them with the dancing. If the *ichisungu* has taken place in the afternoon this dancing will be performed the next morning; and if the relations and friends to be called are at a great distance, the women of the girl's village may wait for them first to arrive. Should it have taken place early in the morning, as is normally the case, the women, together with the *ŵanyinafimbela*, gather at the *umwenje*-tree for the dance. The women stand in a circle, with the covered girl lying in the midst. Usually but one woman dances, while the others sing and clap to give her the rhythm for the dance. On this occasion special

149

songs are sung ; they are songs which are used on no other occasion. First of all the girl who first discovered the initiate at her place beneath the tree sings:

> *Imfuko yanji natola !*
> *Nemwine nshilile-po !*
> *Nechiŵanda nshilile-po !*
>
> " My mole, I found it !
> I myself did not eat of it !
> I, a demon, I did not eat of it."

Then all the women join in song after song, of which the following are but representative:

> (1) *Kwasunta chyungu, ŵanyina-kamwale yo !*
> *Ŵanyina-kamwale, iŋanda yapya !*
>
> " The flames have shot up, O mother of the maid !
> O mother of the maid, your house is burnt ! "

> (2) *Ŵanyina-kamwale, inongo yalala, inongo yalala !*
> *Ngailale !   Nkaŵumba imbi !*
> *Ukuŵumba temilimo !*
>
> " O mother of the maid, the pot is cracked, the pot
> is cracked !
> Let it be cracked !   I'll mould another !
> Moulding is not work ! "

> (3) *Uyumwana nimwanani ?*
> *Nimwana-chitondo !*
> *Ŵawishi ninkalamu !*
> *Wishi alaŵuluma !*
>
> " This child, whose child is she ?
> She's the child of male lion !
> Her father's a lion !
> Her father roars ! "

The women and initiated girls (*ŵamoye*) who have come from a distance have their special contribution to the singing. They sing:

> *Ichisokosoko chali mwiyamba,*
> *Chyaumfwa'kawele !*
>
> " The Sokosoko bird was in the forest,
> And it heard the shouting ! "

It is the shouting, dancing, and singing which have brought them together.

Sometimes the girl goes to sleep, covered up as she is all day under the *umwenje*-tree   The *nyinachimbela* will turn her so that she lies comfortably. This *nyinachimbela* is generally the *nyinakulu* (grandmother) who has the duty of confining (*fundika*) the girl, but some one else may be appointed.

If the *ichisungu* takes place in the afternoon the girl eats nothing until the next day ; if it takes place in the morning she must be without food until she reaches the village in the evening.

When evening comes the covered girl, who is now called *moye*, is carried pick-a-back (*ukupaapa*) by the women to the village. On the road, as they come to the outskirts of the village, all the women sing:

> *Unomushi waŵani?*
> *Tuwinjile Somale !*
> *Amaombe Somale e !*
>
> " Whose is this village ?
> Let us go into it, Somale !
> The double-drums, Somale *e* ! "

Then they enter the village.

When they reach the house of the one who is going to confine and instruct the girl there is assumed difficulty in taking the girl in. The one who is carrying her on her back goes backward (*ubwifutenuma*) a little way through the doorway, comes out again, and then goes inward and outward, keeping up this swinging motion for a considerable time. Meanwhile the assembled women outside sing:

> *Mumpela'mapapula-nguŵo, nemwine-mwana !*
> *Kasolo, nemwine-mwana !*
>
> " Give me the baby-cloth, me, the owner of the child !
> O little mouse, me, the owner of the child ! "

The one carrying the *moye* sings in reply:

> *Intululu yainjila,*
> *Yainjila mumuchyembo, yainjila !*
>
> " The mungoose has entered,
> It has entered the hole, it has entered ! "

She sings this as she sways backward and forward, and then as she ceases singing she enters the hut and sets down her burden on the bed behind the screen (*ichipembe*). The screen was arranged while the girl was still beneath the *umwenje*-tree. *Amasasa* (grass mats) were hung in front of the bed, so that the girl is hidden and in the dark.

THE LAMBAS OF NORTHERN RHODESIA

Akasela Dance

During the night following that day, and on the two succeeding nights, men and women dance the *akasela*. When the village headman or some responsible elders are not present—and these older folk seldom stay the night through at such a dance—the *akasela* degenerates into all types of immorality. Excited by the suggestiveness of the dancing, the men and women no longer dance apart, but, getting nearer and nearer, the men catch at the breasts of the women, until passions are inflamed. During the dance, or while 'sitting out' around the fires (*amashiko*), pairs arrange to go off to some vacated house and commit fornication. They will never go into the bush or the long grass for such a purpose, for that is deadly taboo (*umushiliko*). Often a woman will refuse the suggestion of her dancing partner, and afterward report him to her husband; the would-be seducer will have a heavy fine to pay.

On such an occasion as this *akasela* songs are sung, of which the following are examples:

(1) *Muyaya-ngoma kanchiliwo,*
Inshiku shilalala,
Shyangalula ŵuchyakuukwa.

"For ever and ever I have been.
The days cause change.
They have made me an old man."

(2) *Neŵo kuŵuko bwanji taŵanjeŵa-po;*
Waŵulo'kukweŵa, ulenda naŵo?
Musalamba kainama!

"Me, at my wife's home they do not revile me;
Wouldn't they talk about you, do you live with them?
The talker bows in shame!"

Some of these dance songs are of very recent origin, as, for instance:

(3) *Munshilo'mwila'makalichi,*
Nechyani chyaye'li chyambuka!

"In the path where the railway coaches go,
The grass too goes catching alight!"

(4) *Chyaŵakatuŵile ŵalukuŵalaya*
Kuŵoma wo! muŵila!

"It belongs to Katuŵile. They are summoning them
To the Boma, *wo!* It means a wailing!"

After this the people who gathered together scatter to their various homes.

ICHISUNGU—INITIATION

Ukufundika

From this moment the *moye* has entered a period of seclusion. She is under the supervision of her *nyinachimbela*. There are many prohibitions she has to observe at this time. She may not drink *ubwalwa* (intoxicating beer). She may not see any man. She may not see the roofs of the huts, for she must forget the old life, she is entering upon an entirely new one. She may not speak but in a whisper, lest bad luck should come to her. Whenever she goes abroad it is beneath a pall!

Early in the morning she may be taken out of the hut. Completely covered over, she is carried on the back of one of the girls until she is some distance from the village, where she may throw off her pall and play openly with her playmates, all of whom, naturally, are girls. In the hut, too, she may sit uncovered, but no man or boy may enter. Women and girls may come in and see her, but it is significant that, apart from her *nyinachimbela*, no grey-headed woman may see her uncovered. Should such a one desire to see the girl, she would have to give some money to the *nyinachimbela*, who would then uncover the *moye* for her to see. If she finds her sitting carelessly the old woman will pinch the girl and say, *Tolukututiina fweŵakulu?* "Don't you fear us old people?" This is just to warn her to behave in a seemly manner.

No work is given to the *moye*, except that she may accompany the other girls when they go to bail out fish and bring to her *nyinachimbela* the proceeds of her catch.

Ukufunda

But all during this period of seclusion and confinement the *nyinachimbela* instructs (*funda*) her initiate (*ichisungu chyakwe*). She will teach her some of the details of special cooking, as, for instance, how to cook the different kinds of relish. But her instruction is principally upon points of behaviour, which will have a bearing upon her future married life. Here are listed a number of the things which are taught.

(1) *Pakulala nemwalalume koti komusumuna, sombi kani waseesa akasuŵa kakushile'milopa pakulala nemulume woŵe liŵili tekumusumuna yo, ukaŵone'milandu.* "Quoties cum viro concubueris, penis tibi detergendus est: sin autem menstruaveris, et quo die sanguis effluere cessaverit, cum viro [marito] iterum concubueris, penis non est detergendus ne tibi obsit."

In the first case if the injunction is not obeyed it is considered that the woman despises her husband, as though he were a dog, in the second case *amakowela muntiŵi* (severe pains in the chest) are feared when running. Disregard of these injunctions provides grounds for divorce and the payment of beads.

(2) *Kani waseesa tekwinjila umuli umulume muŋanda; kaŵili tekwikata kumuchele, tekwikata kumulilo; koti umulume katanga kafuma muŋanda eli ungenjila.* "If your periods are upon you, don't enter the hut in which your husband is; further, don't touch the salt and don't touch the fire; first let your husband come out of the hut, then you may enter." In practice, if a woman in that condition finds her husband already in the hut she will call out, *Fumeni, nyinjile,* "Come out, that I may enter!" He will come out; then she may enter, and he will re-enter after her. A woman in that condition is further instructed, *Tekwipika neli fyakulya koku,* "Cook no food at all!" If a husband and wife are on a journey the husband will do all the cooking while his wife is unwell.

(3) *Tekulukusooŵola, kani ŵanoko ŵafuma-mo muŋanda, ŵakushya-mo wenka.* "Don't take food from the pot on the fire if your mother has gone out of the hut and left you alone."

(4) *Kani wakutumo'mukulu umwanakashi tekukana; kani masaka komupelela; kani kunika koya.* "If an older woman sets you some duty, don't refuse; if it is corn, grind it for her; if it is to water, go."

(5) *Kani wasangano'muntu alukwiŵa mwenu, tekumuŵepela, pakuti kani ŵakamwipaye, fikaŵa koti mulandu woŵe; koti komuchyenjeshya lukoso.* "If you detect some one stealing at your home, don't report him, because if people kill him you will be to blame for his death; just warn him."

(6) *Umukulu kakukumanya nesaŵi, komupela-po, tekumutana.* "If an elder meets you when you have fish, give some to her; don't refuse her."

(7) *Kani waupwo'mwalalume, kani waŵona mufila, tekweŵa'ti mukane nkopwe naumbi, pakuti imilimo yaŵalalume yinji, alishi ukuchita naimbi.* "If you marry a husband and find that he is lazy, don't make up your mind to get a divorce and marry another, because men's work is of many kinds. He will be able to do some work well."

(8) *Kani waupwo'mwalalume, usangane alukulye'fyakutoŵela muŋanda, tekuya ili ulaŵila kuŵaŵyoŵe, koku.* "If you marry a husband and then find that he eats the relish in the house, don't go and talk about it to your companions."

(9) *Kani umulume aŵuuko'ŵushiku, afwaye'nshima, komutekela-*

po, tekuya kuŵuula'ŵaŵyoŵe ati aŵalume ŵalafwayo'kulye'nshimo' ŵushiku. "If your husband wakes up in the night and wants *inshima*, make it for him. Don't go and tell your companions that your husband wants to eat *inshima* in the middle of the night."

(10) *Ŵanokofyala tekukulaŵishya naweŵo koŵalaŵishya, koku, kawikele lukoso ichishinshi.* "If your mother-in-law reviles you, do not answer back; just keep silent."

(11) *Kani waumfwa'ŵantu ŵalukulaŵishya ŵanoko, tekuya kuŵaŵuula ŵanoko, koku.* "If you hear people reviling your mother, don't go and tell your mother."

(12) *Tekulukuchita ŵumenso-menso, pakuti ŵumenso-menso taŵaŵona-po nepo ŵafwa.* "Don't practise harlotry, for the harlot knows not where she is going to die."

(13) *Kani waseesa tekulala nemwalalume ukufika kukushila kwakuseesa.* "When you menstruate, have no connexion with a man until your periods have finished." A woman who hides from her husband the occasion of her periods is looked upon as an *imbifi*, an immoral woman, and is driven away.

(14) *Kani umulume akutwala mumpanga, kawisa, kolaŵila, mulandu ukulu.* "If your husband takes you into the veld, come and report; it is a very grave charge." Copulation anywhere but in a hut is a deadly taboo.

(15) *Kani umulume akulya, kawisa, kolaŵila, nekumutwala kumfumu, imfumu kaimwipaya.* "Si vir te ederit [*i.e.*, inguen, ut canis, lamberit], veni et rem indica, et duc eum ad principem ut hic eum interficiat." This also is a deadly taboo.

During this *ichisungu* period of seclusion the *moye* will join the other girls at the *amansanshi* (play huts). Here her initiated companions teach her concerning marriage, and how to behave when a suitor comes to ask her to marry him. Here also she begins the daily operation of stretching her vagina with her fingers in order to ensure safe delivery at childbirth. During this period, too, *ichileŵeleŵe* medicine is given to the girl to ensure her bearing a child. She is further instructed that, when she becomes pregnant, she must call her *nyinachimbela* to "imitate the expulsion of the head of a child" (*ukweshyo'mutwi wamuntu ukufuma*). The *nyinachimbela*, when called, inserts her hand into the vagina of the pregnant woman, closes the fist therein, and then pulls it out. This operation is repeated several times for two or three days, and the same is done again shortly before the woman is delivered. Its purpose is obvious.

Ukukunga

The initiate is kept *muchyumbo* (beneath the pall) for three or four months, the length of time being decided by her *nyinachimbela* ; "if she commences at the time of the floods [*pamuŵundo*], she will emerge when they have harvested the corn." Meanwhile her hair has been growing long, for it may not be cut during this period. When the time for release approaches the girl's father, or her suitor if there is a young man who has previously been giving her calico as his affianced wife, will bring beads to the *nyinachimbela*. Then a woman skilled in making the headdress of beads (*ukukunga*) is sent for to adorn the girl's head. This woman used to be paid in bark cloth for her services; if she were a friend the value of the cloth would be about two shillings, if a stranger, about five shillings. A piece of thin cloth is placed over the hair, and with a needle and bark thread a covering of beads is worked into this, sewn through and connected to the hair beneath. The result is a complete head-covering of beads attached to the hair.

Ichimbwasa

After this the girl's mother brews beer (*kumbo'bwalwa*), and there is a great gathering of men, women, and children. Then, while the girl is still within the hut, they hold the *ichimbwasa* dance. Sometimes they dance outside the father's house, sometimes outside that of the *nyinachimbela*. One woman— sometimes two or three—will dance, while the rest, men and women, sit round and sing. At times an old man of social standing will don the *insangwa* (rattles) and *uŵuyombo* (dancing fringe) and dance a solo dance in the ring. This dance is kept up through the night. Here are some examples of *ichimbwasa* songs :

(1) *Muɲombo'fuŵeto'mulomo mwalwa naŵani?*
Nalwa naŵangabwe ŵampandawile'ngala!

   " Ground-hornbill with closed mouth full, with
        whom have you fought?
   I have fought with Ngabwe, and he tore to bits
        my feather headdress ! "

(2) *Lileele lileele, ndino lyamwela,*
Ngaŵakandasa'katemo,
Kampita kunuma kandele.

   " 'Tis withered, 'tis withered, here it is the winter
        leaf.
   Though he wound me with his axe,
   I'll pass behind him and lie down."

ICHISUNGU—INITIATION

(3) *Ndi katele kaluŵumbe,*
Ifi mulukulaŵila ndukumfwa!

" I'm a fragile calabash.
What you say, I hear."

(4) *Aŵalamba kubwalo,*
Shyani ŵalamba Chikwangala?
Nkalambe Chikwangala!
Kwa! Kwa! Chikwangala!

" Those who do obeisance at Court,
How do they do obeisance, O crow?
Let me do obeisance, O crow!
Caw! Caw! O crow!"

On the morrow the *ichimbwasa* is continued during the morning.

In the afternoon, at about 4 P.M., the *moye* is brought out from the hut of confinement with the calico over her head. A girl, called the *kanshya*, carries her on her back, and comes and kneels on a mat (*isasa*) put in the courtyard; the *moye* keeps her head buried in the back of the *kanshya*, and the *ichyumbo* is over them both. Then the *ichyumbo* is taken off by the *nyinachimbela*, but the *moye* keeps her eyes covered and her head buried in the other's back. As soon as the calico is removed the assembled people all bring gifts and place them on the *isasa*. These gifts consist of beads, bracelets (*iminkonka*), and cash. The *moye's* maternal uncle (*mwinshyo*) brings a fowl. The gifts which her father, her uncle, and her sisters bring belong to the girl herself, but all the other gifts are collected together and appropriated by the *nyinachimbela*.

The *kanshya* now takes up the *moye*, carries her to her father, and kneels with her on her back in the doorway of the father's hut. The *moye's* father makes her a present, maybe of calico, and again she is taken up, and this time carried to the hut of her maternal uncle. He too gives her some calico. She is then carried back to the hut of her *nyinachimbela*. The next morning the girl emerges as an ordinary villager, to take her part in village life, no longer the girl she was when she entered, but a woman, with all the responsibilities which that entails. It will be her father's duty now to pay the *nyinachimbela* an *ichilundo* (a four-yard strip) of calico for her services.

After her initiation the *moye* continues to share her grand-mother's hut, unless she is immediately claimed in marriage.

Sometimes several initiates go through the ceremonies at the

157

THE LAMBAS OF NORTHERN RHODESIA

same time. They will all be housed in the one house, under
the guidance of one *nyinachimbela*. With the Lambas there is
no harsh treatment of initiates such as is found among the
Lenjes. Before initiation a girl is not supposed to have any
sexual dealings with a man, but after initiation she is immediately eligible.

CHAPTER X

MARRIAGE

Sexual Behaviour

EXAGGERATED statements have often been made concerning the looseness of the morals of the natives of Central Africa. Some of these statements may be true of certain tribes, when applied to persons outside the marriage bond, but even with those persons, in certain tribes, the statements are either entirely false or grossly exaggerated. There are certain contributory causes to a belief in these statements. The fact that the Lambas have no word for 'virgin' has been interpreted as meaning that there are no such things as virgins among them. It must be remembered, however, that their women marry early—at the age of fourteen often—and that, owing to the custom of polygyny, there are no unmarried adult women, unless they are diseased or temporarily divorced. In villages, among people of their own clan, are to be found many girls who remain virgins until their marriage after the *ichisungu* ceremony. There are, of course, in native society, as in more civilized communities, those who go astray or are led astray before this period. It must also be remembered that in these days the introduction of European customs and mode of life, with all the contacts which that means, has undermined tribal control, throwing the social fabric into the melting-pot. There are not now those restraints which were potent a few years ago, with the result that to-day there is certainly a tendency to moral looseness. But we cannot put this down to the Lamba social organization, which is definitely opposed to moral laxity. In this chapter we deal with the true Lamba conception of marriage and its obligations and with the relations of the sexes.

Imbuli

A girl before her initiation is called *imbuli*, and if a man violates an *imbuli* the act is regarded by the tribe as one of *uŵuchyende*, adultery. In such a case there is no fine imposed, but the man is warned and severely spoken to (*laŵishya*). But if a man has

159

chosen an *imbuli* to become his wife, as soon as she has gone through the *ichisungu* ceremonies he may have intercourse (*lalika*) with her as often as he pleases. The two may cohabit in the same house, the girl drawing water for him and performing other duties. People say, *Aliupile akaŵuli*, "He has married a little girl," but such marriages are not looked upon with great favour. When they take place, however, they are confirmed after the initiation of the girl. Naturally, during the initiation confinement the man is not permitted to see the girl. He will at this time give to the girl's mother an *insalamu* (ring) as a pledge that the girl is his wife.

Moye

If a man who is not her betrothed violate a *moye*, an initiated girl, there will be a serious lawsuit. A *moye* after her initiation is looked upon as *umuseesa*, a woman in her menstruation, until such a time as her chosen man "takes her *ichisungu*"—*i.e.*, deflowers her. Should another take it, her glory is gone.

Selection of a Wife

It is the general rule that the parents, especially the mother, of the young man choose his bride when it is considered that the time has come for him to marry. When she has decided upon a likely girl, the first inquiry the mother makes is as to whether the girl is unmarried (*umushichye*). If the answer is in the affirmative, the mother visits the girl's mother and tells her that she wants her son to marry the latter's daughter. The answer will be, "I shall ask my daughter this evening." Some days afterward the mother of the youth comes for her answer. If the answer is satisfactory, she goes to her son and says, "We have found you a wife. You find the calico." This calico is for the *ichyupo*, the necessary bridal pledge. The young man now procures the calico (*inguŵo*) and goes to see the girl. He gives it to her to take to her mother, and tells her that on the next day he will come to begin the building of a house in her village. When he has completed the building of the house he procures further calico to take to the woman, so that she will come to his new house as his wife.

In the old days the *ichyupo* given to the prospective mother-in-law by an ordinary commoner was *ichilundo chyamusompo uŵakupashila*, a four-yard piece of bark cloth, sewn to make it double the width and half the length. The value varied from two to four shillings. More well-to-do persons would give four or five

MARRIAGE

hoes to the mother of the girl, to be taken to her brother (the girl's maternal uncle) for him to distribute. The value of a hoe was about two shillings. In these days more is generally given as *ichyupo*, the amount varying from ten to twenty shillings, according to the desire of the suitor; and cash, calico, or blanket may be the medium in which the payment is made. In the case of cross-cousin marriages, which will be discussed later, the *ichyupo* is not insisted upon, though it is customary to send a present of calico to the bride and something to the *mwinshyo* if he is in rags. The passing of *ichyupo* cannot be looked upon as purchase. In the first place, the value of a slave is always many times greater than any *ichyupo*, and a wife is reckoned as of far more value than a slave. Then the terms under which the *ichyupo* is returnable are such as cannot imply that the wife is in any way bought. The term 'dowry' cannot be used in this connexion, for a dowry is what the bride brings to a marriage, and the *ichyupo* is always provided by the husband or his relations. The *ichyupo* seems to be a marriage pledge deposited with the clan of the bride as a guarantee of satisfactory behaviour.

When a grown man of his own desire is seeking a wife he visits different villages until he sees a woman who attracts his fancy. He then inquires from some one whom he knows in the village as to whether the woman is married or not. If she is unmarried (*umushichye*, a term indicative of living out of wedlock, whether widowed, divorced, or not yet married) the next question asked is, *Mbamwinando?* "What is her clan?" For a man may not marry a woman of his or his father's clan. If all is satisfactory, the suitor will tell his friend that he wants to marry the woman, and will ask him to speak to her. The friend will speak to the woman, and persuade her to come and see her suitor and speak to him. Sometimes from bashfulness a woman will refuse to go and speak direct to a suitor, but sometimes she will go. The suitor will then make his proposal plain, *Ndukufwayo'kuupa weŵo*, "I want to marry you!" If the woman is not impressed, she will answer, *Tachili chyeŵo chyanji; mwipushye ŵatata naŵamamo' luchyelo*, "It is not my business. Ask my father and mother in the morning!" Some are blunt enough to say right out, "No, I do not want you!" Others again, not desiring to offend, will say, "I cannot, for I am already betrothed," or "I am not one ever to marry!" Sometimes the girl, when sending to her father, will instruct him to refuse the suitor for her.

If the girl decides to accept her suitor's proposal she will some-times sit silent and give him no answer. Then she will get up and

THE LAMBAS OF NORTHERN RHODESIA

go to her house. The friend of the suitor will follow her to her house to get her definite answer, and she will say, "I consent. In the morning let him ask my father and mother."

In the morning the friend, who acts as go-between, visits the prospective father-in-law and says, "My friend who has come here desires your daughter!" The other asks, "Have you asked the girl?" On receiving the affirmative answer, he says, "All right. We agree if she is willing." The next day the suitor returns to his home to procure the necessary calico. He then brings to his prospective wife's village the *indalama shiŵili ishyansalamo*, the two shillings for the ring. This goes to the girl's mother, who takes it to her brother, the *ŵamwinshyo* of the girl, and, showing it to him, says, "See what your son-in-law has brought. Are you pleased?" His answer is, *Chiweme, ifiŵakumana kulya!* "All right, what is sufficient for the people [*i.e.*, all of us] is food!" meaning "Let him come and work and cultivate in the village and give us food!" Herein lies the man's greatest contribution to the marriage expenses, his practical enslavement for a considerable time. The man further brings the calico for his bride, and then is free to take her to wife. At the marriage the husband's maternal uncle (*ŵamwinshyo*) may give his niece by marriage (*umulokashi*) some four shillings for calico, or maybe only a fowl.

Cross-cousin Marriage

A common form of marriage among the Lambas is that of cousins of a certain relationship (*aŵafyala*). The *umufyala* of a man is the daughter of his father's sister or of his mother's brother—his cross-cousin. She is therefore of a different clan (*umukoka*) from the man. Polygyny is not so common among the Lambas as is generally considered, and though both wives of a polygynist may be *aŵalukoso*, persons in no way related to him, it is often the case that one of them is her husband's *umufyala*.

Betrothals are often arranged by the parents between a boy of about thirteen and his *umufyala* when she is maybe only five years of age. A Lamba girl matures early, and by the time she is thirteen or fourteen the marriage will be consummated. Meanwhile she will be regarded as her cousin's wife, and the boy's father will supply the calico for her clothing. Sometimes, if the girl is older, and she matures before the boy is sufficiently grown up for marriage, her mother will say to her brother, the boy's father, "Your son is still a child, and I want my daughter

162

to marry now." Permission will be given, and the girl will become the wife of some other man. The boy, when he grows up, will marry another woman in the usual way. As this is a matter which concerns relatives, there is no return of any clothing which may have been supplied. Parents are often keen on these marriages, since they ensure that their children do not go away to live at a distance.

From the point of view of the contracting parties, cross-cousin marriage has both its advantages and its disadvantages. The advantage is that if the wife dies the death-due payable to her mother's brother (often the man's own father) is naturally very small in comparison with that which would be payable on account of a wife from a non-related group. The same holds good if the husband dies, for the man's *ŵamwinshyo* regards the widow, if an *umufyala*, as *umwana waŵo*, his own child. The disadvantage of cross-cousin marriage is that the man fears to quarrel with his wife! He dare not strike his *umufyala*, for his father is her *ŵamwinshyo*. His father will say, *Tekulukupama wiso, ulishi ati mukwasu, ali koti nineŵo!* "Don't strike your father. You know that she is my relative, she is like myself." The women, on the other hand, welcome the possibility of the freedom of speech they might enjoy, but they fear the slighting they might experience from a husband who treats his wife as a child.

Marriage of Chiefs

Members of the chief's clan, *aŵenamishishi*, whether men or women, observed special customs in connexion with marriage. In the old days with them it was always 'marriage by capture.'[1] Not only did the chiefs capture their wives, but the chieftainesses also captured their husbands.

(1) **Women Chiefs.** Women of the chief's clan are especially protected from any interference from the time they are girls. A young man would fear a serious seduction charge if anything should happen to a girl of the chief's clan through his misbehaviour. When, however, the girl reaches maturity she herself chooses the man whom she wishes to marry, and then commissions the people in her village, or one of her male relatives, to catch (*ikata*) the man whom she has chosen. The people take lion's fat and set off for the village where the man is living. If they do not find him in his hut they sit down under the eaves and wait for him. When their victim returns and enters his hut they

[1] Except in the case of cross-cousins.

follow him in, smear the lion's fat on his shoulders, and seize him. He is then dragged off to the village from which his captors came, struggling and wailing at the hardness of his fate. Sometimes his friends may come to the rescue, but they desist, and put down their weapons, when it is said, *Tekukomo'muntu wamfumu, mwikesa kwikatalwa nekupooswa kuŵambundu,* "Don't injure a servant of the chief's, lest you all get seized and sold to the Mbundu slavers!" The man is then taken to his future wife. In the morning clothing is given to him, and sometimes a red blanket (*ichimbushi*) is given to the man's father. The marriage is then complete. The husband of a woman of chief's clan is called *lumbwe*, consort.

Men fear to marry women of the chief's clan because of the risk they run of lawsuits and of constant criticism and blame. If, for instance, a child is born, and then dies, which is by no means an uncommon occurrence, the *lumbwe* is charged with being the cause of death by means of his *ichiŵanda*, or attendant demon. The members of the chief's clan, *aŵenamishishi*, pride themselves on the privilege they have of making such a charge: no commoner dare do so. Another of the *uŵuleme* (glories) of the *aŵenamishishi* is the privilege of delayed burial, if they can afford to pay the necessary *aŵenamilenda* (undertakers). The *lumbwe* also fears being insulted for being but a commoner and the ridicule attendant upon his having been caught like a slave. Despite this, the husband has the right to order his wife about and to beat her for any misbehaviour.

Lamba men nowadays are by no means eager to marry *aŵenamishishi*, for though there is no capture, the members of the chief's clan still persist in their right to make vilifying accusations, because this is their *uŵuleme*. This is why many women of chief's clan among the Lambas are married by Ŵemba men, who, being strangers, take no notice of the charges which might be made against them.

(2) **Male Chiefs.** Prominent chiefs, such as Mushili of old, had the power of taking a woman whom they desired, even if she was already married. Such an act might cause the outraged husband to turn *akapondo* (murderer), and kill people in the chief's village in attempting to get at the chief himself. Such *utupondo* are of course not regarded as *imfwiti* (wizards), but as *ifita* (fighters). A man thus deprived of his wife may become an *imfwiti* and attempt the life of the chief by witchcraft.

MARRIAGE

The Capture of Nkandu

The following description of a particular case of 'marriage by capture' was given by a nephew of the woman concerned. During the great famine consequent upon the locust visitation which took place about 1892 many Lambas went to the Lenje country, and when the people of Nsensa's village returned to their homes they went to live in brushwood shelters (*imitanda*). Shiŵata, one of

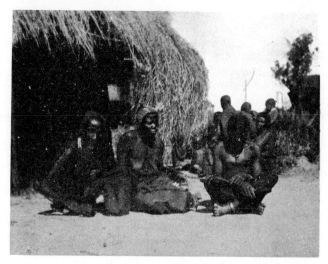

FIG. 64. MUSHILI I AND HIS TWO WIVES, 1913
Nkandu is next to him.
Photo by C. M. Doke

the elders, went to pay his respects to Mushili, whose village was not far distant, and returned in the evening with corn which Mushili had given him. That evening Shiŵata told his wife that Mushili had spoken of coming to Nsensa's village for a visit, and added, "What does he want here?" The wife suggested that it was just a friendly visit, but Shiŵata said, "No. Mushili does not travel without a purpose." The next morning, when all the elders had returned from their hoeing, Mushili and his people arrived. All gathered to greet the chief. Mushili said, *Aŵene- tata ŵali kwisa?* "Where are the clansmen of my father?" Mushili's father was a member of the goat clan, and Mushili wanted the *aŵenambushi* (goat clan people) of Nsensa's village to reveal themselves. The headman, Nsensa, and Shiŵata, his

165

brother, who were *aŵenambushi*, knew then his purpose, though the others did not. All the members of the goat clan then showed themselves, and when they had finished talking the visiting party returned to Mushili's village. When night came a raiding party (*ifita*), consisting of Mushili himself, Mwalo, the present Mushili, and others, arrived at the house of Nkandu, the sister of Nsensa and Shiŵata and a member of the goat clan, and demanded that she open the door. Some immediately entered and said, *Waikatwa, uli musanu!* "You are arrested. You are a wife of the chief!" Nkandu began to scream, but they smeared her with lion's fat, a sign that she belonged to the chief, and Mushili called out, *Tekufuma tata, nemata muno mumushi; nineŵo naisa mukwikato'musanu!* "Don't come out with your weapons here in the village. It is I who have come to capture my wife!" Nsensa and Shiŵata now came out with loud complaint. "Why is it, Mushili, that it is always from this village that the choice is made? For your brother Nkana married here too!" But Mushili replied, "That is no matter, for we ourselves prefer it here!" And they took away Nkandu, crying, and she became Mushili's wife.

Lamba women used greatly to dread marrying chiefs, and even to-day they do not like it. In the old days on the death of a chief his wives were all caught, bound, and charged with having killed him by witchcraft. The chief's brothers charged them with having selfishly used everything the chief had, without having given them anything. Then, when the remains of the chief were taken away for burial, some of his wives were killed that they might accompany him. Of the remaining ones, some became slaves to his brothers, others were sold into slavery. Even to-day the widows of a chief suffer great indignity and persecution.

If the chief had, say, twenty wives, two would perhaps be killed to accompany him to the spirit world; his heir would then distribute some of the remainder to certain of his sub-chiefs, while reserving the fairest for himself, to add to the number of his wives. Care is, however, taken if one of the wives is *umufyala* to the chief; the new chief may marry her or give her to some other relative of the dead chief.

Chiefs marry within the Lamba tribe only. The *aŵenamishishi* of Mushili's district cannot get a wife except by compulsion, and they could not exert that upon a foreign woman without bringing about war. At a distance from Mushili's, at Katanga's, for instance, the *aŵenamishishi* are able to choose (*salulula*) their wives and marry as ordinary people. In these days Mushili's *aẁenamishishi* can only choose women in their immediate vicinity; women further off are still afraid of the consequences of marrying a chief.

If a chief marries his cross-cousin, *umufyala*, she is not taken by capture. She is chosen, and there is no smearing of lion fat in her case. This is because the *umufyala* is child of a chief; her father was smeared when he was caught.

The Marriage

Except in the case of initial marriages, especially those of *ifisungu* (initiated girls), there is no ceremony beyond that of passing the necessary *ichyupo*. When this is done, it is usual for the sister of the man's father (*wishinkashi*) to go and fetch the bride in the afternoon before sunset. She brings her into the man's house, and sets food before her. Sometimes this provision is made by the mother of the man. While the bridegroom is elsewhere, his sisters and other women of the village have conversation with the bride. When they have finished eating, some of the women go away; then the bridegroom comes, and when his sisters have gone each to her house he remains and closes the door. When the marriage is thus consummated, the man begins to fell timber, prepare the *ifiteme*, and burn them. He then goes to his own home to fetch seed, and sows it. When the foodstuffs have come to fruition the man again returns to his own home, leaving his pumpkins and maize to his wife's relatives (*aẁenaẁuko*), who see to it that they use them all. When these crops are consumed the man returns again to his wife's village. This initial crop which is passed over to the wife's relatives is called *ichiluẁulantumbe*, the redemption of the basket, a compensation for the baskets of food he has had from his wife's relatives.

The Marriage of Ichisungu

In the case of a newly initiated girl, *ichisungu*, the marriage ceremony takes on special features. Very often a young man has chosen for his wife an uninitiated girl, *imbuli*, and as soon as she has passed through the initiation he desires to marry her. First he obtains certain beads, which he puts aside. He then builds his house, and when that is ready he goes to the *nyinachimbela*, the old woman who has initiated the girl, and takes to her some of the beads, saying, "To-day I have come to beg for my wife, that you should bring her to me." The old woman replies that she will bring her that night. After nightfall, while the young man is away with his companions, the old woman brings the girl to the hut prepared, and makes her lie upon the bed, and instructs her, *Kani akufilwe umulume uluchyelo winwa-po umufuŵa*, "If your husband fails to deflower you, in the morning don't drink the meal and water!"

The old woman now goes to call the young man. When he comes he brings two strings of beads; one he hangs at the foot of the bed and the other at the head. He may now complete the marriage, but if he fears failure in an attempt to deflower the *ichisungu* he will fly from the house and go elsewhere to sleep. Early in the morning the *nyinachimbela* will come and say, *Mfumine muŋanda*, "Come out of the house for me!" There will be no answer. She will then enter and ask the girl where her husband is, and the girl will say, "He was afraid and ran away." The old woman will then say, "He is a worthless fellow; he has failed!" It is asserted that many men after such an experience have gone away and committed suicide, fearing the ridicule which would be heaped upon them. Many are said to fear, because their elders tell them that an untouched *moye* is 'hard,' and difficult to penetrate (*pushya-mo*), and that if he fails he will die. If a young man tries and fails the marriage is considered null and void, and another may espouse the girl.

If, however, all is successful, and the marriage is consummated, when the *nyinachimbela* comes in the early morning and asks, *Tufumine muŋanda*, "Come out of the house for us!" the young man answers, *Nimwanji muno!* "It is my place in here!" Then the *nyinachimbela* stands outside the hut, and sounds the *ulumpundu*—that shrill whistling—in the early morning. She then enters the hut, gives the young couple *umufuŵa* (meal and water) to drink, and takes for herself the beads which have been hung at the foot and at the head of the bed.

When it is fully daylight the young man's mother comes with a cock and a basket of meal, while the girl's mother brings a hen. Both the fowls are killed, and *inshima* porridge is made from the meal. A crowd of friends gather round as the elder sister of the bride stirs (*nanya*) the *inshima*. The fowls are roasted, and while this is being done the bride takes hold of her husband's arm; at the same time he takes salt with that hand and sprinkles it on to the fowls. Similarly, when the *inshima* begins to boil the man takes the stirring-stick, while his wife grips his arm. When the fowls are eaten no one gnaws the bones (*kokote'fupa*), all eat meat only; the bones are given to the bridegroom (*umwine*

168

wachisungu), who throws them away. After the marriage feast, *ichitenje chyaŵuufi*, the assemblage breaks up, each one going to his own hut. Of this it is said *Ŵaŵakapa*, "They have introduced them into a new state."

That same morning the bride and bridegroom leave their hut and go into the veld with certain of their companions, *ili ŵatando' tuuluka*,[1] "chasing everything which flies." All day long the young people play about in the bush and on the plains, driving off anything they see that can fly, such as flies, gnats, tsetse, butterflies, etc. This is said to be *akeshiŵilo kakutamfye'nsoni*, a token of driving off the bashfulness, for a young man when first married fears to go back to his companions because of the chaffing he will get. They will say to him, *Kamwikala'pa mwemfumu, mwe mwaupa*, "Sit here, O chief, thou who hast married!"

In the evening the young people return to the village, and the bridegroom goes straight to his companions, his bashfulness all gone.

The custom of *ukutando'tuuluka* (chasing away things that fly) is carried out in the case of every woman who has never married before and in the case of every man on his first marriage, even if he is marrying a divorced woman.

The *ichitenje* (feast) is carried out in the case of two hitherto unmarried persons, even if they should be of advanced years, but in such a case there would be no visit of a *nyinachimbela* to the house.

The *moye* only on the first copulation is excepted from the rule to *sumuna*,[2] but she must on all subsequent occasions carry this out.

Observances of Married Life

The condition of marriage entails certain observances which are peculiar to the Lambas and some other Bantu peoples.

It used to be the duty of every wife to *nukulo'mulume amaso pachinena*, to pull out her husband's pubic hair. When this was done she would hold the hair in her two hands together and present it to her husband. He would receive the hair in one of his hands, whereupon his wife would clap her hands together. The husband would then take the hair and throw it away secretly. This action on the part of the wife used to be considered respectful to her husband. Nowadays shaving has taken the place of pulling out the hair, and the woman shaves both her husband and herself.

---

[1] This is a Lenje phrase used by Lambas in this connexion only.
[2] See Chapter IX, Rule (1).

THE LAMBAS OF NORTHERN RHODESIA

But even this practice is fast dying out, and most of the men shave themselves.

If a marriage is fruitless, and there is argument between husband and wife as to which of them is barren, they will agree each to take another partner. The marriage thus becomes null and void. If after this the woman gives birth, and the man fails to become a father, he usually feels such shame that he either leaves the territory or even commits suicide.

An old Lamba custom observed by many men was to allow no one to approach the house lest a stranger should see the wife. A visitor had to stand afar off and call, when the owner of the house would come out and talk with him. Such marks of jealousy, *uŵukwa*, are looked upon with disapproval in these days, though the practice is persisted in by the present Mushili.

Marriage Matrilocal

Lamba marriage is matrilocal. The man always builds a house in his *uŵuko*, the village of his wife and her mother, and usually lives there for at least two years. When this time is completed the husband's desire to go back to his old home will be conveyed by his wife to his mother-in-law, and she will in all probability make the suggestion to her son-in-law that the days of his servitude have been sufficient. He will then be free to take his wife and go back to live at his own village. There he may stay for good, or if his life there does not prove to be happy he may return once again to his *uŵuko*, and settle down there altogether. Men say that they are respected and treated well at their wife's village, despite the fact that in many a proverb and many a folk-tale they bemoan their harsh treatment at the hands of the mother-in-law. There are instances of unfair advantage being taken of a son-in-law, but the bad treatment is more proverbial than real. It is when a man is son-in-law to an *umwinamishishi*, a woman of the chief's clan, that his lot is really unenviable. Being a commoner, he is at the beck and call of all of his brothers-in-law as well, and is expected to supply inordinate demands for calico and to help in providing their tax money. The lot of the ordinary married man in Lambaland is not so bad as it is sometimes painted. An unconscious tribute to the value of the *uŵuko* is contained in the proverb *Umwau wansala nakuŵuko ŵaliutelele*, "The yawn of hunger, and even in your wife's village they heard it!" The man knows where to go when hungry—there will always be some food prepared for

170

him. Nevertheless, a man must behave himself discreetly in his *uŵuko*. If there is a brawl or quarrel on in the village he will be wise to keep out of it, since, being a stranger, he will be liable to get the blame, as all the other participants will be brethren.

There seems to be no definite law concerning the place of residence of children. They are often left with their grandparents when the parents move, but the decision rests with the parents. If a marriageable girl is residing with her maternal grandparents it is they who have the disposal of the *ichyupo*, or marriage pledge.

Polygyny

Polygynists are comparatively few in Lambaland, on account of the difficult lives which such husbands have to live. There used to be a few who had as many as three wives at a time, but there are none known now. Many villages have not a single polygynist in them. The wives of polygynists are called *impali*. The old Mushili had five wives. When I met him in 1913 there were only two left; the others had gone home for good. The present Mushili has but two wives, and they are said to be continually at loggerheads. In Lambaland a wife never desires her husband to marry a second in order to lighten the amount of garden work, as is sometimes asserted. One man, a Ŵulima, by name Kashyonka, is regarded by most natives as singularly fortunate, because his two wives live so amicably together. Even Mushili's wives when they quarrel treat Mushili himself with contempt as though he were a commoner.

If a man is going to marry *impali* he first lives his term of two years at his first wife's village, and then gets permission to go back to his own village. On his taking a second wife he goes to live at her village for two months in order to fell timber for his new wife's relatives. He then brings his new wife home, and both wives live in the same village—naturally each with a hut of her own.

There is usually considerable domestic trouble with the first wife before a man is able to bring home a second one. The man will broach the subject to his first wife, saying, "Wife, I want to marry another wife, for you get too tired with the work, and at times when you are ill I feel the burden of having to do the cooking myself." The woman may answer, "You may marry, but I shall go home to-morrow!" Her husband will retort, "All right. And I shall come to get a gun in compensation for desertion."

The woman is equal to it, and will say, "All right. My relatives will procure one and give it to you."

After such a quarrel the husband will take a ring to the woman whom he has chosen for his second wife. If she agrees, the first wife will hold back until the marriage is consummated. But as soon as this is done the first wife will go and fight with her rival. She will belabour both her husband and the new wife with a big stick, and the second wife will not dare to retaliate, for she fears the first wife, who is considered as *umwine wamulume*, the owner of the husband. In Lambaland domestic differences are not settled in private, and such an assault is carried out in public, and persists until the villagers come and take away the stick from the enraged woman, to prevent her from killing one of her victims. It is said that on such an occasion a chagrined husband has been known to go off and hang himself. After the assault the first wife usually goes away back to her mother's village. She may stay for some considerable time with her mother, until one day her husband arrives, and with violence upbraids his mother-in-law for harbouring his wife. In all probability the woman will quietly return with her husband, and settle down more or less amicably under the new conditions.

Sometimes the first wife refuses to come back to her husband. If he really desires to keep her he will send home the new wife and return to the *status quo*. If, however, he desires to keep the new wife, he can demand from the relatives of the wife who has deserted him the payment of a gun.

Sometimes, after such a definite separation has been effected, the man has found out that he cannot get on with the new wife, and even though his first wife may have married again he will send word that he wants her back. His elders will warn him— *Wemwana akabwelela kalalya*, "Son, what comes back, eats!" If he is persistent he will retort, *Ngakakandye nemwine*, "Well, let it eat me then!" They will say, *Ichyukawona chyowe wenka*, "What will happen to you is your own doing!" It is believed that if a man returns to the wife whom he has once divorced his death will be hastened. The *ichiwanda*, attendant demon, of the woman will, they believe, kill him. Unless the woman were married to a stranger from a distance she would never consent to give up her new husband for the one who had divorced her.

In the family of a polygynist the children having the same father but different mothers are always called *awanawankashi*, brethren, though they belong to different *imikoka*, taking their clan from that of the mother. Naturally marriage between such persons is forbidden.

The first wife of a polygynist is the *umukashi - mukulu*, the 'great' wife, the principal wife, and her hut is referred to as the *iŋande'kulu*, the 'great' house. The subsequently married wife is called *umukashi-mwanichye*, or child-wife, and her hut is referred to as *iŋande'nini*, the 'small' house. The eldest child of the *iŋande'kulu* will always be reckoned the eldest of the family, even if born after the eldest child of the *iŋande'nini*. For instance, A. married two wives, B. in 1900 and C. in 1905. The first child of B. was not born until 1908, whereas the first child of C. was born in 1906; nevertheless, B.'s child was called *umwana umukulu-ẁantu*, the 'eldest' child, and C.'s child was termed *umwana umwanichye-ẁantu*. In this way the Lambas call Isaac the *umukulu*, elder brother, of Ishmael, who was not the son of Abraham's principal wife.

Divorce

The marriage tie among the Lambas appears to be considerably looser than among a cattle-keeping people, with whom a considerable pledge of cattle is necessary on marriage. This looseness has been increased in the country since the advent of goods and money and of foreign natives who can offer more attractions to the Lamba women than their husbands can. Many cases are to be found of men and women who have had four and more marriages. Nevertheless, it must be recorded that there are very many cases of real love between husband and wife, and of a lasting affection which holds them together throughout life.

In the Lamba social system there are definite grounds for divorce, with a definite recognition of liability with regard to restitution of the *ichyupo* (marriage pledge) or additional payment of compensation. The following are the commonest grounds for divorce:

(1) **Divorce of the Wife.** (*a*) If the parents-in-law continually harass the man he can claim restitution of the *ichyupo* and, if he has made a marked contribution to the village life, also of a gun as compensation.

(*b*) If the wife has committed adultery the husband can, should he divorce her, claim from her *ẁamwinshyo* money or a gun in addition to the restitution of the pledge. This will be additional to his having killed the co-respondent or obtained a gun as his redemption.

173

(c) If the woman develops leprosy, syphilis, or yaws. There is no restitution of pledge in this case, and many men would continue to look after their wives.

(d) If the woman becomes a thief. This would mean restitution of the pledge, and sometimes payment of a gun.

(e) If the woman is nagging, disrespectful, and quarrelsome. Restitution as for (d).

(f) If the woman refuses to remain when her husband desires to marry another wife. Payment of a gun is demanded, as the woman has acted according to her own desires.

(2) **Divorce of the Husband.** (a) If he fails to clothe his wife. No restitution of pledge.

(b) If he fails to prepare a garden. No restitution of pledge.

(c) If he continually beats his wife. No restitution of pledge.

(d) If the man proves to be impotent (*shyamawawa*). No restitution, the man usually taking it upon himself to leave the district from very shame.

(e) If the woman ceases to care for her husband. This entails restitution of the pledge and payment of a gun, for the Lambas say, *Uwaŵipa aŵipa netwakwe*, "He who becomes bad, becomes bad with all his belongings too!" That is, "If you don't like me, you've no right to like what you have got from me."

(f) If the man develops leprosy, syphilis, or yaws. No restitution of pledge.

Divorce is so common among the Lambas that they say, *Ŵalakokola pakwambishya, pakulekana taŵakokola*, "They delay over their courting, but when getting divorce they do not delay." In all cases of divorce the children remain under the care of the mother, to whose clan they belong.

Marriage Restrictions

According to Lamba social law, a man may not marry a woman belonging to the same clan as himself, such marriage being regarded as incest. But the restrictions go even farther than this. A man may inquire of the woman whom he wants to marry as to her clan, but it is necessary to find out whether the clans of their fathers are different also. If they are the same the woman would call the man *indume*, brother, and should he marry her he would be said to have married his *umwana muŵyakwe*, his fellow-child, which is prohibited. Nevertheless, there are many *aŵapupa*, lawless persons, who overlook this prohibition in these days, and are merely ridiculed for their action. They quote a current proverb in excuse, *Akasaŵi ukulyo'mukwaŵo ekunona!* "The little fish that eats its mate is the one that gets fat!" In such a case, if it were found out that the fathers belonging to the same clan knew one another, a divorce would be insisted upon. If the mother of one party and the father of the other belong to the same clan there is no restriction, for this is the condition for the accepted cross-cousin marriage.

CHAPTER XI

DEATH AND BURIAL CEREMONIES

Cause of Death

AMONG the Lambas it is very seldom that death is attributed to natural causes, though often in cases of newly born babes and very old persons no other cause of death is imputed. In warfare death is often accepted as the direct result of the fighting, because the men fighting are, as a rule, volunteers; they go to war of their own accord. Should a man have been compelled to go, the responsibility for his death would not rest upon the actual person who inflicted the wound, but on the person who insisted on his going to fight.

In certain cases death is attributed to the direct action of Lesa (the deity), especially when a man is struck by lightning or smitten down by smallpox. This latter affliction is believed to be the direct result of breaking certain taboos, and it is considered the deceased's own fault if he has incurred this punishment.

Death is also at times attributed to a person's being struck by an *ichiŵanda* (demon) or an *ichinkuwaila* (goblin), that weird denizen of the forest which is believed to take possession of certain persons. The *aŵalaye* are believed to be able to treat persons affected by *ifiŵanda* and the *ŵamoŵa* those who have come into contact with *ifinkuwaila*, but they may be called too late, and the sick man may die.

Apart from such special cases, however, all death in Lambaland is put down to witchcraft. It matters not that a lion has devoured the unfortunate victim; it could not have been an ordinary lion, but one produced or induced by witchcraft. Even if a man commits suicide his action must have been induced by witchcraft.

During a holiday time at the mission school at Kafulafuta a few of the schoolboys remained at the mission to earn a little money by holiday work. In the late afternoons, with some of these boys, we missionaries were in the habit of going to the river to bathe. One day while bathing a lad named Chyola dived into the pool and disappeared. We could not recover his body until the next day, when it was evident that he had died of heart-

176

failure. His parents eventually laid a charge of witchcraft against his companion, one of the senior boys, who had persuaded him to stay with him at the mission instead of going home for his holidays.

Death and Burial

When a man is taken ill the *umulaye*, doctor, is sent for to diagnose, not his illness, but the cause of his illness, and to prescribe the necessary treatment for the removal of this cause. We shall consider the methods employed by the *awalaye* in a later chapter.

When, however, all the efforts of the doctor have proved unavailing, and it is seen that the illness has got such a hold upon the man that his recovery is despaired of, his relatives decide to move him to a little hut *mumpanga*, in the veld, a little distance from the village, because of the noises which go on in the village. They do this as a last resort to give the sick man a chance of recovery. This removal has been misinterpreted by many as a callous and selfish procedure, to prevent his dying in a good hut, but it is not so, for his hut, even if he has not died in it, will not be used again. If the weather is clement, an *umutanda*, a shelter of branches and leaves, will serve the purpose of sick-room, but in the rainy season an *inkunka*, or thatched lean-to, will be erected. Notice will be given to the villagers that they must not go there to worry the sick man with their presence.

When the dying man realizes that the end is near he calls his relatives—brothers if he has any—and commits to them the care of his children. They then know that he is dying. Men usually show concern for the future of their children, but few consider the wife who is left; nevertheless, there are some who will instruct their relatives to treat their wives with kindness, because they have been faithful and dutiful throughout their married life. If the man has any possessions, such as goats, for instance, he may instruct his relatives to give some to his children; the rest will naturally go to the relatives, as goods are inherited within the clan. He may further inform them that he leaves no debts, and tell them that, should demands be made upon his estate, they are to refuse to pay anything. He may even think of some little detail such as this: "So-and-so gave me some tobacco to smoke, and I promised him sixpence; if he comes for it, give it to him."

Relatives and friends now gather from all directions; some sit inside the house and others outside, where they light fires to await the death. As soon as it is known that life has left the body the relatives begin to wail. A brother now closes the eyes of the

dead man, for a man must not die with his eyes open—*tekufwe'*
ntunami. It is the women who do most of the wailing. At
first they roll themselves in the dust as they wail. The men soon
cease from wailing, and then stop the women's cries, saying,
Tanje tupopele'mfwa, "First let us enshroud the dead!"

His relatives now bring beads and put them round his waist,
and maybe two strings of beads around his neck and others on
his arms above the wrists. These are looked upon as a sign of
farewell. The body is now prepared for burial by being folded
up (*ukupeta*). The knees are brought up to the chin, the arms
also doubled up, with the hands upon the respective shoulders
and the elbows brought to
touch behind the knees, as in
the accompanying illustration.
The native puts no other in-
terpretation upon this position than that it is to assist in
the type of burial which they
observe, a type employed on
account of its economy in the
size of the grave and the
amount of digging necessary.
The folding of the corpse is
carried out with the corpse

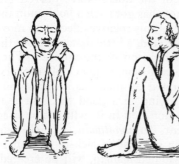

FIG. 65. METHOD OF FOLDING A CORPSE

lying on its side, it being immaterial upon which side it lies. The
body is held in this position for a few minutes until rigidity sets
in, when it remains in that position. If for any reason the folding
has been delayed until the body is already rigid, force is used to
bring it into position, but no binding of a corpse is ever resorted
to. The next thing done is to enshroud the folded body in white
calico (*imbafuta*) if it can be procured. A further covering of
bark cloth (*umusompo*) is put over this, or a blanket if the deceased
owned one. After this the body is laid upon a mat (*impasa*)
placed on the floor against the wall of the hut; another *impasa*
is placed as a screen in front. Were the deceased a wealthy man,
a further strip of white calico would be placed over the screen.
Several guns, loaded merely with powder, are now discharged,
and the wailing breaks out afresh, with added intensity. The
guns are said to be merely a sign to distant people to let them
know that the death has taken place.

Meanwhile the widow of the deceased has been lying on the
floor of the hut against the screen which separates her from the
corpse. As she wails she rolls about on the ground.

178

DEATH AND BURIAL CEREMONIES

In the morning the *awenamilenda*, undertakers, come forward for the work of conducting the funeral. These men may belong to any clan. They are usually elders (*awakulu*), and are paid for their work. Among the Lambas there are no people who regularly do undertaking work, but maybe, on hearing the guns, some men from a neighbouring village will come, enter the death hut, and sit down. If the deceased is not to be buried early they will sit there all day, and the people will thus know that they have elected to do the undertaking.

One of the deceased's relatives will now say, "Give the widow some water to drink, a pipe to smoke [*ukupeepeshya*], and some *ifisunga* [mild beer]," for neither a widow nor a widower may eat,

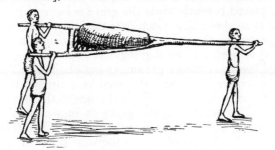

FIG. 66. IMISEEẀA FOR THREE CARRIERS

drink, or smoke until helped to do so by relatives of the deceased. This is termed *ukukapa*, a rite of initiation into a new state, into that of widowhood.

When the time for burial has arrived the corpse is brought out into the *uluẁansa* (court), bound with calico round the body and the head. The brothers and children of the dead man now come and throw meal (*uẁunga*) upon the shrouded body, to bid him farewell (*mukumulaya*); it is considered that he is undertaking a journey, and he needs to carry the meal. The body is now set upon an *impasa*, and two men carry it.

If the corpse is heavy the *awenamilenda* prepare a bier (*imiseeẁa*), resembling a machila, and two carry it, being relieved at intervals. Another kind of bier is composed of a large pole forked and branched at the one end. Three carriers convey this, one taking the end of the pole in front and the two others the ends of the forking at the back. Bark rope between the forks gives the support for the body.

A machila (the usual hammock of conveyance) is not used, for the death bier is never brought back to the village.

179

Maybe about ten men will go off with the body, five of these probably relatives, the other five paid *aẁenamilenda*. Directly the bier is taken up there is a great outburst of wailing. The bearers carefully avoid all paths when going to the burying-place (*umulyashi*). Each village has its own burying-place, and even if the village is moved to a considerable distance that same burial-ground is used. When a village is moved care is taken not to go close to a burial-place or to make the gardens too near one.

If the distance to the *umulyashi* is considerable, the bier is put down several times on the way.[1] When the spot is reached the bier is set down and the corpse laid on a mat (*impasa*). If it is during the rainy season a small shelter (*insama*) is erected, and the body placed beneath while the grave is being dug. Some of the relatives sit down and watch over the body, while the younger men begin to dig the grave. One hoe (*akalonde*, an old worn-down hoe) is used for the digging. It must not be restored to the village, hence economy prescribes but one hoe. The digging takes considerable time, and the men take turns with the hoe. First of all a stick is broken off and the size of the shrouded body measured. The length of the grave is measured accordingly. The hole is dug down until it is waist deep. When that depth is reached a shelf is hollowed out on the west side. This they call *iŋanda*, the house, in which the body is to be laid. When this is all hollowed out the mat (*impasa*) on which the body is lying, or another one brought from the village, is placed on the floor of the *iŋanda*.

Two men now take their positions in the grave, and two others hand down the body to them. One man now gets out, leaving room for the remaining one to place the body properly in the *iŋanda*. The body is laid on its left side, facing eastward; the head of the body is thus toward the north and the feet toward the south.

The reason for the facing eastward is explained by the natives as follows: "If the face is turned to the west the spirit cannot return to be reborn, but if a man faces the east his spirit will return. If a man is buried facing westward the *aẁenamilenda* [undertakers] would be considered *imfwiti* [wizards] for denying to the spirit the joy of return. In looking eastward he also looks for the return of Luchyele."[2] The Lambas have a saying,

[1] For burial from Katanga's village it is not put down at all, as the distance is short; from Nsensa's it is put down once. Generally an overgrown spot not likely to be visited by hunters is chosen.
[2] See Chapter XIV.

Kumbonshi takuya ubwela, "To the west he does not go who would return again." A dead man thus buried would 'go for good.'

After the body is laid in position the bier is cut up and the pieces of wood used to form a screen between the *iŋanda* and the *ichilende* (the hole first dug). The axe used for this purpose may be restored to the village. Against the screen (*ichipembe*) is placed another mat, and then the filling-in operation begins. First, big clods of earth and stones are handed down to the man

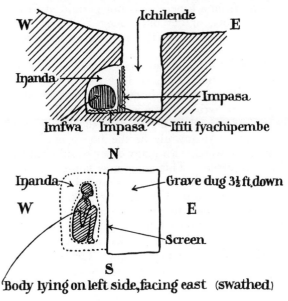

FIG. 67. PLAN OF A LAMBA GRAVE

in the grave; these he sets against the screen, which he holds in position and fixes firmly. When the screen is firm the man comes out from the grave. All the members of the burial party now assemble round the grave; they kneel down, and in concert push forward the earth with their elbows into the grave, chanting together *Yo!* "No!" After a time two of the men get into the grave and tread down the earth with their feet. The grave is then completely filled up; every bit of earth excavated is put on the mound, and any that has been carried some distance away is carefully swept on to the grave. A large mound is thus formed, and this is beaten and smoothed with the hands.

A plate belonging to the deceased is now brought; a hole is

driven through it, and it is placed on the mound—"as a sign to warn people that there is a person there." In the old days an *ichilukwa* basket was used for this purpose. The hoe-head is now knocked from the haft and thrown on to an anthill among the graves. Many such hoes are to be found in the *imilyashi*. Should the hoe be returned to the village, it would be considered equivalent to bringing back the dead body. Nowadays calico is torn and pierced, and set on a long pole at the grave as a flag to mark that it is a grave.

On returning from a funeral it is not permitted to shoot meat, pick fruit, dig roots, or cut out honey. This is an important taboo, and in the breaking of this is believed to have originated many of the Lamba clans.[1]

After the funeral all who have taken part go to the river and bathe completely. Before this is done they are said to have the death (*ulufu*) still upon their bodies. Then they all go to the village. On their arrival there is a great outburst of wailing. The *aŵenamilenda* stand in a row near the house in which the death took place. Meanwhile in the house one of the village elders has been on watch with many other people, talking over the affairs of the deceased. This elder now comes out and lights a torch of dried grass, which he carries round the group of *aŵenamilenda*; when this is done they all enter the deceased's house. *Inshima* porridge is now prepared, and a grilled (*iyakochya*) fowl, which they eat. They then separate, to go to their own houses. It is now the duty of the heir of the deceased (*umwine waufwile*) to arrange the pay of the hired undertakers. The two who receive the body in the grave will be paid about five shillings each, the others about three shillings each. The relatives of the deceased now shave their heads as a sign of mourning, but this privilege is denied for the present to the relict.

Amalilo

In the evening the undertakers are called, the principals being paid first and then the juniors. Every one then sits down for the night of singing. Dancing by single dancers is indulged in at this stage, but there is no community dancing. The songs used at the *amalilo* (mourning rites) are generally chosen from the *ifinsengwe*[2] (hunting songs); others are those composed by the *aŵayambo*. The *aŵenamilenda* have rattles (*imiseŵe*) and calabash drums (*imbila*), which they sound in the hut, while the men and women sit about outside and assist in the singing. The following are examples of the songs used:

---

[1] See Chapter XII.   [2] See examples in Chapter XV.

DEATH AND BURIAL CEREMONIES

(1) *Chingalika umunamusanga mumilamba,*
    Wapapa neŵana ŵakwe mumilamba!

> "The male zebra, where I met him in the track,
> Carried his children on his back, in the track."

(2) *Shyakaiwa, Shyakaiwa, walila Mumba, Shyakaiwa.*
    Walukoshi ŵakantwalila mwana,
    Kwenda kandila! [1]

> "Shyakaiwa, Shyakaiwa, Mumba has cried, Shyakaiwa.
> Mr Eagle has carried off my child.
> I wail as I go!"

(3) *Kaŵombwe, kaŵombwe, pamwala kalukulila:*
    Kaŵule kalile, lelo amenda apwa, twapelelwa.

> "Little frog, little frog, was croaking in the vlei.
> Can it help croaking? To-day the water has dried
> up.
> We are bereft."

(4) *Kako, kako, mwimbileni, kako,*
    Yaweyawe [2] *mwimbileni!*

> "That one, that one, sing ye to him, that one,
> Yaweyawe, sing ye to him!"

Preparations for the Beer-drink

In the morning corn is set in soak for the beer-making. While they wait for the malt to set the people begin to dance the *ichinsengwe* dance. This dancing is done during the night only; there is no drumming, and only solo dancing. During the daytime the people sleep or go about their usual occupations. Maybe four days will pass before the *amamena* (malt) is dry. When this is ready the young people will say, "We too ŵant to mourn with the drums. We do not know the *ichinsengwe.*" So they begin to dance to the accompaniment of beaten drums, keeping this up each night until the beer is brewed. These young people dance various dances, such as the *akashimbo*, the *akasela*, the *ichipelu*, and the *umusakasa.*

On the night before the beer is brewed the *aŵenamilenda* come again, and again begin to sing *ichinsengwe* songs in the deceased's hut. Meanwhile the younger folk still dance the *akasela* outside. The women and the older men spread their sleeping mats outside

---

[1] The construction is Lenje; the song is said to have originated in the Lenje country from the crying of the *akatuutwa* bird when the eagle caught her young.

[2] *Yaweyawe* is a term applied to the dead man, and only used in this connexion. It is possibly derived from *ukuyaŵa*, to sing mourning songs. As this song is sung all stand, and then go round and round, following in a line the *umutatwishi* (song-leader)

and lie down watching the dancing. On this occasion the dancing is necessarily strictly moral. The dancers continue thus right through the night, and both *akasela* and *ichinsengwe* are kept up into the next day. The beer is now in the house with the *aŵenamilenda*. By midday the drum is stopped and the beer-drinking begins. When all are seated one pot of beer is given to the younger people who have been dancing the *akasela*, and the others are given to the older mourners. In the evening, when the beer-drinking is over, the hut of the deceased is closed and a white log of wood leant against the door. This house is never opened again, even if the deceased died in a shelter outside the village. In the house

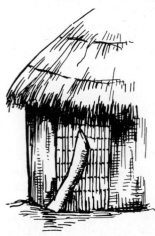

are left only the bed cross - poles on which his mat used to lie. The house is left to rot of its own accord. If the village is deserted and the houses burnt, this one will be left; *it must rot and fall by itself.* The white log against the door is a sign to everybody, from wherever he may come, that it is a house of the dead (*ichituuka*). In all, about ten days cover the time from the death to the shutting of the house.

FIG. 68.   ICHITUUKA

When the period of mourning is completed, a month or maybe two months after the death, the relatives of the deceased shave the head of the widow (or widower if a woman has died). This sign of mourning is denied for so long in order that the relict may realize that she (or he) is not a free person until the death-dues are paid.

Burial of a Woman

In the case of the death of a woman the preparations for burial are carried out usually by the husband if she has one, or otherwise by one of the *aŵenamilenda* (undertakers), assisted by an old woman, *nyinachimbela*, who will put on the beads. There are no female undertakers, and a man always swathes the corpse. While the undertakers who convey the corpse for burial are all men, some female relatives may accompany them merely as witnesses.

When a pregnant woman dies the husband is forced to accompany the undertakers to the burial. If the husband is afraid he will have to find a village elder as substitute, and pay him as much as a gun for his services. When they go they prepare a sharp stake of an *umutoŵo*-tree called *ichinsonta* to take with them. On reaching the place of burial the husband rips open the woman with the *ichinsonta*, stabs the unborn child through, and, holding it up in the air on the end of the stake, shouts, *Lesa walya ŵaŵili*, "God has eaten two!" He then throws it down and rushes away from the gruesome ordeal, returning alone to the village. Headman Kalimbata was forced to do this when his younger brother's wife died and her husband ran away. After this is done the mother is buried in the usual way by the *aŵenamilenda* and the child laid against her in front, the *ichinsonta* being withdrawn and used to prop up the screen.

If a substitute has gone in place of the husband, that very evening, when the people are gathered, the bereaved man takes a gun and in the presence of the people gives it to the village elder, saying, "You have helped me in a difficult task!"

Should the husband refuse to go, and should there be no substitute, he would be caught by the *aŵenamilenda*, taken along forcibly, and compelled to perform the deed, for the Lambas fear that if the woman is buried in child it will mean that other women of the same clan will die pregnant. There is thus a fear of the working of sympathetic magic. This is only done in cases of advanced pregnancy, known to everybody.

Burial of Children

When a baby dies two of the relatives take the little body, one of them carrying it on his shoulders, trussed and wrapped in calico. A small grave of the same pattern as an adult's is made. Wailing is indulged in only by the mother and her relatives, who remain in the house for one day. There is no dancing, nor is the house abandoned.

In the case of children from two to eight years of age four people may go to the burial, of whom two will be *aŵenamilenda*. There will be one night of *ichinsengwe* singing, but no beer-drinking or regular dancing.

Lepers

The Lambas never bury those who die of leprosy. They build a high platform and place the body on top to decay, so that it will not pollute the ground and cause fellow clan members to contract the disease. An *umushitu*, or swamp-forest, is generally chosen for this purpose.

Burial of a Chief

When an important chief becomes ill, and the people know that he is seriously ill, they send to the *aŵenamilenda*,[1] telling them not to go away, because the chief is seriously ill and may not recover. The chief's wives are watched, to prevent their escape. Directly the chief dies his relatives send to fetch the keepers of the spirit-huts, the *aŵenamilenda*, without letting the villagers know. Meanwhile the chief's relatives take all his wives and shut them up in a house, making the door fast. The younger members of the chief's clan guard the house, while the women of the clan and the daughters of the *aŵasanu* (chief's wives) take them food. The women of the clan act as wardresses when it is necessary for the imprisoned women to go into the bush to relieve nature. The wives are looked upon as witches who have killed the chief.

On the arrival of the *aŵenamilenda* the news is published abroad, that every one may know that the chief is dead. Then all the people gather together to mourn. The other members of the chief's clan arrange the payment of the *aŵenamilenda*, according to their station, and when a quantity of goods has been brought payment of the younger *aŵenamilenda* is made, the chief *umwinamulenda* only being left unpaid.

Wearing a huge headdress of guinea-fowl and *mukuta* feathers, the *aŵenamilenda* now take charcoal and pound it with red ochre (*ulushila*). On one side of the face they smear the red ochre, on the other charcoal, and in the middle of the forehead they smear flour. Then they set about catching fowls in the village. These fowls they bring back and eat. They are feared by everybody. They sleep in the house with the corpse, but no one will enter for fear of punishment should he spit on the floor.

The body of the chief is laid on an *umusengelo* (reed mat) on cross-poles very near to the ground; it is stretched out, not trussed up at all. A trench is dug encircling the bier, and earth is heaped up to touch the bier all round. The rotted remains and the water poured on will go into the trench.

When the body of the chief has begun to swell the *aŵenamilenda* heat water and keep sprinkling it on the body. When they eat they burn the feathers of the fowls they have killed in order to counteract the stench of the corpse. This pouring on of water is continued day by day, and the chief's slaves are kept hard at it drawing water and grinding flour for the *aŵenamilenda*. When

---

[1] In the case of Mushili the chief *umwinamulenda* was Chinguŵe, Mukupe and others assisting him.

DEATH AND BURIAL CEREMONIES

decomposition is practically completed the undertakers inform the people that "the chief wants to take his journey" and that they must grind much flour. When they are ready to begin the long journey to the burial-place the *aẁenamilenda* again don their headdresses and decorate their faces with ochre, charcoal, and flour. The people prepare for them a fine house elsewhere in the village, and bring them baskets of meal and fowls.

Dancing and beer-drinking go on while the body is decomposing, and on the last night the people indulge in *akasela* dancing all night and into the next day.

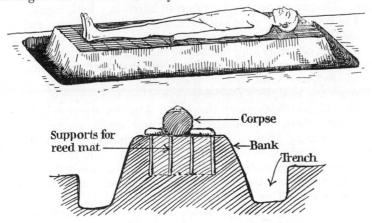

FIG. 69. HOW A LAMBA CHIEF IS PREPARED FOR BURIAL

Now in the *akaẁungo*, as the *ichituuka* or house of the dead chief is called, mere bones are resting on the stand. The *aẁenamilenda* take out the teeth and toe- and finger-nails of the chief, and hand them over to Lyala [1] from Mwema's district, who has arrived to take charge of them. If all the teeth are not there, Lyala, on counting them, will say, "The teeth are not all here!" And one will answer, "No. One he had taken out!" Lyala keeps the teeth and nails of each chief in a separate packet of cloth in a closed calabash, which is placed on a stand in a small lean-to hut (*inkunka*). People from Mushili's village will never sleep at Lyala's, as they consider it as though it were *kumulyashi*, at the burial-place, as part of the chief's remains are kept there. The presence of the teeth and nails is a sign that the chief is still in the village. Is there any significance in the fact that these are the only bony parts of the body visible during life?

[1] *Ilyala* means 'nail.'

After the removal of the teeth and nails the bones are bound up, as in the case of an ordinary death, the dry tendons still being there so that they do not come apart. They are then wound round with calico print. Beads have already been placed upon the waist, neck, and wrists.

At the end of two months the *aŵenamilenda* go and prepare an *ichikondo*, a bark canoe, and the *imiseeŵa*, a single long white pole. They make a fire, heat to redness an axe, and burn markings upon the pole. Great Lamba chiefs never cross a river in a bark canoe, because they know that they will one day 'sleep' in one. No commoner can be taken to burial in a bark canoe.

The remains are placed in the canoe, cloth is put over, and the canoe is secured beneath the long carrying-pole. As the procession starts off on its long journey to the resting-place of the chiefs many people accompany it, to see off the chief, sounding the shrill *impundu* cries, while the younger *aŵenamilenda* range through the bush on either side pretending to be hyenas. Four of the *aŵenamilenda* carry the bier. The two wives whom the chief loved best, tied round the waist with cords, are taken with them, weeping bitterly. One of the undertakers goes ahead, clanging an *ulusonsolo*, a heavy double bell, while those behind keep up a noisy shouting. When a village is reached the people fear the procession, but the principal *umwinamulenda* says, *Tamutaile'mfumu?* "Don't you make gifts to the chief?" Everybody comes and brings gifts of beads and metal armlets, while the village headman brings a length of cloth. Everywhere the people greet the *cortège* with shrill *impundu* whistling, while the men come and take their turn at carrying the *imiseeŵa*. At the village where they spend a night, if there is no drum they sleep without any singing or dancing. A good house in the midst of the village is swept for the 'chief' to sleep in, and fowls are brought to the *aŵenamilenda*.

On the day before they reach the *umulyashi* the 'hyenas' go on ahead to visit the spot, and then return to meet the chief. The principal *umwinamulenda* asks them, *Shyani ukomwaile?* "How is it where you went?" And they answer, *Yo, ŵaŵasumina!* "No. They accept him!" meaning that the chiefs buried there before are prepared to receive the recently deceased chief. Then they all go on to the burial-place.

The burial-place of the Lamba chiefs of Mushili's country is in an *umushitu* (rank forest) on the Kafinga river, near Kashise's village, in the Belgian Congo.

The *cortège* enters the *umulyashi*. This is a sacred *umushitu*;

DEATH AND BURIAL CEREMONIES

there is no water here, not even in the rains. The principal *umwinamulenda* enters with a shout of triumph, *akasemo*, used only by a man who has killed his foe. *Wahe! wahe!* he shouts, and all make shrill response. The younger ones cry like hyenas, and the rattle bell is violently rung.

Now the two widows of the chief are killed with spears, and the chief is buried in the way in which ordinary persons are. When this has been done the slaughtered wives are cut up, their limbs and portions of their bodies being hung about on the trees throughout the *umushitu*. Numbers of vultures assemble to the feast as soon as the people leave the spot. Ntenke and Mushili were the first chiefs to be buried without this taking of life; when Nkana was buried women were slain, but it is not certain whether they were wives of his or not.

When the people return home they recount to the new chief everything that happened along the road. He then pays them for their services.

The hut in which the chief's body had rotted is shut up and left to fall to pieces by itself.

When the *awenamilenda* have departed there comes Kaŵalu, the guardian of the chief, to receive from the new chief the spears, axes, and bows and arrows which the old chief used to use himself. These he takes and cares for in his shrine, *umulenda*. Kaŵalu preserves these relics of all the chiefs, keeping them and their various ornaments in order. At Shichyuŵa, near Kombe, also bows, large spears, and "wonders of the past" are preserved. Here, too, an inventory of all these things is made at the end of each month.

Kaŵalu and Lyala are paid for the work they do. The new chief, the heir, takes charge of the *inkombo* (calabashes) of the deceased chief, and is responsible for their care.[1] Lyala is paid a gun at the reception of each chief. Kaŵalu is paid at first about ten shillings, but he has the privilege from time to time of getting money from the people by begging rain for them from the chief.[1] In the olden days also, at the new moon, Kaŵalu would go in the morning to his *umulenda*, take out a bow, wrap it completely in calico, and carry it, ringing his *ulusonsolo*, from village to village. At his arrival in a village all would utter the *impundu* cries, and shout, "The chief has come!" They would then catch fowls and make offerings, while the *ifilolo* (headmen) of the chief would present calico. In this way Kaŵalu regularly made a considerable sum. The *awenamilenda* who attended for the dissolution of the

[1] See "Spiritism," Chapter XV.

189

body were paid as follows: the principal a gun, and the younger men about £1 each.

Death-dues

In the case of an unmarried person, *umushichye*—that is, a person not living in wedlock, whether in English parlance a bachelor (or spinster), widower (or widow), or divorced person—the Lambas say, *Alafwa lukoso*, "He merely dies," meaning that his death involves no payment of death-dues by anyone. But the death of one partner in married life involves an *umulandu wamfwa*, a death responsibility, dischargeable only by payment of a death-due by the surviving partner. This payment has to be made to the relatives of the deceased. That this payment has nothing whatever to do with the *ichyupo*, or marriage pledge, is evident from the fact that it applies both to the widow of a deceased husband and to the widower of a deceased wife.

After the period of mourning has passed the relatives of the deceased approach the relict and say, "If you have means [*uŵuŵoni*], bring them and redeem yourself [*luŵuka*]." The usual price of redemption nowadays is a gun, of value about fifty shillings. If the relict can raise the amount necessary—maybe by borrowing from relatives—and it is accepted by the relatives of the deceased, they bring a string of white beads and tie them above his left wrist. They then bring meal (*uŵunga*), throw it all over his body, and utter the shrill *lulululu* cries, saying, *Pano wemukwasu fuma-po waluŵuka koyo'kope!* [1] "Now, brother, go—you are redeemed; go and marry!" He is then once more a free agent (*umwana-waŵene*), and may consider taking another wife; in the case of a woman, she may consider another husband. The throwing of the meal is always a sign of redemption, in this instance from the spirit of the departed, which is no longer in his charge, dependent upon him, but free to pass into the care of one of the relations and be represented by an *ulukombo*,[2] or calabash.

These death-dues originate in the Lamba belief in the guardian demon (*ichiŵanda*) looking after the interests of each individual.[2] The payment is out of respect to the deceased, and it is believed that, if payment is not made and the relict marries again, the *ichiŵanda* of the deceased will wreak vengeance on the defaulter. This *ichiŵanda* is regarded as the *inkalamba yamukoka*, the messenger of the clan of the deceased.

There was the case of a man named Makaka, who became a Christian. His wife died, and he procured the necessary amount

---

[1] To a woman they would say *Koyo'kopwe*, "Go and be married."
[2] See Chapter XV.

to redeem himself, but refused to undergo the heathen rite of *ukupooswo'ẁunga*, having the meal thrown over him. At the time the matter was waived, and he married again. When, however, his second wife died there was a great outcry against him. The *ichiẁanda* of the first wife, people said, was not appeased, as no meal had been thrown, and it had therefore caused the death of the second wife.

In the case of the death of a woman the gun would be handed to her *mwinshyo* (maternal uncle), or, failing him, to her brother. In the case of the death of a man the gun would go to his *mwinshyo*, or, if there was one living, to his elder brother. Should the *mwinshyo* already have a gun, he may give the gun of the death-due to the younger brother of the deceased. If money is paid it is usually divided out, and this division is carried out by the *mwinshyo*.

It is said that many *aẁongwa*, people of low moral and social standing according to Lamba standards, say that they do not want to marry again, and so refuse to pay the dues. They leave that particular district and marry again elsewhere. But if they are found out they will be driven away from their new home, lest they should act in the same way there.

When the man is in favour with his parents-in-law, and they do not want him to go and marry elsewhere on his wife's death, they will offer him his wife's younger sister. If he agrees he will marry her, but will still have to pay the due for his first wife's death. In this case he may marry before the redemption is completed. The younger sister is termed *impyani*, heir.

Similarly, when a man dies his younger brother may inherit the widow before she has redeemed herself. Many years may pass in this way, but the husband will fear that if she does not pay the amount due to him he will not have wherewith to pay the due to her relations should she predecease him; he will therefore press for payment. Should she die before paying, he will have to pass over a small amount, say £1, in order to free himself from the *ichiẁanda chyamukwaẁo*, the demon of his brother. On the other hand, should the woman's second husband, her first husband's brother, die before her redemption, she would never be redeemed, but would become a slave to the relatives of her husbands.

An interesting point arose on the death of the chief Mushili in 1917. He left two wives, one of whom was Nkandu, whom he took by capture from Nsensa's village. The new chief, Mushili, first of all took Nkandu for his own wife, but on account of her age sent her back home to Nsensa. He then demanded payment, because she was of no more use to him. Mwendo, by the hand of Joshua Kamwendo, sent him a gun and thirty shillings. Mushili refused so small an amount. It was argued that Nkandu was now very old, and that she had served the old Mushili for many years. From that time Mushili has said nothing further concerning the matter, but the people of Nsensa expect that he will try to get something before Nkandu's death.

Ukulule'mfwa

In some cases the announcement of a death is made in an indirect way, for fear of assault. If a man has taken his wife to his own village (*ubwinga*), and she is taken ill there, and he does not notify her relatives immediately, he will fear for his personal safety if he goes and tells them of her death. He will send a substitute with a gift. When this man reaches the outskirts of the village he climbs an anthill, and shouts out, *Ichyamwachetekele nsansa nsansa*, "What you believed in is all scattered!" The villagers call out in reply, "What are you saying, you who shout in the veld?" And he calls again, "What you believed in is all scattered. So-and-so is dead!" They then tell him to approach, but he fears to do so, and does not trust their assurances until the village headman himself goes to the anthill to fetch him down, when he explains the whole affair. This procedure is called *ukulule'mfwa*, the announcement of death.

Imilao

Among the Lambas dying men sometimes give instructions, which are as a rule carefully carried out, for they say, *Tekupufyo' mulao*, "Dying men's instructions are not to be disregarded." He may say, "When I am dead, do not trouble my widow; if you do, you will see ill-omens; but let my younger brother inherit her, and care for these my children."

The Uncleanness of Death

Touching the dead produces a ceremonial uncleanness, and the *awenamilenda* are said to have *ulufu* (death) upon them until they have completed the ritual and bathed ceremonially. In the same way widows and widowers have *ulufu* upon their bodies until they have paid the death-dues and have had the meal thrown upon them as a sign of their release from the *ichiwanda* (guardian demon) of the deceased.

CHAPTER XII

IMIKOKA—THE CLAN SYSTEM

Imikoka

EVERY Lamba belongs to one or other of the thirty-two exogamic clans, which are called *imikoka*. The child derives his *umukoka* from his mother, and as property must remain within the clan this system ensures that inheritance is in the main matrilineal. While clan descent is purely matrilineal, its importance is reflected in the spiritual conceptions of the people. Children of a different clan may be named after a certain ancestral relation, but the spirit of that deceased relative, or the afflatus from his spirit, can only be reincarnated in a child belonging to the same clan.

The Lamba clans can no longer be regarded as totemistic, though they bear totem names, half of which are those of animals. It is possible that they have moved away from an original totemistic regard for the animals whose names they bear. As will presently be observed, the native tradition has it that many of the clan names originated from particular behaviour on the return from a funeral. To this day it is taboo for anyone to shoot game, pick fruit, cut out honey, or otherwise procure bush food on the return journey from a funeral, "lest," they say, "the very food procured be named as your *umukoka*." Nevertheless, this prohibition is so far lifted that the *aŵalembo*, members of the bee clan, may cut out honey; the *aŵenachyowa*, members of the mushroom clan, may pick mushrooms, and so on; but on no account may any animal, bird, or fish be killed on such an occasion, not even by members of the clan representing such an animal, bird, or fish.

In ordinary circumstances there is no totemistic ban on meat-eating; for instance, a member of the goat clan may eat goat flesh. Naturally the members of the chief's clan, the *aŵenamishishi*, have the highest honour, and it is conceded that the *aŵenambushi*, who were ousted from the chieftainship, have more honour than any of the other clans of commoners.

In the following pages is given a list of the thirty-two Lamba clans, with details as far as the Lambas know them.[1]

---

[1] About several of the clans the Lambas can give no information further than the meanings of their names.

THE LAMBAS OF NORTHERN RHODESIA

(1) *Aŵenamishishi*, the clan of the hair of the head. The origin of this clan is traced back to the story of Chipimpi and Kaŵunda, when Kaŵunda bathed in the blood of a human being. The hair of the human head, *imishishi*, is considered by the Lambas to be their 'glory,' "for," they say, "if a man has no hair he is a bald-pate." They further maintain that the *imishishi* distinguish man from the beast. The importance of the hair is recognized on several occasions:

(*a*) Men, women, and children shave during mourning.

(*b*) During the *ichisungu* initiation of girls beads are woven in the girl's hair (*ukukunga*).

(*c*) The changing of the hair to grey and white heralds full age, and *aŵamfwi*, grey-headed persons, are greatly respected.

(*d*) On going to war *ubwanga bwankondo*, the war charm, is worn in the hair.

It is asserted by some that the term *imishishi* is a euphemism, and that the real totem is either *amaso* (pubic hair) or *amankuluk-wapa* (hair of the armpits), but this is vigorously denied by most Lambas, who look upon the assertion as libellous. This is the one 'non-commoner' clan of the Lambas, the clan of the *imfumu* or chiefs; all other Lamba clans are those of *aŵachyete* or commoners.

(2) *Aŵenambushi*, the goat clan. By tradition this was originally the chief's clan, before the chieftainship was assumed by the hair clan. Hence it is the most respected of the clans of the *aŵachyete*. Despite the evidence of the story of Chipimpi and Kaŵunda, many members of this clan maintain that their totem is not the goat, but the water-beetle, which bears the same name, *imbushi* or *imbushi yapamenda*. This species of water-beetle is held in considerable respect, because when a pool dries up it flies up and searches elsewhere at a distance for water, while goats are despised for their dirty eating.

(3) *Aŵenatembo*, the wasp clan. This is the clan of the Lenje chiefs, but with the Lambas it is a clan of commoners. The origin of the clan is traced to the following story. Some people returning from a funeral went into the bush to eat honey. As they were getting out the honey their faces were badly stung by bees. On their return to the village they were asked, "What has stung you?" Desiring to hide the fact that they had honey, they replied, "Wasps!" But a child had accompanied them, and when he was questioned he told what actually had happened. In derision the nickname of wasp, *itembo*, was applied to them.

(4) *Aŵenaŋanga*, the clan of the 'doctor,' also called *aŵena-nsumbi*, the clan of the fowl. Here the term *iŋanga* refers, not to

the ordinary doctor, but to a black and white bird called the *shiwakota*, or *iŋanga yakwe shiwakota*, a bird which is called "the doctor of all birds." Another name of this bird is *umukuta*. It catches fish, and in Lamba folklore was the master of the original fowls [1] (*insumbi*). These slaves of the *umukuta* were sent to the village to trade his fish, but, finding corn on the ash-heaps, they stayed there, and became domesticated. They now fear to go near the river lest the *umukuta* should catch them, and he still calls loudly for his fish.

(5) *Aŵenambeŵa*, the mouse clan. As they returned from a funeral some people found a large buck dead. They brought it secretly to the village, and while they were cooking some of it their friends asked them what meat it was. Their reply was, "Mice!" When their deception was found out, however, they were dubbed with the nickname, which has clung to them.

(6) *Aŵenanyendwa*, the needle clan, the clan of the Ŵulima and Lala chiefs. The term is derived from *inyenda*, a large needle used in basket and mat work.

(7) *Aŵenansofu*, the elephant clan. The origin of this is like that of the *aŵenambeŵa*. People eating freshly killed meat tried to deceive their companions by saying that they were eating a piece of elephant-hide!

(8) *Aŵenaŋandu*, the crocodile clan.

(9) *Aŵenansoka*, the snake clan. It is sometimes said to members of this clan, "Why is it that your kinsmen the snakes bite you?" And they reply, "They do not realize that we are their relatives." This is said in sport, however, for there is no serious thought in the Lamba mind connecting the person with the clan animal.

(10) *Aŵenakaŵundi*, the galago clan. On the return from burying their brother certain men caught a galago in a tree-cleft. Their attempt to deceive their fellows at the village regarding this dainty earned for them the clan name.

(11) *Aŵenansanje*, the blue monkey clan. This was originally a Lala clan.

(12) *Aŵenambwa*, the dog clan, also called by the Lenje name of *aŵenankuwa*. Members of this clan indignantly deny any relationship with the dog when teasingly accused of it.

(13) *Aŵenankulimba*, or *aŵenakunda* (the Lala term), the pigeon clan.

(14) *Aŵenanguni*, the honey-guide clan. Members of this

---

[1] See *Lamba Folk-lore*, by C. M. Doke (American Folk-lore Society, 1927), p. 121.

clan are teased by being asked, "Since your brother the honey-guide lives in the bush, why don't you go to him and get him to lead you to honey?" And they reply, "He is not our brother; he is a chief of the country, and gives food to all alike."

(15) *Aŵenanguluŵe*, the river-hog clan, the clan of certain Aushi chiefs, also called *aŵenakauluŵe*, the little river-hog, and *aŵenanama*, or *aŵanyama*, the animal or meat clan. It is said that people eating meat they had procured on returning from a funeral were dubbed *aŵanyama*. Members of this clan are teased by being told that "Your clan is not a nice one, because when we work and work at our gardens your brethren [the pigs] come and steal!"

(16) *Aŵenamaila*, the sorghum clan. *Amaila* is the Lenje term for the Lamba *amasaka*.

(17) *Aŵenachyowa*, the mushroom clan. The original members of the clan are said to have picked *uŵowa*, mushrooms, when returning from a funeral.

(18) *Aŵenakani*, the grass clan, originally a Maswaka clan. This clan is praised, since grass, when thatched on the roof, is a protection from rain.

(19) *Aŵenachyulu*, the anthill clan.

(20) *Aŵenanswi*, the fish clan, also called *aŵalonga*, the running stream clan, the clan of Kaonde and Aŵenambonshi chiefs. This is held in respect because of the value of fish as relish. The origin is said to have been in the bringing of fish to the village by those returning from a funeral.

(21) *Aŵenaluwo*, the wind clan, from the Lenje term for wind, also regarded as the small elephant clan, as opposed to the *aŵenansofu*.

(22) *Aŵenamulilo*, the fire clan. This clan is held in considerable respect, on account of the value of fire.

(23) *Aŵenamfula*, the rain clan, also held in great esteem, on account of the value of rain for growing the crops and for quenching thirst. The members of this clan have no special power over rain.

(24) *Aŵenankalamu*, the lion clan, also called *aŵenango*, the scorpion clan, and *aŵenakasonga*, the scorpion sting clan. In jest the members of this clan are taunted with being *uŵulwani*, wild beasts who eat people. Their reply is that that cannot be so, since lions kill them as well as other people.

(25) *Aŵenampumpi*, the wild dog clan, the clan of the North-west Lenje chiefs.

(26) *Aŵenakaloŵa*, the earth (soil) clan.

IMIKOKA—THE CLAN SYSTEM

(27) *Aŵenakalungu*, the bead clan, the clan of Ŵemba chiefs.
(28) *Aŵenamumba*, the clay clan. The originators of this clan
are said to have broken taboo when returning from a funeral by
bringing moulding clay to the village.
(29) *Aŵenaŵesa*, the plain clan.
(30) *Aŵenachyela*, or *aŵenambulo*, the metal clan.
(31) *Aŵenakashimu*, or *aŵalembo*, the bee clan, the clan of the
Kaonde chiefs. It is held in esteem on account of the value of
honey. The name is said to have originated through the cutting
out of honey on the return from a funeral.
(32) *Aŵashishi*, or *aŵenamusamba*, the bark rope clan. The
former word is derived from *ulushishi*, bark rope, and the latter
from the *umusamba*-tree, which produces the best type of bark for
rope. This clan is held in esteem because of the usefulness of
ulushishi, and because this is used in making the *imiseeŵa*, or
funeral bier.

With the Lambas the chieftainship is with the *aŵenamishishi*;
all the other clans are composed of *aŵachyete*, or commoners.
Nevertheless, certain of these *aŵachyete* clans are the clans of
chiefs in neighbouring territories, but not in Ilamba proper.
The clans of the immediately surrounding chiefs are as follows:

Lenje—*aŵenatembo*.
North-western Lenje [1]—*aŵenampumpi*.
Ŵulima and Lala—*aŵenanyendwa*.
Aushi (first division)—*aŵenanguluŵe*.
Aushi (second division)—*aŵenambushi*.
Kaonde and Aŵenambonshi [2]—*aŵalembo*.
Ŵemba—*aŵenakalungu*.

The Lamba clans are paired off in opposites,[3] which are called
aŵalongo. Should an *umwinachyowa* be seen talking to an
umwinachyulu, it is said, "He is talking to his *umulonga*." It is
probable that originally some of these clans were violently opposed,
though to-day the opposition is confined to jesting. The opposites are as follows:

Hair clan *v.* goat clan (on account of the chieftainship).
Wasp clan *v.* honey-guide clan (because the honey-guide eats
the young bees and wasps).
Mouse clan *v.* snake clan and wild dog clan (for snakes and
wild dogs eat mice).

[1] As in Mukubwe's territory, and such chiefs as Lupumpala.
[2] As Shiŵuchinga.
[3] *Cf.* Melland, *In Witch-bound Africa*, pp. 251–253.

197

Elephant clan *v.* metal clan (for with metal the elephant is killed).

River-hog clan *v.* lion clan and dog clan (for it is hunted by them).

Crocodile clan *v.* fish clan.

Galago clan *v.* bark rope clan (for bark is used to tie up the galagos).

Mushroom clan *v.* anthill clan (for certain mushrooms grow on anthills).

Grass clan *v.* (*a*) fire clan (for the fire burns the grass), (*b*) all other clans (for everybody is hidden by the grass when going *kuchisompe*, to relieve himself).

Rain clan *v.* fire clan (for the rain puts out fire).

Lion clan *v.* (*a*) river-hog clan, (*b*) all other clans (for every one fears the lion).

Clay clan *v.* all others (for every one eats out of a clay pot).

Bark rope clan *v.* (*a*) galago clan, (*b*) all other clans (for every one needs it on the bier when he dies).

Some Clan Customs

The most important feature of the Lamba clan system is that it is exogamous—that is, marriage between members of the same clan is regarded as incest; every man must marry a woman belonging to some other clan than his own. Chiefs, therefore, *must* marry wives belonging to the commoners' clans, and, similarly, women of chief's clan must take husbands who are *aꞷachyete*. Obviously, since descent is matrilineal, the children of Lamba chiefs belong to the clan of their mother, a commoner, and cannot inherit a chieftainship. The children of chieftainesses, on the other hand, are of chief's rank, and are within the possibilities of inheritance.

There is a custom called *ukuꞷombola*, or *uꞷuꞷomboshi*, by which a child can claim a gift from a grandparent, *ꞷakapa*, of the same clan as the child's father or mother. The child on a rainy day may go and stand outside the grandparent's house, and say, *Nqisa kuꞷombola*, "I have come to crave!" It is customary to give the child a fowl, but should he enter the house he would get no gift.

When one sneezes it is customary to say *Kuliꞷatata*, "To my father," or to mention the clan of the father—e.g., *Kumbushi* ("To the goat"), *Kunguni* ("To the honey-guide"), as the case may be. An ordinary healthy sneeze is thus acknowledged as the gift of the father.

IMIKOKA—THE CLAN SYSTEM

The Kinship System

Besides understanding the clan system, it is necessary to realize that the Lamba kinship system is radically distinct from that which obtains in European countries. The commonly accepted terms 'father,' 'mother,' 'brother,' 'sister,' 'cousin,' etc., have, in Bantu kinship systems, entirely different boundaries of significance from those to which Europeans are accustomed. The following is an analysis of the system obtaining among the Lambas.

(1) **Blood Relationship.** (*a*) GRANDPARENTS AND GRAND-CHILDREN. There is one term, *kapa*, for grandparents on either side, irrespective of sex. The plural prefix, *ŵa-*, is used always as a sign of respect. There is but one reciprocal term, *umwinshikulu*, grandchild, used irrespective of sex. Other terms are used for maternal grandmother, indicating second and third person possession—viz., *nokokulu* (thy maternal grandmother), *nyinakulu* (his, her, maternal grandmother), *nyinakulufwe* (our maternal grandmother), *nyinakulunweni* (your maternal grandmother), and *nyinakuluŵo* (their maternal grandmother). Similarly, the paternal grandparents are called *shikulu* (= sir, master, mistress); e.g., *ŵashikulu ŵanji* (my paternal grandfather), with possessive forms *wisokulu* (thy paternal grandfather), *wishikulu* (his, her, paternal grandfather), *wishikulufwe* (our paternal grandfather), *wishikulunweni* (your paternal grandfather), and *wishikuluŵo* (their paternal grandfather).

(*b*) PARENTS AND CHILDREN. There is no general term to indicate 'father,' but varying terms are used containing the idea of the possessor; e.g., *tata* (my father), *wiso* (thy father), *wishi* (his, her, father), *wishifwe* (our father), *wishinwe* (your father), and *wishiŵo* (their father). The terms for 'father' are used also for the father's brothers, and for anyone belonging to the father's clan, the term *umwana* being reciprocated. *Tata-mukulu*, *wiso-mukulu*, etc., are used for the father's elder brothers, and *tata-mwa-nichye*, etc., for the younger brothers.

Similarly, there is no general term for 'mother,' but possessor-including forms; e.g., *mama* (my mother), *noko* (thy mother), *nyina* (his, her, mother), *nyinefwe* (our mother), *nyinenwe* (your mother), and *nyinaŵo* (their mother). The terms for 'mother' are used also for the mother's sisters, and in a general way for members of one's own clan, provided they are elders (as one's mother) in grade. *Mama-mukulu*, *noko-mukulu*, *nyina-mukulu*, etc., are used for the mother's elder sisters, and *mama-mwanichye*, etc., for the younger sisters.

There is one reciprocal term, *umwana* (plural, *aŵana*), meaning child, which is used by all the persons called 'mother' or 'father.' A woman also calls her brother's children *aŵana*. When it is necessary to distinguish the sex of a child the words meaning male and female are added; e.g., *umwana umwalalume* (son) and *umwana umwanakashi* (daughter).

The father's sister is addressed as *tata* or *tatankashi*, the terms *wisonkashi* and *wishinkashi* indicating second and third person possession. The mother's brother is called *mwinshyo*, usually with the plural prefix, *ŵa-*, of respect.

The term for a brother's child, when a woman is speaking, is *umwipwa* (plural, *aŵepwa*), irrespective of sex. She may also call him *umwana*. The term for a sister's child, when a man is speaking, is *umwipwa*, irrespective of sex; in this case there is no alternate term which can be used.

(*c*) BROTHERS AND SISTERS. There is one term which means brother when a man is speaking and sister when a woman is speaking, and which may be used of any 'brother' by a man and of any 'sister' by a woman, irrespective of age; viz.,

> *umukwasu* (my, our, brother—man speaking),
> (my, our, sister—woman speaking).
> *umukwanu* (thy, your, brother—of man),
> (thy, your, sister—of woman).
> *umukwaŵo* (his, their, brother),
> (her, their, sister).

There is another set of terms used by brothers in speaking of brothers, and by sisters of sisters, which stress age, one term being used by an older brother or sister of a younger and the other by a younger of an older; thus *umwanichye*, a younger brother of male or younger sister of female, and *umukulu*, an older brother of male or older sister of female—e.g., *umukulu wanji*, my elder brother (man speaking) or my elder sister (woman speaking).

A sister calls her brother *indume*, and a brother calls his sister *inkashi*. These terms are used for older and younger alike.

These same sets of terms are used for the children of the father's 'brothers' or the mother's 'sisters,' the terms for older brothers and sisters being applied to the children of the older brothers of the father or sisters of the mother, and the terms for younger brothers and sisters being applied to the children of the younger brothers of the father or sisters of the mother. These terms are also used for members of one's own clan, provided they are of the same age grade.

IMIKOKA—THE CLAN SYSTEM

(*d*) CROSS-COUSINS. While parallel cousins are addressed as own brothers or sisters, cross-cousins are addressed by quite a different term. Thus *umufyala* is used by both man and woman for the father's sister's child or the mother's brother's child, irrespective of sex. Cross-cousin marriage is a common form of marriage among the Lambas.

(2) **Relatives by Marriage.** (*a*) PARENTS-IN-LAW AND CHILDREN-IN-LAW. *Tatafyala* (with variations as for father) is the term used for father-in-law by both man and woman.

Mamafyala (with variations as for mother) is the term used for mother-in-law by both man and woman.

Umuko is the term used for son-in-law by both man and woman.

Umulokashi is the term used for daughter-in-law by both man and woman.

(*b*) HUSBAND AND WIFE. The husband is *umulume*, the wife *umukashi*, while *muka-* may be prefixed to a proper name to indicate "the spouse of"—e.g., *mukakatanga*, Katanga's wife, *mukachyalwe*, Chyalwe's husband. *Mukolo* is the term used for the 'great wife,' all of whose children are considered 'older' than any others, irrespective of their real age. Thus Isaac is considered to be *umukulu wakwe* Ishmael, for his mother, Sarah, was Abraham's *mukolo*. Any wife of a polygamist is called *umusanu*, while the second wife is called *mutepa*.

When two men have married sisters, the man calls his wife's sister's husband *umuufi-muŵyanji*, my companion in marriage. When two women have married brothers, the woman calls her husband's brother's wife *umuufi*. Wives of polygamists call one another by the term *umukashi-muŵyanji*, my fellow-wife.

(*c*) BROTHERS-IN-LAW AND SISTERS-IN-LAW. A woman terms her husband's brothers and sisters *umulamu* (plural, *aŵalamu*) or *ŵukwe* (plural, *ŵaŵukwe*), irrespective of age. *Umulamu* is used by a man of his wife's brothers and sisters, irrespective of age.

The *mwinshyo*, mother's brother, has considerable power over his sister's children; he to a great extent makes the decision regarding his nieces' marriages. It is the father's duty to clothe and feed his children, but the *mwinshyo* will often supply food. If a married nephew (*umwipwa*) dies, the *mwinshyo* has the disposal of the death-due payable by the widow; similarly, if a married niece dies, the widower's death-due is at his disposal. Generally a father is allowed full control over his children, and it would be very seldom that his wishes regarding their marriages were thwarted, but at his death the authority of his wife's brother over the children is reasserted. A nephew is usually very familiar with the wife of his *mwinshyo*.

The *tatankashi* (etc.) is held in respect. If her brother is dead, she will have part of the marriage pledge upon the marriage of her brother's daughter. She is treated by her brother's children as they would treat their father. The bond is close, for she is of their father's clan. Her children may marry her brother's children, for they are cross-cousins, and in this case no 'fear' of her is felt by her sons-in-law. The usual taboo of approach to or converse with a mother-in-law is very strong; this is dealt with in Chapter XIII.

Two men or two women who are cross-cousins, *awafyala*, would treat one another as brothers or sisters, because one is the child of the other's *mwinshyo* and the other the child of the *tatankashi* (etc.). There is no joking or teasing between them.

In a family the eldest-born child is called *umuŵele* and the youngest *kaŵinda*, and the latter name is often assumed by the child as his own name for life.

The Lambas have no system of age grades such as obtains among the Kikuyus, but those who are born at approximately the same time are called *aŵali*, contemporaries. True *aŵali* are only recognized in the immediate neighbourhood of their birth-place. Nevertheless, all belonging to the same clan and of the same generation are generally considered 'brothers' and 'sisters,' and those of the same clan, but of the generation above, would be considered as 'mothers' (*ŵamama*, etc.), even though they were men.

Orphans

Owing to the clan and kinship organization of the people, there is practically no problem when children are orphaned. An orphan, *umwana-wanshiwa* or *umushyala*, if he has been living with his parents in his father's home village, will be taken by his father's brother (*ŵawishi*) and handed over to the sister (the child's *wishinkashi*); failing that, the *ŵawishi* himself will look after him; failing that, the child's *inkashi* (sister); failing that, *umukulu wakwe* (an elder brother); and, failing that, word will be sent to the home village of the dead mother, that he may be sent for to reside with her relatives. Failing any such relatives to look after the child, an *ichimbela* (an old woman beyond the age of child-bearing) belonging to the same clan will be sought, to adopt and rear the child as her own. Failing anyone of the same clan—an almost impossible supposition—the chief of the village would adopt the child.

There is thus no need for orphan houses in Ilamba. Instead of having to look for protection when orphaned, the child is immediately claimed, as a natural course, by the nearest relative responsible. Even if the mother and father should both die in the same day, as happened repeatedly during the influenza epidemic of 1918, the aunts and uncles, who regard him as their *umwana*, at once take him in and provide for him.

If the child has been living with his parents in his mother's home village, his *ŵanyinakulu* (maternal grandmother) will take him; failing her, his *nyina-mukulu* (mother's elder sister); failing her, his *nyina-mwanichye* (mother's younger sister); failing her, his *inkashi* (her *umukulu*, if the orphan is a girl); failing her, his *umukulu* (elder brother, *indume* of a girl orphan); and, failing any of these, some relative of the same clan, of whom there are likely to be many in the village.

Arrangements regarding the adoption or wardship of orphans are usually mutual, and no cases of quarrelling are known over this disposal. In many cases of orphans residing in the father's home village the wife's relatives, when they came to mourn, have taken the child back with them to their village, despite the fact that there were father's relatives to look after the child.

The following table of relationship illustrates a case in point:

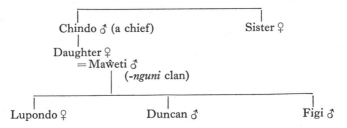

On the death of the daughter of Chindo, wife of Maŵeti, the sister of Chindo tried to get the children, but Maŵeti refused to part with them, and brought them up himself.

Inheritance of Property

(1) **On the Death of a Man who left Wife, Children, and Property.** The whole property will belong to the brothers of the deceased. The widow has no claim to anything, but the brothers may give certain articles to the children, and will see that they are

well provided for. The garden will belong to the widow, for it is her own property, the results of her labour. Should the deceased have left much property, his brothers might provide the widow with clothes until such time as she is able to redeem herself. The wives of 'wealthy' men have sometimes been able to put aside sufficient of their own to pay the death-due at once. Hoes, pots, mats, and baskets belong to the widow, but the brothers take axe, gun, spear, bow, tongs, money, calico, and any other valuables.

(2) **On the Death of a Wife.** *Aẁenaẁuko* (*i.e.*, the wife's relatives living in her home village) will take pots, baskets, mats, and hoes. Should the husband have put away in safety any money which he had given to his wife, he would hand it over to her relatives; he would fear the anger of the deceased should he hide and keep anything he had given to her. Sometimes husbands put aside money for their wives to pay the death-dues and avoid being kept in servitude. The wife's relatives— *aẁalamu* to the widower—may give some of this money to their deceased sister's children. Of fifty shillings they might give twenty. Again, when the widower pays his death-due and frees himself (*luẁuka*) his *aẁalamu* may give the children something. If the children are grown up, and their father has not sufficient to pay their maternal uncle's demand, they might say, "Pay us what you have, and we shall see that our maternal uncle does not worry you." They will then bind white beads on his arm and throw the meal over him, *lululu*-ing and saying, *Fumeni-po mama, ẁatata pano waluẁuka, twalya-po!* "Go away, O Mother, Father has now redeemed himself. We have eaten of the death-due!" For the customs and reasons of the death-dues see Chapter XI.

Genealogical Tables

The first table, on p. 205, shows a family of the goat clan. The head of the family was Nsensa. His reincarnation is seen in the youngest child of Makanchye, daughter of his sister Nkandu, and his name is carried on by the child of Mwanali-ẁanika, his great-nephew, who married a goat clan wife. Nkandu, the eldest woman of this family of the clan, first married Munyeke, an *umwinamaila*, but she was later taken by capture by the paramount chief Mushili, smeared with lion fat, and thus became his wife. Munyeke fled to Momboshi in the Lala country, and did not return, fearing Mushili. The children remained at Nsensa's village. Here Nkandu's daughter

GENEALOGICAL TABLE I

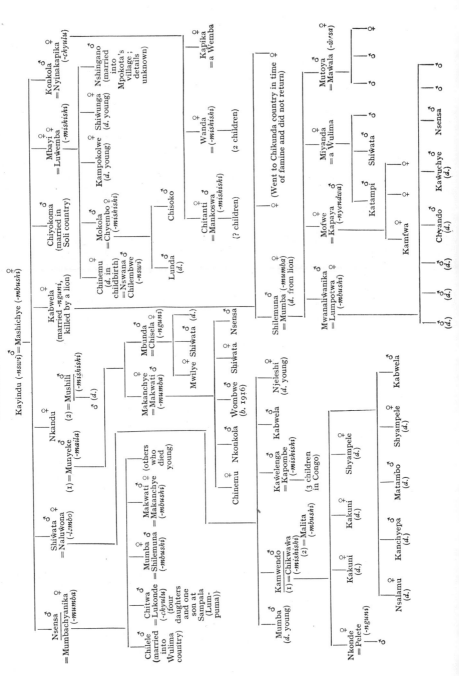

GENEALOGICAL TABLE II

(*awashishi*)

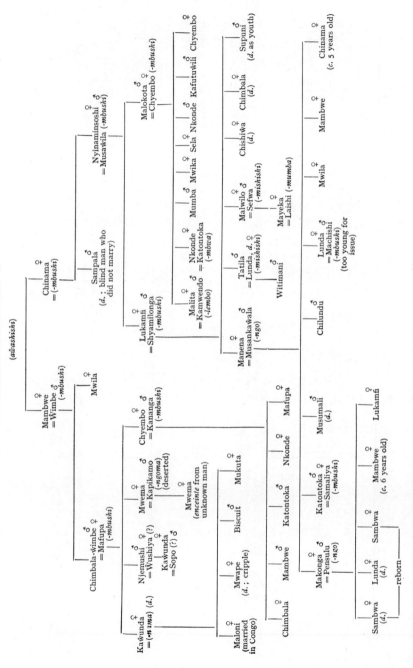

Makanchye married, and in 1916, when visiting the village, I jokingly dubbed her latest baby Ŵombwe ("Frog"), a name which his mother at once adopted, and had confirmed by presents on both sides.

The high infant mortality is best seen by the list of Kamwendo's children. This is a complete list, given to me by Joshua Kamwendo himself. Most of the other families can be taken as having a similar history, but as unnamed babies and those dying very young are seldom mentioned by Lambas when recounting their children, details concerning them were unknown to Joshua Kamwendo. Mumba and Makwati, daughter and son of Nsensa, show instances of cross-cousin marriages. Makwati was also married elsewhere.

The second, on p. 206, shows a family of the *aŵashishi* clan, given to me by Malita, one of the members, and wife of Joshua Kamwendo. It is noticeable that a blind man or cripple girl would not get married. Tatila, whose wife died, has not yet redeemed himself from the death-dues. An interesting case of the rebirth of one child, who died as an infant, in another of the same family, born shortly afterward, is shown in that of the Sambwas.

CHAPTER XIII

TABOO AND BEHAVIOUR

Umuchinshi

THE Lambas have almost a recognized code of polite behaviour, which they call *umuchinshi*. The breaking of any of the rules of behaviour constitutes ill-breeding, rudeness, lack of manners, and is treated in much the same way as similar breaches would be in our own society. Ill-mannered children are cuffed or beaten, older people reprimanded or ostracized.

Little children are taught these rules from infancy. If they do not accept gifts in the proper way the gifts are taken away from them.

The following are some of the most important of these rules:

(1) When receiving a gift take it with both hands extended, in this way expressing gratitude. (This is equivalent to the English "Don't forget to say 'Thank you!'")

(2) When a child finds an elder sitting down he must sit down cross-legged, and when answering his greeting he must clap his hands. This will please the old man, who is sure to turn to his wife and say, *Munanyineni uyumwanichye, kukanwa kwatuŵuluka*, "Make some *inshima* for this child; his mouth is whitened [with the dryness of hunger]."

(3) When a child overtakes his elders on the road, going in the same direction as he is, he should take their load, if they have one, and carry it. If this is done the journey will be a fortunate one.

(4) When eating *inshima* with one's elders, never get up to go until the elders have finished.

(5) When travelling at a time of food-shortage, give the village headman some assistance in his work if you desire him to provide you with a meal. The usual free hospitality cannot be expected in time of famine.

(6) If your mother sends you to fetch firewood, go without gainsaying her.

(7) If your father sends you on an errand, go silently, without a single question.

(8) When people come before the chief they sit before him

208

cross-legged and clap. He does not answer. Again they clap, and then the chief says, *Mitende mweŵame*, "Greeting, friends!" And they all reply, *Mitende kasuŵa*, "Greeting, O sun!" for do they not all come to him to warm themselves?

(9) When the elders are talking over cases the younger people leave them alone, and go to their own place of meeting at a distance.

(10) When a great chief comes to the village the young boys and girls hide themselves; only the elders meet and converse with the chief.

(11) When an *umulaye* (diviner) has been summoned to the village he expects to find a hut swept, bed arranged, water drawn, a pot of *ifisunga* (light beer) ready, a basket of meal, and a fowl. He will also find all the people in a state of nervous apprehension, due acknowledgment of the dread and fear which he inspires.

(12) When a *mukamwami*, or spirit-medium, has been summoned, the same preparations are expected as for an *umulaye*, but there is no fear at his approach.

(13) When an *umupalu* (professional hunter) has been summoned to hunt by a chief he expects to find a hut prepared and *ifisunga* ready.

(14) Greeting used to be done by hand-clapping, but intimate friends would *sunsana*. This was done as follows: A. grips with right hand B.'s right wrist and shakes it; then B. does the same to A. This is no longer seen, but *ukupakana* has been introduced by the Ngoni. Right hands are gripped, and moved from side to side; then thumbs are gripped, and similarly moved; and when the hand grip is released each party claps, or strikes his palm on his breast.

(15) When the husband departs on a journey his wife claps her hands. In these days there is a modern innovation by which young people show their affection. After shaking hands in the ordinary way (*ukupakana*), the fingers are run up the companion's fore-arm, to tickle the upper arm. This is only done by persons who are very intimate.

(16) If you meet a great chief on the path when travelling, lie down on the left side and clap the hands.

(17) When you receive a gift from the chief, clap your hands, then take up a little dust (*iloŵa*, earth) and rub it on the shoulders and chest, placing the arms crosswise. Some rub the dust on the forehead. This is called *ukulamba*.

(18) When making a request to the chief, clap.

(19) When a chief upbraids you, remain silent, answer not a word, and his anger will pass.

(20) When at a gathering for an *umulandu* (case) before the chief, if it is necessary to relieve yourself, leave quietly, but on returning to resume your place clap your hands.

(21) When a commoner is eating or drinking with the chief the chief is the first to wash his hands, the commoner following him, but the commoner is the first to partake of the food or drink. This applies whether the chief or the commoner is the host, and was evidently intended to guard the chief against poisoning.

(22) When sleeping in the bush the chief must be in the middle, with the *awachyete* (commoners) around him (this a protection from wild beasts), but when sleeping in the house the *umuchyete* must be near the fire, the chief well away from it (this to prevent his clothes from being burnt).

(23) On a journey the youngsters must precede their elders. There are several reasons for this. The children act as *awapupwishi*, dew-driers, shaking the heavy showers of water from the long grass, that their elders may pass in comparative comfort. They also save their elders from walking into wild beasts or an enemy ambush. In all this the value of the elder is in marked contrast to that of the child. A child is despised until he can win his position as a man.

(24) It is the husband's duty to open the door in the morning and to shut it at night.

(25) When sleeping, the wife sleeps behind her husband against the hut wall, while he lies facing the door. The Lambas say, *Tafipusa kuchiwi*, "The enemy does not miss the door!"

(26) Should a child be witness to irregular proceedings between a man and the wife of another, he must say nothing. A witness in a charge involving a death is liable to be killed in revenge.

Taboo

Apart, however, from the various prohibitions and commands which govern ordinary good social behaviour, the Lambas are hedged in by a strong and binding system of taboo. There are two terms used in Lamba to indicate different types of taboo, *ukutonda* and *umushiliko*. The first term is indicative of social prohibitions and other actions such as would bring risk, trouble, personal harm, ostracism, or even a law-case upon the breaker or others. The rules under *ukutonda* are much stronger than those which govern *umuchinshi*, etiquette. The second term, *umushiliko*, is perhaps the real equivalent of taboo. The breaking of *imishiliko* would make the offender a social outcast; punishment is seldom inflicted by chief or people—it is the work of the *ichiŵanda*, the attendant demon of the offended, to bring disaster, generally death, upon the offender. Alongside of the *imishiliko* are *imbiko*, omens of imminent disaster. The breaking of an *umushiliko* constitutes an evil omen, but, apart from this, the attendant *ichiŵanda* helps his 'ward' by arranging for *imbiko* to appear in his way, and so dissuade him from a course which would lead to his death. The almost automatic working out of the results of broken taboo has by some[1] been attributed to the action of an impersonal dynamistic power. Among the Lambas, however, it is very clear that it is brought about directly by the action of the *ifiŵanda*. The Lamba belief in *ifiŵanda* is discussed in Chapter XV.

In order to make clear the differences between *ukutonda*, a breaking of which is punishable by people, and *imishiliko*, a breaking of which is avenged by demons, lists of the more generally recognized taboos under these headings are now given.

Ukutonda

(*a*) **Regarding Marriage and Family Relations.** (1) The daughter-in-law must not use the name of her father-in-law in his presence or in the presence of his relatives. When she has borne two or more children she may use the name in speaking to her children. The daughter-in-law must not use the name of her mother-in-law in her presence. Should this taboo be broken, the woman would be considered *ichyungwa*, or *umupupa*, a lawless, irresponsible person, a hooligan. No such prohibition is placed on a man toward his parents-in-law. This is comparable to the Zulu-Xhosa custom of *ukuhlonipa*.

(2) The Lamba woman holds in awe (*ukutonda*) her father-in-law (*ŵawishifyala*), her husband's mother's brother (*i.e.*, his *mwinshyo*), and her husband's male nephews of different clan (*aŵepwa aŵalalume*).

(3) The Lamba man holds in awe his mother-in-law (*ŵanyina-fyala*), whether in the presence of others or not. He must not meet her or speak to her. The awe seems to be mutual. Should the woman see her son-in-law coming along the path, she would turn off into the bush and pass him at a distance. Should his mother-in-law be in his house, the man may not enter. The taboo is relaxed in so far as a man often converses with his mother-in-law if one of them is in the house and the other out of sight

---

[1] See Smith and Dale, *The Ila-speaking Peoples of Northern Rhodesia*, vol. ii, p. 79 *et seq.*

behind the house. It would be considered extremely unbecoming for a man to be seen eating by his mother-in-law or to see her eating. All this they explain by saying, "Is it not she who gave birth to the wife?"

The Lamba man also holds in awe his nieces of a different clan from himself (aŵepwa aŵanakashi) when in the presence of others.

(4) The father must not sit on a child's bed, whether a son or daughter, and the mother is only permitted to sit on her unmarried daughter's bed.

(5) A grown son must not sit or lie on his mother's bed.

(6) The father's sister (wishinkashi) must not pat the buttocks of her nephew (umwipwa).

(7) The younger wife must not refuse to carry the load for the principal wife on a journey.

(b) **Regarding Death and the Dead.** (8) Don't sit and meditate on the likeness of a deceased relative. Arising from this, there is a natural dread among the Lambas of seeing the photograph of a person who has since died.

(9) Don't approach a burial-place. If an umulyashi is chanced upon when hunting, the hunter runs away as fast as possible. This is in marked contrast to the custom of the Lenjes, who have not this taboo, and bury their dead in the village.

(10) A polygynist must not die in the house of his younger wife, but in that of his principal wife.

(11) Don't step over a corpse.

(c) **Regarding the Village and Village Activities.** (12) Don't pound or cut firewood at night, lest a lion should be summoned.

(13) Don't mention a lion at night or it will appear. The Lambas say, Anuke'nkalamu wisalishye! "Mention a lion and shut tight the door!"

(14) Don't throw a tsetse-fly (akasembe) in the fire or it will call a lion.

(15) When women bathe, men must not go to see, lest it should lead to quarrelling at the village.

(16) Don't look into the pot in which cooking is being done. The cook and owner may of course look in.

(17) Don't step over another's outstretched legs, lest the latter's legs should become heavy.

(18) Don't go naked; it is sufficient to wear a loin-strip (uŵukushi).

(19) Don't send your elders ahead along the path, lest evil befall them. (See under "Umuchinshi.")

(20) If two companies, not mutually known, meet on the path, they must stand separated by a little distance while talking, and then pass on, lest treachery should be practised. Similarly, when meeting at a river where rest is desired, the companies must sit removed from one another by a little distance.

(21) When fish-traps have been set, the first fish caught must be eaten by the husband; the succeeding ones may be taken to his wife. Should the wife eat the first, the fish would *umfwe'nsoni* (feel shame) if eaten by a woman, and refuse to be caught.

(22) Don't go out naked in the village at night, lest you meet an *imfwiti* (witch or wizard) and be taken for one yourself. When an *imfwiti* is caught by the witch-doctor, he will mention your name, saying, "I met him naked."

(23) A stranger to a village must not carry his spear on his shoulder.

(24) A stranger must not hold the string of his bow upward in a village.

(25) Strangers must not approach the chief with their weapons; they must leave them at a distance and approach unarmed.

(26) A stranger approaching a house must sit beneath the eaves and clap to attract attention. Thereupon the owner will come out, and, after inquiries, give him all hospitality. A friend would come to the house, say *Naisa*, "I have come," and then enter. A relative would enter without a word.

(*d*) **Miscellaneous.** (27) Don't use obscene references—e.g., *Apo weŵo tofwite bwino paŵukala!* "So you have not your penis properly clothed!" Such obscenity incurs the anger of the elders.

(28) Don't mock a cripple, blind, deaf, or dumb person, or an orphan. A fine of goods may be imposed for such an offence, and it is also feared that such an offender may himself be inflicted with lameness, blindness, etc. Two proverbs illustrate this: *Taŵaseka-chilema, naweŵo ekwisa kulemana!* "Don't mock a cripple or you will become a cripple!" *Taŵaseka-mwananshiwa, Lesa alikubwene, ekuŵona naweŵo ŵanoko ŵafwa naŵawiso!* "Don't mock an orphan; God sees you, and behold, your mother and father also may die!"

(29) Don't insult your father, even if he is scolding you. Lambas often run off and leave the father scolding rather than run the risk of arguing.

(30) Don't lie on your back if it is raining. Lightning might strike you.

(31) Don't kill frogs. You might skin (*ukuuŵuluka*) like a snake, for the snake eats frogs.

(32) Don't kill a chameleon. For the Lambas say, *Lufunyembe alafwile'nsanso*, "The chameleon dies through a sieve"—*i.e.*, after his case has been sifted, and he has been proved guilty.

(33) Don't spit on anyone, even when fighting with him.

(34) Don't step on or over the shadow of a *mukamwami* (medium) or a paramount chief.

(35) The *umulaye* (doctor) forbids a cured leper to eat barbel (*umuta*), bush buck, zebra, or guinea-fowl, the last three because of their spots (or stripes), the first because when it is put on the fire its skin peels off easily as does that of a leper.

(36) Sufferers from goitre (*iŵofu*) do not eat barbel, because it has a swelling in the neck.

Imishiliko

(1) Menstruating women (*aŵaseesa*) are themselves taboo during the period of menstruation. They have *uŵufungushi* (uncleanness) until they have bathed themselves. The various prohibitions applied to them are considered in Chapter IX. Should one, for instance, prepare food for her husband, he will have pains in his chest when he runs, "as though there is blood there."

(2) Fire must not be transferred from the old village to the new, or from the old house to the new. Fresh fire must be made with the fire-sticks. People who have had misfortune may have warmed themselves at the old fire.

(3) No work must be undertaken in the village while a burial is being carried out.

(4) One who has taken part in a burial must bathe before going to his wife, lest he transfer *ulufu* (the death) to his wife, and she die. Should this taboo be broken, a gift of goods, of value about three shillings, must be made to the woman to ward off the evil consequences.

(5) All hair must be picked up and buried, lest the *ikwikwi* (bird of ill-omen) should use it for nest-making, and the owner die.

(6) If a man is falsely reported at his home as dead, when he returns home he must not go straight into the village. Should people see him, they would prevent him from entering. A doctor must first be called. He will bring medicinal leaves and fire, and place them smoking between the man's feet as he sits; he will then switch the man with the zebra tail he carries, and cause the smoke to reach all parts of the man's body. When the leaves

have finished burning the man and the doctor will go together to the village. The man will wait without until his father comes and throws meal (a sign of life) upon him and his mother sounds the shrill whistle (*ulumpundu*). Then may he enter the house. If these precautions are not taken the man will die.

(7) The hoofs of a zebra must not be brought into the village.

(8) If a hare (*akalulu*) is killed it must not be brought to the village intact with head. The head must be taken off and carried separately.

(9) The skull of an ant-bear, when killed, must be left in the bush; it is taboo to bring it to the village.

(10) When the husband is on a journey in order to seek wealth (*ukunonka*) his wife must not shave her head, for it is a sign of mourning, and he will die.

(11) Sexual intercourse is forbidden (*a*) the day before going to war, (*b*) if smallpox is near, (*c*) the day before going to the *ichintengwa* (smelting-house).

(12) If the husband is going to the war, and his wife catches him by the arm, he must not go.

(13) When you have cut down a branch of a tree, do not drag it through the village, lest a lion should catch a man and drag him off.

Imbiko

As has already been noticed, *imbiko* and *imishiliko* are closely associated. *Imbiko* are omens of death, portents of coming disaster, or warnings to avoid disaster, always involving death. Although most *imbiko* are attributed to the *ichiŵanda* (demon), some are said to be sent by the *umupashi* (departed spirit) which the person is bound to look after—*e.g.*, the spirit of an elder brother. This spirit will send *imbiko* to warn him not to go a certain way or not to do a certain thing. The man on returning to the village will inquire of an *umulaye* the reason for his receiving these omens, and after the divination the answer may be, "It is your spirit which is angry. You did not give him a parting offering before you began your journey." The man will make the necessary offering at the shrine, and then undertake his journey in safety.

The following are examples of *imbiko*:

(1) A millipede coming in summer-time.

(2) A chameleon climbing *down* a stick.

(3) A green roof-snake on the ground.

(4) An adder passing quickly.

(5) A python travelling quickly.

(6) A hare, after running away, stopping to look at one.

(7) Finding a dead hare with head intact.

(8) A lurie flying westward.

(9) A ground hornbill crying *Woh!* at one near by.

(10) A genet crying while being killed.

(11) An *ikwikwi* bird crying by day.

(12) Long delay in the coming of rain (*ichyangama*). This is taken to be an omen of the death of a chief. Sometimes, however, when divination has been carried out, the doctor says, "No, it is the spirit of a certain chief, who is angry because you have not brewed beer in his honour."

(13) Finding maggots on human excrement.

(14) When on a journey seeing a tree or a great branch of a tree fall.

(15) Seeing a stick-insect (*masombwe*) trembling on a stick.

(16) Finding black mamba snakes (*ififiitishi*) fighting.

(17) Meeting a funeral. One must turn back.

(18) A mud-wasp (*inununshi*) gathering clay and sprinkling it on to one when sitting.

(19) A hyena coming along the path to the village in daytime.

(20) A hyena excreting in the village.

(21) A person whose parents are still living eating an *akatuutwa* (bird resembling a small dove).

(22) A twitching (*ukuŵimba*) of the lower eyelid.

(23) Spasmodic twitching (*ukubwitaka*) of the thigh—an omen of the death of one's relatives-in-law (*aŵenaŵuko*).

(24) A blindworm (*ichiŵimbili* or *chilele*) jumping from tree-top to tree-top.

(25) A jackal calling continually in the west, or in the village itself but once.

(26) A cock crowing at night. He is killed and eaten immediately, but even then the death his crowing has heralded is awaited.

(27) A strong house falling down.

(28) The wall of a grave falling in. This is a very serious *imbiko*.

(29) A pot of beer falling over by itself.

(30) The moon looking red, with a red circle round it. This signifies a gathering plotting against a chief, and some chief is sure to die.

(31) The sun with a red circle round it. The meaning is as for (30).

(32) A son throwing down his father. In addition to the severe punishment which this would merit, it is an ill-omen for the father.

(33) Seeing a chameleon digging a hole like a grave (*indili*). Fear for the welfare of an absent relative would at once be felt.

(34) A duiker coming from the east, crossing the path, and going westward.

(35) Squeezing a maggot from one's own body.

(36) Buzzing in the ears. It is thought to presage the death-wailing.

(37) Seeing the shadow of a corpse. The Lambas say, *Uwafwa takwete chinshingwa*, "A corpse has no shadow!"

Other Omens

All omens are not bad according to the Lamba conception. Good omens are called *ifyamushimu*, or in true Lamba *imipashi* (spirits). These—as are also the *imbiko*—are often revealed in dreams, a subject necessarily associated with that of omens by the Lambas. The *imipashi* may be divided into (*a*) *amalya*, signs of coming food, (*b*) *awensu*, signs of visitors coming, and (*c*) *uwuwoni*, signs of coming wealth.

(*a*) **Amalya.** (1) Twitching of upper eyelid.

(2) Fly entering the mouth.

(3) Child eating cinders.

(4) A twitching of the nerves of a double tooth.

(5) A lurie flying ahead eastward.

(6) A leopard eating meat on a tree-branch.

(*b*) **Awensu.** (1) 'Pins and needles' in the feet.

(2) A 'dryness' of the eyes.

(3) Sleeplessness.

(4) Soot falling from the roof (visitors will come that very day).

(*c*) **Uwuwoni.** If you see an insect (*umuchyewu*) passing, and say, "I shall take a good look at it" (*nkachyewuchisya-po*).

Imiloto—Dreams

The Lambas are firm believers in the significance of dreams. Generally the dream is taken to be a portent, good or evil, of what is taking place or about to take place. There are cases, however, of the dream 'going by opposites.' They believe that during sleep the spirit leaves the body, to wander about. What is dreamt is what the spirit undergoes. The spirit returns immediately the person wakes up. If a person is wakened up he may say, "Why did you wake me so suddenly, instead of letting me finish dreaming where I went?"

Dreams are really all omens, and hence one finds the following divisions: (*a*) *imbiko*, (*b*) *imipashi*, whether merely *ukutemwa* (good fortune ahead) or *amalya* (coming food), and (*c*) those indicating witchcraft, *uŵufwiti*.

(*a*) **Imiloto yambiko.** (1) When a man on a journey dreams that there are many people gathered somewhere in a courtyard, he will say, on waking in the morning, "To-day I am going home. There is something wrong there. There is mourning." His companions will ask, "What did you dream about?" He will say, "I dreamt a crowd of people gathered in my courtyard, with fires made everywhere." His companions will say, "Indeed that augurs ill." The man goes home, and when approaching the village inquires of villagers the news, and hears, "So-and-so has died!" He then says, "I saw it where I went. I did not dream well."

(2) If a person dreams that a dog is biting him he will not undertake a journey on the morrow; but if he dreams that a lion is biting him he considers it a good omen, and will undertake his journey or his hunt without fear. It is considered lucky to dream that a spirit has changed into a lion to come and catch a person.

(3) If a person dreams that many people are chasing him, in the morning he will say, "Let us beware in this village, let us hide our possessions, for raiders are coming!" His advice is often followed.

(4) If a man, when away, dreams that his wife has grown very fat he knows that she must be ill and about to die, but if he dreams that she is very thin he knows that she is in good health— this by opposites.

(5) If a man dreams that he is digging holes, while others behind him are filling them in, it is an omen of a relative's death— they have been burying him.

(6) If a person dreams that guns are fired at him it is a sign of impending death, but if the guns misfire it is a sign of good fortune.

(7) If an accused man dreams that he is bound he will escape to a distant part of the country in the morning.

(8) It is unlucky to dream of talking every day with youngsters.

(9) If a man on a journey dreams that another is 'sporting' with his wife he will suspect adultery.

(10) If a person dreams that maggots are eating him some one is going to die.

(11) If people dream that they are eating honey the omen is bad.

(12) If people dream that they are anointing themselves with honey the omen is bad.

(13) If a man dreams that people are carrying sleeping mats (*amasasa*) between them it is a sign of an approaching funeral, but if it is a long white forked pole (*ulupanda*) they are carrying the omens are good.

(14) If a man on a distant journey dreams that he speaks to a relative who will not answer it is a sign that that relative is dead.

(15) If a person dreams of a house with a closed door and a white pole leaning against it, it is the house of some one recently dead.

(16) Dreaming of many people drinking beer indicates mourning ceremonies.

(17) Dreaming one is clothed in oil-softened bark cloth (*inguẁo yamafuta*) is an ill-omen, but it is a good omen to dream one is wearing ordinary bark cloth.

(18) It is an ill-omen to dream one is wearing black, but the opposite to dream of wearing white.

(19) Dreaming of many vultures in the courtyard indicates that they are gathered to a corpse.

(20) Dreaming that a snake has bitten oneself or a relative is an ill-omen.

(21) Dreaming that you continually live with your wife means that she is going to divorce you, while dreaming that she has divorced you means that the marriage will not end early.

(22) To dream of one's mother is bad.

(23) To dream that a dead relative comes and scolds means that another relative is about to die.

(24) For many people to dream of a man recently dead is an indication that an *ichiẁanda* (demon) is at work.

(25) If you dream that the elders are calling you to accompany them, don't answer them, remain silent; it is witches trying to get you to accompany them in their nefarious work.

(26) If you go with your companion to the river, and he has leaves, don't ask him to give them to you to put in your water-pot (to prevent the water from spilling), lest when you sleep at night he should come and ask for them back. This would signify a death, and you would be considered an *imfwiti*.

(27) Dreaming of much food means going to bed hungry, but dreaming of hunger means food.

(28) If a man dreams that he has hurt himself he must not go to hoe the next day.

219

(29) Dreaming of a deceased relative is said to be caused by the spirit of the deceased visiting the sleeper. In order to ward off the evil consequences of this beer must be brewed in honour of the spirit who has been objecting to lack of attention.

(30) Dreaming that one is hoeing *imilala* (raised garden-beds) is indicative of a grave.

(31) Dreaming that he is having intercourse with his wife is to a man a sign that his wife is committing adultery.

(*b*) **Imiloto yamipashi.** In addition to those included in the previous section as contrasts, the following examples may be given:

(1) Dreaming that a man is dividing out (*ukwaŵa*) tobacco is a sign that a buck will be killed.

(2) For a hunter to dream that, in killing a man, he wounds him repeatedly, and he as often gets up again, is a sign that the hunter is going to be successful.

(3) Dreaming of *amawo* (millet) is a sign of long life, for the grains of the millet cannot be counted.

(4) Dreaming you are lying in dung is a sign of coming meat, the dung being a sign of the *uŵufulu*, the chyme or stomach contents of an animal killed.

(5) Dreaming of skinning a snake means that a buck is going to be killed.

(6) To dream that a companion who has gone far away is returning means that, though he will not come soon, he is well.

(7) Dreaming that he is always bathing in the river presages the possession of the man by an *ichinkuwaila* (goblin); he will become a *moŵa* (professional dancer).

(8) To dream that one's relative is dead means that he is well.

(9) If a man dreams that a doctor diagnoses his case and prescribes certain medicine he will procure that medicine, put it on his sores, and be recovered.

(10) If a man dreams that he is beaten he knows that when his law-case is settled he will not be beaten.

(11) If a man dreams that a friend gives him something he believes that he will get it.

(12) If a hunter dreams (*a*) of blood, (*b*) of committing incest, (*c*) of defecating, (*d*) of the birth of a baby, or (*e*) of tobacco he fully believes that his next day's hunting will be successful.

(*c*) **Imiloto yaŵufwiti.** (1) If you dream that your mother-in-law has come to talk in your house, know that *imfwiti* (witches) have come.

(2) If you dream that your house is burnt, it is because *imfwiti* have come to the house.

(3) If you dream continually that a naked man comes to your house, know that he is an *imfwiti*. This is a case for the witch-doctor.

Ukulota Kwaŵami—the Dreams of the Aŵami

All the dreams of the *ŵamukamwami* (spirit mediums) [1] are considered portents of pending evil. They are communicated to the people in order to induce them to bring gifts for the purpose of warding off the evil prophesied.

(1) If the *ŵamukamwami* dream of birds eating the corn, they call upon the people to *ŵomba*, bring gifts to ward off the birds threatening the crops. In doing this the people abase themselves before the *mukamwami*, sing, and make gifts of beads.

(2) Some days later a *mukamwami* will say, "I dreamt that all the people had sores." The people, fearing smallpox, will bring further gifts.

(3) Later on he may say, "I dreamt that all the people were violently coughing, for 'the chief' [*i.e.*, the *umwami* possessing the professor] brought the disease in an arrow-sheath and let it out in the village, for he is angry with you because you do not *ŵomba*." This too will bring more gifts.

(4) In order to get further gifts he will say, "I dreamt that 'the chief' came with locusts in a huge calabash, and wanted to open it in your gardens, for he says you do not obey."

(5) The *mukamwami* may further tell the people that he has dreamt that 'the chief' has shut up water in a calabash, which means that the rain will be withheld, though the people really believe that Lesa alone regulates the rain. The *ŵamukamwami*, however, deceive them by saying that the *aŵami* have access to Lesa.

(6) If he dreams that 'the chief' has set up a high pole all will believe that the rain will be satisfactory, and will only stop "when the pole sinks into the ground."

(7) If the *mukamwami* dreams of things itching over his body the people will expect an epidemic of *impele* (the itch), and bring offerings to ward it off.

Naturally the *ŵamukamwami* only make known such dreams as will bring them wealth.

[1] See Chapter XV.

CHAPTER XIV

THEISM AND COSMOGONY

THE belief of the Lambas in the spiritual world is a very real and potent one, as will be observed later, but their conceptions regarding the universe in which they have their material existence are very vague and hazy, and they do not seem to give much time to pondering upon them. Their spiritual conceptions are bound up with a firm belief in the existence of disembodied spirits, a soul land, and a doctrine of demons, mingled with a belief in various types of spiritual possession. Their conception of the universe is as necessarily linked up with a belief in a supreme being. The Lambas are theists, and withal monotheists, but their theism, as will be seen, scarcely enters into their religious life at all.

The Earth

The earth they call *pano posonde*, "here outside," for they say of themselves, *Tuli ŵantu ŵakwe Lesa aŵeshile pano posonde*

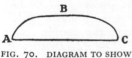

FIG. 70. DIAGRAM TO SHOW THE LAMBA CONCEPTION OF THE EARTH AND SKY
AC, the flat earth ; ABC, the dome of the sky.

mukwandamina-po lukoso, tukabwelelo'ko kwesu! "We are people of God who have come here outside just to sun ourselves; we shall return yonder to our home!" Where *uko kwesu* (our home yonder) is they are very vague; it is evidently not within the earth, but somewhere beyond the heavens.

They believe that the earth is flat, and that the dome of the sky comes down and meets the earth at its confines. At the ends of the earth the clouds come downward (*sesemuka*) to touch the earth; and the dwarf dwellers at "land's end," called *utulya-makumbi* (little cloud-eaters), cut off slices of the clouds, take them to their home, cook them, and eat them as their staple food. The Lambas say that these little people swarm out, men and women, with their baskets and knives, take the cloud slices to their villages, and cook them "as we do mushrooms." There is another version of this, which says that the clouds swing backward and forward at "land's end," and that slices are cut off against the sharp edge of the earth, collected by the little folk, dried in the sun like cassava, pounded in their mortars, and made into porridge.

In the Lamba story of *Ŵamwana-nkalamu na Ŵamwana-ŋombe* we read [1]

> And so it was that he [Cow-child] travelled that great distance, and arrived at where the clouds reach the earth, and they had put up a ladder. Then he climbed up and reached a small house, and saw the daughter of God.

The realm of Lesa is evidently above the dome of heaven, which is conceived as something solid.

The Sun

The sun (*akasuŵa*) travels across the dome of heaven until it reaches "land's end," and then it secretly travels back at night, very high up, behind a bank of clouds. The sun is a huge globe. On it are *aŵantu* (people), of a different creation from humans, who have daily duties. During its night journey, when it has cooled off, they polish it to make it shine brightly, and then they light the fires, so that great heat is given out. It begins to cool down as it gets to the west. There is another army of workers, who drag and push the sun on its daily journey; and yet another, who take it back at night. When the sun begins to rise the Lambas say, "The fire has only just been lighted." In the same way, when it sinks red in the west they say, "It is because the fire is beginning to go out." In winter-time (*pamwela*) the people on the sun do not make the fires up so strongly, "lest we should burn up the crops of our friends down below," and they sprinkle water on to it to damp down the fires; the steam given off is seen in the overcast days. In summer-time they pour on no water, for they want to dry up the earth's *ifisompe*, tracts of long grass.

Regarding eclipses of the sun, the Lambas merely say, "They have covered the sun over," referring to the *aŵantu* on the sun.

The *insasamyenje*, or rays of the sun, often seen as he sinks in the west, are called by the Lambas *imimpe*, being likened to the branching tunnels made by the *imfumbe* mice.

The Moon

The moon (*umwenshi*) does its work by night. It too has *aŵantu*, workers, who wash it clean. Every day they wash and rub it over. It is very big—"too big to be picked up!" It also

[1] See *Lamba Folk-lore*, by C. M. Doke, p. 19.

returns back to its starting-point every day, and in its journey at times it barely misses the sun. By some it is called *aŵepwa* (nephew, sister's son) of King Sun. The sun is therefore *ŵamwinshyo*,[1] maternal uncle to the moon.

The Lambas have a saying—they call it *ichityoneko lukoso*, merely a myth—that the sun and the moon are striving over the kingdom. The moon hurls his darts at the sun, and they are seen sticking into him; then the sun retaliates and throws mud at the moon, the dark patches being clearly visible on him.

The Lambas have the following folk-tale of the sun and the moon. While at a meal the two had an argument. Said the sun, "When I, sun, come out, all in the country, people and birds, begin to walk about." Said the moon, "When I too come out all the people walk about." So the moon first appeared, and the people came out and said, "Let us go to work." But when they reached their gardens they could not see how to work. When, however, the sun came out they all greeted him, saying, "The sun is the Great One," for the forest was white and the grass was visible. Then did the moon agree to be the nephew of the sun.

Full moon is called *umwenshi uŵulungene*. When the moon is only half-full the Lambas say it is hidden in its house and is peeping out, only the *amasengo* (horns) appearing. Of the new moon they say, *Lelo mufiso mwanaka, umwenshi ulukwikala*, "To-day [our] legs are weakened, the moon is settling down." At new moon the position of the moon is watched. If it is standing upright, its horns pointing westward, they say, "Our fellows out west are unlucky; they are going to perish." If its two horns point eastward they say the same of their fellows out east. But if the moon lies evenly upon its back they look upon it as a good sign, and say, "The moon is standing well!"

The Stars

The stars (*utuŵangaŵanga*) are the favourite attendants (*aŵapanga*) of the moon, who is their chief. All are round (*utuŵulungene*), and the twinkling of some is due to the making of fires on them. They all have *aŵantu* on them to make up the fires. In a fanciful way some Lambas speak of the starry sky as God's village, with the fires showing in the doorways, Venus being the hut of the principal wife. But others say this is but fancy, and it is not generally believed in. The Milky Way (*umulalafuti*) is merely looked upon as a sign of approaching dawn, for then it is

[1] Note the respectful plural used here.

at its brightest. *Iŵuushya-nama* (the rouser of the buck) is the first star to appear at early dawn, a sign to the animals to go and graze. It is followed by *intanda* (Venus), the real herald of dawn.

Rain

Above the dome of the sky is a great lake of water, kept back by a bank or weir, *ichipanda chyakwe Lesa*. There are guardians of this lake, and it is their duty to guard the bank. It seems that Lesa does not desire to give much rain to the earth, for the Lambas say that sometimes he sends youngsters to guard the bank, who begin to play, and make holes through which the water pours down as rain (*imfula*). But when there is no rain they say that Lesa has now sent grown men to guard it, who respect the will of their master.

Lightning

The Lambas always use the term Lesa in connexion with lightning (*akampeshimpeshi*). *Lesa wapata*, "God is scolding," they say. The lightning is believed to be caused by the people guarding the weir. They swing round the *imyele yakwe Lesa*, the knives of God, and the flashes from these knives at times go very far. The Lambas say that the *imyele* do not fall themselves, but should they do so *ichyalo chingatoŵeka*, the country would be destroyed. When a flash appears there descends to the ground an animal like a goat, with beard and horns complete, but with feet and tail like a crocodile. It comes down on the end of a strong cobweb. Should the cobweb break, the animal, remaining, cries like a goat, and the people run together to kill and burn it. They fear that the animal might kill them, and those who destroy it must have *ubwanga bwayamba*, protective medicine. Usually the web does not break, and the animal returns into the sky.

People fear a tree struck by lightning, and will not use any such for firewood, for they think that 'power' has been left in it.

Thunder, *ukululuma*, is said to be a noise made by the guardians of the weir. They shake huge metal drums.

Theistic Belief

The Lambas believe that there is a "high god." He is generally called Lesa, but there are various other names by which he is called. They give him the name Nyambi, used also by the Kaondes, and in oath-taking use Mulungu and Shyakapanga. He is often designated as Lyulu, which means in the first place "the heaven." This term is also used out of respect for

225

prominent chiefs. Then there is the name Luchyele, in all probability connected with the verb *ukuchya*, to dawn. The derivation
of Lesa is not known. It seems likely that it is connected with the
root *isa* (come), and some natives explain it by saying, *Pakuti
alesa panshi*, "Because he comes down to earth!" *alesa* being the
habitual tense. This is very doubtful. Another possible derivation connects it with the verb *lelesa*, which means to have tender
compassion.

Lesa is believed to be the creator of all things, of the *aῶantu*
who live in his realm, those working on the sun and the moon,
those in charge of the abode of the dead, those guarding the
animals under the name of *ῶakaaluwe*, and of the *aῶantunshi*,
human beings, those on the earth, who are subject to *imikoka*, or
clan distinctions. In addition to the material creation and that
of the different types of *aῶantu*, he is said to have created the
ifiῶanda (demons) and the *ifinkuwaila* (goblins) which play so
large a part in the people's spiritistic beliefs. The creation of all
things is attributed to Lesa. The Lambas say that he created the
sun before he created the moon, and that the stars were created
later still. Under the name of Luchyele, as we have noticed, he
arranged the whole country, rivers in their places, mountains,
anthills, grass, trees, and lakes. He came from the east, and went
to the west, where he climbed up by a ladder into heaven. It is
said that he left word with the communities of people whom he
placed in the land that they were to remain and await his return,
even if it were to be long delayed. He will come down again in
the east, and then, as he passes, will take all the people with him.

It may be thought that this belief in the return of Luchyele is
due to missionary influence, but when one takes into consideration the whole belief of the Lambas regarding *ichiyaῶafu* (the
abode of the dead), the two conceptions are found to fit, and I
cannot but feel that the natives are correct when they affirm that
this is the belief which has been handed down to them from their
fathers. They maintain that Luchyele will really come again,
because he promised the people that he would send them the sun
every day; he has done this, and so he will fulfil the other promise
too. The dead, they say, are waiting in *ichiyaῶafu* for Lesa to
take them out—otherwise of what value is *ichiyaῶafu*?

Ichiyaῶafu is conceived as being within the earth, but the abode
of Lesa is *kwiulu*, in the heaven. When God descends to collect
the people he will blot out all rivers and trees; the people he
carries will have to be changed to conform to those who are in
ichiyaῶafu, who have no sex or clan distinctions. The *imipashi*

(spirits) who were originally left by Lesa to help and care for the people are earthly beings and cannot leave this abode; they, together with the *ifiŵanda* and the *ifinkuwaila*, will be left behind when the people are taken.

Lesa is conceived as living in his great village, seated on a metal throne (*iteŵe lyachyela*). The 'village' is so great that the ends of it cannot be seen. There are many *aŵantu* there, but no gardens. Lesa is said to sit alone on his throne—he has no wife. This is in contradiction to the common talk of the stars being lights in the houses of the wives of Lesa; serious Lamba thinkers say "that is only conjecture." All the people in the village of Lesa eat food from the *ilonga*, or great eating-trough of the chief; and the food is so nice that if any drops on to the ground they pick it up and eat it, not minding the earth adhering to it!

In Lesa's country there is no river, nor is there any grass in the *uluŵansa* or courtyard, which is smooth and made of metal. There is no water, only honey (*bwenko'ŵuchi*). Only at night does Lesa leave his throne to enter his house. There is no sleep there; sleep will end when Lesa takes the people from the earth. The Lambas say, however, that there are both day and night.

The part played by Lesa in present matters is said to be as follows:

(1) He sits on his throne judging the affairs of the people in his country—*aŵantu ŵakwiulu*. He has *impemba* (councillors) who assist him in these cases and *ŵamulonda* (watchmen) who carry messages to his *ifilolo* (headmen).

(2) He appoints *ifilolo* to the work of guarding the weir and the rainfall. They have to *alule'fiŵeshi fyakwe Lesa*, flash the knives of God, and thus send lightning when the rain falls. He gives and withholds rain.

(3) He sends *amanata* (leprosy), *akapokoshi* (Kafir pox), *ichingwali* (smallpox), and such epidemics as the influenza of 1918.

(4) When death occurs it is said, *Ni Leso'mwine wamutwala*, "It is God himself who has taken him."

There is no worship of Lesa, no *ukuŵomba* (gift to avert disaster) as to the *aŵami* (spirit mediums), no *ukupupa* (ceremonial offering) as to the *imipashi* (spirits of departed), and no *ukupaapatila* (prayer). People fear him too much, and consider him beyond their reach; they can but say, *Lesa mutofwe-ko*, "O God, help us!" Only one prayer to God has been identified. When going to *pupe'mipashi* and to throw meal on the ground in the *utupeshi* a person may pray, *Lesa, mutupele'mfula, fweŵantu ŵenu!* "O God, give us rain, us, your people!" Otherwise

227

they make offerings to the *aŵami*, for it is they who are able to speak to Lesa. They therefore say to them, *Mutupaapatile kuli Lesa mweŵami, fweŵantu twaloŵa!* "Pray for us to God, O spirits of the chiefs, for we people are done for!" And the *ŵamukamwami* will give them assurance that the rain will fall.

It is said that God is angered when people sin deeply, when they commit adultery, steal, or murder, and that he punishes by sending leprosy and smallpox. But there is no way of approaching him for a cessation of these judgments; the people have just to bear them.

Of thunder the Lambas say, *Ninyambi ulukululuma lelo!* "It is God who is thundering to-day!" In oath-taking they say, *Shyakapanga wopelo'yo andye lelo!* "Let the very God devour me to-day!" or *Kani nachite'chichyeŵo Mulungu wopelo'yu apone anjipaye!* "If I have done this of which I am accused, may God himself fall and kill me [by lightning]!"

There are two folk-tales, to be found throughout Bantu Africa, which give the native conception of the origin of death and its certainty. They are connected with the conception of the "high god." The following are the Lamba versions.

How Death Came into the World

Long ago the chief on earth used to travel from place to place, but eventually he desired to settle down; he therefore sent some of his people to God to fetch seeds, that he might sow them and have his own gardens. When his messengers reached God they were given some little bundles tied up, and instructed not to undo a certain one of the bundles, but to deliver them to their chief. "Of these bundles, don't undo this one," he said. The messengers had to sleep on the road, but their curiosity overcame them. One said, "Mates, let us see these parcels that the King has given us!" And they began to undo them. When, however, they undid the forbidden package—the package of death—death spread abroad. In fear and trembling they went to their chief, and confessed to him that one of their number had opened the little package and let death escape. And the chief was angry, and said, "Catch him, and let us kill him." And they killed him. And death entered the world.

The Story of the Chameleon and the Lizard

God sent the chameleon to the people with this message: "Tell the people that when they die they will return again."

The chameleon set off on his journey, stepping slowly and deliberately, *kamu kamu kamu*, rolling his eyes around at every step. After some days God sent the lizard with another message : "Tell the people that when they die they will die for ever!" It was not long before the lizard overtook and passed the chameleon, reached the people, and delivered his message. Sadly late, the first messenger arrived with his message of life, but the people would not believe him. They hated him for his delay, and, taking nicotine (*ikondyo lyafwaka*), made him eat it, and so killed him. And that is why the chameleon is to this day held in hatred.

CHAPTER XV

SPIRITISM

The Spiritual Conception

To the Lamba the spiritual world is one which has daily contact with almost every phase of his life. In order to understand his conception of this spiritual world it is necessary to ascertain his beliefs concerning what happens after death; and it is amazing to find how clear and concise these are.

One man briefly stated the commonly accepted belief to me as follows:

"When a person dies his body is buried; he himself goes to *ichiyaŵafu* [the abode of the dead], and his *umupashi* [spirit] returns to the village to await reincarnation." Thus, then, we find that the Lambas believe definitely that the living person is made up of body, person, and spirit. These three entities are naturally bound up together and interdependent in life, but are separated completely by death. Much in the burial rites can only be understood and explained by a study of Lamba belief in the origin or destiny of the person and the spirit, which, together with the body, constitute the living being. As was noticed when dealing with the burial rites, the body faces east, to facilitate the return of the spirit in reincarnation, and also so that it may look for the return of Luchyele. Death means the end of the body. But why is it that witches and wizards are invariably burnt? It is because fire, when medicinally treated by the *umulaye* (doctor), is the one thing that can destroy the spirit as well as the body. Nothing can destroy the 'person.'

The Person

The body is the visible portion of the living being, but the 'person himself,' *umuntu umwine*—I hesitate to use the term 'soul' to indicate this, as the Lamba conception is so different— is only perceptible through his speaking, and that he has not left the body is indicated by his breathing. The Lambas use the term *umweo*, life, as synonymous with *umuntu umwine*, and when

SPIRITISM

a person dies they commonly say, *Umuntu waleko'mweo*, "The person has let go his life." The *umweo* is that which lives in the heart and causes it to beat. They say, *Umweo eupema*, "It is the life which beats." It is further significant that *umweo* is practically synonymous with *umutima*, heart, a word derived from *tima*, which is equivalent to *pema*, to breathe.

Ichiyaŵafu

At death the person himself, *umweo* or *umuntu umwine*, freed from the body, *umuŵili*, and also unlinked from the spirit, *umupashi*, goes away to the west, to *ichiyaŵafu*. This term means "the place where go the dead," being derived from the words *ya*, go, and *aŵafu*, dead people. The person, then, according to the Lamba conception, is rigorously differentiated from the spirit. No spirit, they say, ever reaches *ichiyaŵafu*. The charm of *ichiyaŵafu* to the Lamba is that it is the place of rest. An old Lamba may sometimes be heard to say, *Kamfwa bwangu nkatushye kuŵaŵyanji*, "Let me die soon that I may rest with my companions"; and on hearing that some one has died he will say, *Lelo umuŵyesu waya kutushya-po*, "To-day our friend has gone to take his rest." This thought is carried so far that in the past many have been known to commit suicide in order to reach this abode of rest more quickly.

Ichiyaŵafu, according to Lamba conception, is described as a large country, situated somewhere in the west—some say underground—ruled over by a king who is not and never has been a human being. This king must not be confused with the deity, Lesa; he is set over the realm of the departed by Lesa. He is assisted by numbers of officers, *ifilolo*, whose duty it is to introduce to him the visitors as they come, and to assign to them their various places in the midst of their relatives.

It is only the persons of departed human beings which go to *ichiyaŵafu*; no dogs or other animals are to be found there. It is only the human being which has a 'soul,' or person, and this belief is quite naturally found in the Lamba conception of the spiritual.

Ichiyaŵafu is the great place of levelling. The dead of all tribes and nations go there, and live in perfect harmony. There is but one tongue, which each person acquires immediately he is greeted by the king. In *ichiyaŵafu* there is no distinction of social status; no distinction is made between the persons of chiefs, commoners, or slaves. Even the persons of witches and wizards go to *ichiyaŵafu*, for their witcheries have been left behind them. Entrance to *ichiyaŵafu* is not in any way dependent upon moral excellence, for any such attributes or lack of them are connected with the body and the spirit, and do not, according to Lamba ideas, affect the person himself. *Ichiyaŵafu* knows no clan distinction. As we shall see later, the clan is inseparably connected with the spirit, but has no connexion with the person. Sex is another distinction foreign to the self, and thus unknown in *ichiyaŵafu*. Sex is but a bodily distinction in Lamba belief, foreign to both spirit and person. The distinction of age is similarly unknown in the spiritual realm. The Lamba crudely expresses these various beliefs. Says he, "At death the person is immediately transported to *ichiyaŵafu*, where he takes on another body, different from that which was laid in the grave, for that was dissolved, but one in which the *ichiwa* [face or features] is the same, one which is recognizable and has a voice which is recognizable. This new body is material, but there is no possibility of disease or death coming to it, for is it not in order to rest that these bodies are given? All there are males; there is no female. When a woman dies she leaves her womanhood in the grave, and appears as a man in his prime. If a baby dies, when he goes over there he appears as a grown person, and can talk. A madman, when he dies, appears in *ichiyaŵafu* sane; and a very old man will appear there as one at the height of his manhood."

The Lambas have very hazy ideas as to what *ichiyaŵafu* is like, but they say that there are no houses, no trees, no grass, no dust, but everywhere it is clean and beautiful. There is no need to arrange a sleeping mat; all may lie comfortably on the soft ground. It is not thought that they sleep, but they rest and rest, and hold pleasant conversation one with the other. This period of rest in *ichiyaŵafu* is not to go on for ever; Lesa is to come and take out these departed when he comes again to gather the people.

Umupashi—the Spirit

The spirit, *umupashi*, as we have noticed, does not go to *ichiyaŵafu*. At death, when the body is buried, the spirit returns to the village to wait. It seems that the spirit haunts the body until the burial has been completed, and then hovers around the village where its previous activities have been centred, awaiting the opportunity for reincarnation. Meanwhile, it needs certain attention, and looks for the *ifiŵaya*, or drinking-gourds of beer and gruel, and for the *imilenda*, or spirit huts, in which to dwell. If these necessaries are not provided, and the spirit is left uncared-for and uncomfortable, its state will be reflected in sickness coming upon *awene wamupashi*, the 'owner' of the spirit, or upon some member of his family. The doctor will have to be called in, and his diagnosis will be, "It is your spirit which is causing this."

The Owner of the Spirit

The 'owner' of the spirit is some relative of the deceased, a child, maybe, or a younger brother, but of necessity not husband or wife. If the deceased were a male, the owner of the spirit, responsible for its welfare, would be decided in order of preference as follows: (1) *umwanichye wakwe*, his younger brother, (2) *umwana wakwe*, his son or his daughter, and (3) *umwipwa wakwe*, his sister's child. The owner of the spirit is then said to inherit the spirit of his elder brother or of his father; and a daughter may even inherit the spirit of her father. If the deceased were a female, the inheritance of the spirit would be decided in the following order of preference: (1) *umwanichye wakwe*, her younger sister, (2) *umwana wakwe umwanakashi*, her daughter, and (3) *umwinshikulu wakwe umwanakashi*, her granddaughter. Thus it is seen that no male can *pyano'mupashi wamwanakashi*, inherit the spirit of a female.

Umulenda

When some time has passed after the death of a man his mother will say to his younger brother, "Do you, his younger brother, build the *imilenda* for your elder brother; it is you who have inherited his spirit. Inherit, then, his name, and build for him the *imilenda*." The young man will then adopt his elder brother's name. This, however, does not mean that he has become possessed by the spirit of his brother; he is but the guardian, and that spirit is still at large, awaiting an opportunity of reincarnation.

After some days' further delay the heir, *impyani*, will have beer brewed, and summon his friends. Before the beer is touched there is the work of building the *umulenda*. A space is cleared *muchitumbo*, in the garden-clearing, a little distance from the hut which the deceased had occupied, and one hut is built. All the men gathered to the beer-drink assist in the building, bringing the sticks, grass, and bark rope. The *umulenda* is a very small hut, made of sticks and grass in the same way as is an *inkunka*, the temporary lean-to erected on a new village site. At times the

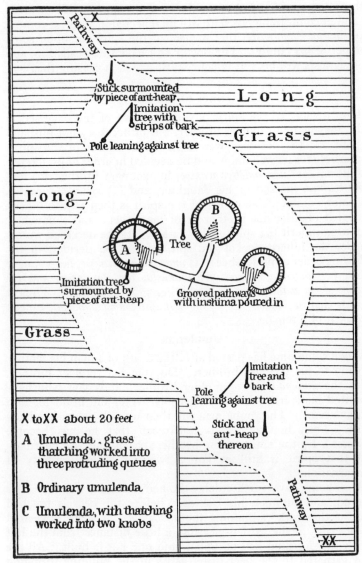

Stick surmounted
by piece of ant-heap

Imitation
tree with
strips of bark

L—o—n—g

G—r—a—s—s

Pole leaning against tree

Long

B

Tree

A

C

Imitation tree
surmounted by
piece of ant-heap

Grooved pathways
with inshima poured in

Grass

X

Pathway

Imitation
tree and
bark

Pole
leaning against tree

Stick and
ant-heap
thereon

XX

Pathway

X to XX about 20 feet

A Umulenda, grass
thatching worked into
three protruding queues

B Ordinary umulenda

C Umulenda, with thatching
worked into two knobs

FIG. 71. IMILENDA

234

umulenda is as much as 4 feet 6 inches in height. A small platform of sticks, *akapingwe*, is constructed within before the hut is finished. This platform consists of four *impanda*, forked sticks

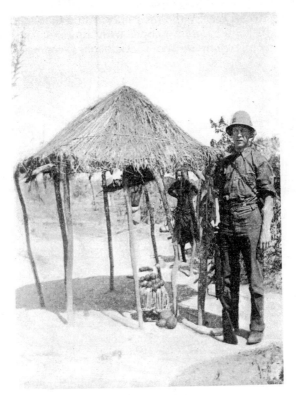

FIG. 72. UMULENDA OF A MOWA, WITH AUTHOR
See p. 255.
Photo by the late Rev. J. J. Doke

planted in the floor, two *imitanti*, transverse sticks joining the pairs of forks, and a number of *ubwalangwe*, or sticks laid across the *imitanti*. This platform is erected to support the calabashes of beer; they are not placed on the ground for fear of the termites. Finally a small grass door is made to fit the doorway.

Ichinsengwe

When the building is finished all who have helped sit down to drink the beer. After the beer-drink they begin to dance the *ichinsengwe.* This dance, which is usually connected with hunting celebrations, is also carried out when honouring the *imipashi*. Men only build the *umulenda*, and men only drink the beer at first, though sometimes a few women participate later. The dancing is carried out by the men only, while the women *lishyo' lumpundu*, make the *lululu* sound with lip and hand. Both men and women join in the special songs composed by the

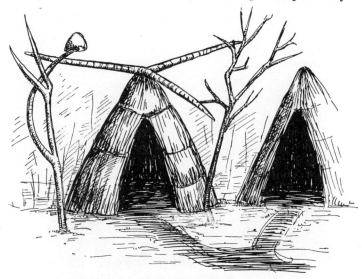

FIG. 73. SPIRIT HUTS

Erected in a pathway near a village, about seven miles west of Kafulafuta Mission. Height, 1 foot 10 inches. See Fig. 71, huts marked A and B.

aŵayambo, those professional dancers of whom more anon. I give but two examples of this type of song:

    (1) *Akana kali kamo, chyenjelo'kuleya'malambo !*
        Kalalenge'nkaka, chyenjelo'kuleya'malambo !
        Pakukane'nshima, chyenjelo'kuleya'malambo !

        " The little child is one,
            Mind you avoid the death-places !
        It brings anxiety,
            Mind you avoid the death-places !
        When it refuses food,
            Mind you avoid the death-places ! "

    (2) *Mama, mbangule umunga,*
        Ne chyende-ende ulitemenwe !

        " Mother, extract the thorn for me,
            For me, the wanderer you love ! "

So the dancing and singing go on, and the owner of the spirit rewards those who have come to help him with payments of beads. The company does not break up till the late afternoon.

Meanwhile, while the beer-drink is still going on, the owner of the spirit brings some new drinking calabashes, *ifiŵaya* or *inkombo*, two or three of which he has specially prepared, dips out some beer from the pot at which the assembled people are drinking, carries the *inkombo* to the *umulenda*, and places them on the *akapingwe* within.

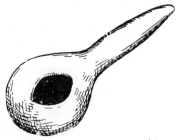

FIG. 74. ULUKOMBO, OR ICHIŴAYA

When all the people who had gathered have dispersed the owner of the spirit utters these words: *Ubwalwo'ŵu namupeni, kanyenda nemakosa*, "This beer I have given to you. Let me travel with strength!" After that, while he is alone, he will drink up the beer he has placed in the *umulenda*, and restore the *inkombo* to their place on the platform. From time to time he will take beads and place them within the *umulenda*, saying, *Ubwalwa bwenu twanwa, twamuŵichileni-mo uŵulungu, twaula*, "Your beer we have drunk, we have put in beads for you, we have bought it." These beads are left there indefinitely; they are *ukutonda*, forbidden things, because they belong to the spirit.

Ukupupa

All this is called *ukupupe'mipashi*, or *ipupwe*, and is designed to give due and expected honour to the spirit of the departed. If this honour is not paid the spirit will vent his annoyance by causing illness in the family of his heir. One of the prime causes of the carrying out of this *ipupwe* is to prevent such illness, or to restore health to one so afflicted. From this point of view the *ipupwe* may be considered propitiatory. The translation of the term *ipupwe* by 'worship' thus hardly seems adequate.

The building of the *umulenda* is the only occasion on which *ubwalwa* (intoxicating beer) is brewed in honour of the departed spirits. When the firstfruits ripen, however, *ifisunga*, non-intoxicating beer, is brewed before the *umulenda*, where all gather to drink it; some is then placed in the *inkombo* which are within the hut.

237

Spirit of a Chief

For the spirit of a paramount chief, after the funeral ceremonies (described in Chapter XI) have been completed, an *umulenda* is also constructed. The chief himself goes to *ichiyaŵafu*, and his spirit returns to his home village to await reincarnation, though some say that the *ŵamukumbe*, maneless lions, are reincarnations of departed ancestral chiefs. This is especially believed if the lions are met with at the *umulyashi*, burial-ground of the chief. This belief is extended to an ordinary lion if it is met when it is devouring a kill. Hunters will try to drive the lion off, and will flatter (*totaishya*) it by calling it by the names of various chiefs, begging it to give its people some meat. The chief's successor, *uwalye'shina*, he who has 'eaten' his name, becomes the owner of that spirit. He it is who brews the beer, summons the people, and builds the *umulenda*, in the same way as has been described already in the case of a commoner. The new chief thus becomes the guardian of the *inkombo* (calabashes) of his predecessor.

When an ordinary *umulenda* rots the owner will take out the *inkombo* and place them under the eaves of the *insense*, veranda, of his house. He may later on build another *umulenda* and restore the *inkombo*, but often this is left until sickness comes to a member of his family. The doctor, when called in to diagnose, will say, "Build the spirit hut, for the spirit is angry at having to sleep outside!"

The *imilenda* are kept shut, except when the owner wishes to see whether the termites have been at work. Anyone else would fear death should he meddle with an *umulenda*.

Umulenda of a Chief

The *umulenda* of the paramount chief at Kaŵalu's village is much larger than the ordinary spirit hut of the *inkombo*, and in it are stored the *amata*, weapons, of the deceased chief. This *umulenda* is immediately replaced by a new one when it becomes rotted. The *umwinamulenda*, Kaŵalu, calls together his friends, some of whom go for poles, others for grass. As they return to the village with their loads of poles and grass the men chant, *Kumilenda takupito'we'ŵele, ŵalipinika-ko!* "None with a breast passes the spirit huts; one cuts it off!" This is believed to be but a refrain, and is never seriously carried out against any woman, though at such a time women are strictly forbidden to go near the building. If there is no beer ready *inshima* porridge is cooked and a white cock killed. The cock's feathers are pulled out and stuck in all over the hut. The *inshima* is eaten, and with it the fowl *iyakochya*, grilled (literally, burnt), never *iyakwipika*, boiled. This procedure is similar to that followed by the undertakers in the death-hut.

Imilenda are not built to the spirits of children or youths, but in honour of those of elders only. It is said that a young man could not have a younger brother or a child old enough to carry out the duties required. Great care is taken to preserve the *imilenda* from grass fires, and I have not heard of any cases of their getting burnt.

Help of the Umupashi

It is believed that the spirit will help the owner in various ways if honoured and housed comfortably. When a man is going on a journey he will take some meal and go and throw it into the *inkombo* in the *umulenda*, and say, *Ndukwimo'lwendo, naisa kumulayeni*, "I am starting on a journey, and have come to bid you good-bye." This is done that the spirit might go before him and assist him on the way. Again, when a dead antelope is found the fortunate man will say, *Umupashi wanji wampela*, "My spirit has given it to me"; and there is a common saying used to a person of sharp tongue: *Ulukulawila koti mupashi utapa-nama*, "You speak like a spirit that does not give meat."

Akapeshi

There is quite a different type of spirit hut, erected only in honour of chiefs and renowned village headmen. This is the *akapeshi*, erected for the purposes of bringing rain.

When the rain holds off and the prospects of a harvest are endangered, Kaŵalu, the guardian of the chief's *amata*, will call a young doctor, *umulaye uwamipini*, a doctor of axe-handles, one who divines to detect the interference of the spirits, but has not yet learnt to probe the world of demons or to exorcise *ifiŵanda*. He will say to the doctor, "Divine for us, that we may see what is holding back the rain." And the doctor's verdict will be, "It is the chief who is angry, because you have not built the *utumimba*." *Utumimba* is but another name for *utupeshi*, the small spirit huts of the crossroads.

When Kaŵalu is alone again he will go to his chief, and tell him that the (dead) chief is angry, because they have not built him any *utumimba*. Then early the next morning men will carry meal and go and erect two *utumimba*, sometimes even four, at the crossing of the ways where the undertakers had rested and set down the bier when on the way to bury the remains of the chief. Men usually go in pairs to build these miniature huts at all the places where the corpse had rested. When the huts are completed meal is placed in lines on the ground before the *utupeshi*, and the men rub some of it on their faces. If one of the men, while on this work of building the *utupeshi*, finds something—*e.g.*, honey or meat—he does not conceal it, but takes it to the *umwinamulenda*, saying, "This is what the chief has given us." All then partake of it, and say, "The chief has prepared us a meal to-day."

If it rains on the day on which they build the *utupeshi* no one will go to work in the gardens; all will stay at home in order to honour the chief for having given them rain on that day.

Afterward passers-by will place small offerings of meal, honey, meat, etc., in the doorway of an *akapeshi*, saying, *Fyamfumu*, "They belong to the chief." This is to prevent the chief from getting angry.

Utupeshi are similarly erected in many villages at the crossroads in honour of the spirits of the chiefs of those villages. All this is called *ukulombe'mfula kumfumu*, begging rain from the chief, and is considered a surety of abundant rains.

Firstfruits

The *utupeshi* (spirit huts) also play their part in the recognition of the firstfruits. Before the people partake of the new season's food tiny pumpkins, cucumbers, and maize are carried by the village headman to an *akapeshi* in the pathway. Little furrows are made in the doorway, and the offerings are placed therein, with these words: *Ifyakulya mfi twaleta mukumusomweshyeni, pakuti nafweŵo tulukufwayo'kulya*, "Here is food, which we have brought that you may taste the firstfruits, for we too desire to eat." These offerings, which are by no means " of the best of the flock," are left there to rot or dry up. In the same way, when the *amasaka* corn ripens the headman of each village goes through a similar act, and thus all members of the village are free to partake of the new corn.

The *utupeshi* are not revered as highly as are the *imilenda*. They do not house the departed spirit, and when grass fires destroy them nothing is thought of it. The *akapeshi* is temporary in its use, while the *umulenda* serves its purpose as long as the spirit is awaiting reincarnation.

SPIRITISM

Reincarnation

The Lambas state that more than one spirit may be housed in one *umulenda*, provided that the spirits are all of one *umukoka*, or clan. The denoting of the clan is one of the most important functions of the *umupashi*. The Lambas say, *Ichikulu kumipashi mukoka*, "The great thing with the spirits is the clan." In this the spirit is most unlike the person. We see from this, too, how inseparably totemism, as far as it applies to the Lambas, is bound up with spiritism.

Afflatus. The spirit can only be reincarnated in a member of the same clan as the deceased; and when a baby is born it is usually the duty of the maternal grandmother to decide upon the child's name, which is that of the deceased whose spirit is believed to have entered the babe. As has already been said when dealing with the naming of the child, if the name decided upon by the grandmother is not the correct one the displeasure of the spirit is shown in the child's falling sick. Then follows the necessity of a doctor to divine, in order to ascertain what spirit it is that is reborn. All this goes to show that in addition to the reincarnation of the spirit there is the power of the spirit to hold himself aloof and show displeasure. It seems that it is not the entire spirit which is reincarnated at a birth, but a kind of afflatus from it. This view is borne out by the fact that the spirit of one ancestor may be born into more than one babe at the same time. This is further confirmed by the fact that the spirit is still honoured and propitiated after a child bearing the same name has been born. The child in whom the spirit of a chief is reborn is accorded a certain amount of respect, and may, on attaining manhood, eventually be chosen to the chieftainship.

Imipishi

The Lambas' belief in the spiritual world goes very much deeper than an acceptance of the existence and potency of the *umupashi*, the spirit of the departed. They have a firm belief in the existence of apparitions and ghostly forms and visions, which they designate generally by the terms *imipishi*, *imichishi*, or *ẃamukupe*. These terms, which are synonymous, signify something evasive, which one has seen indistinctly, but which disappears entirely when one would investigate it closely. This general term of *imipishi* is of very wide significance, and is applied in the following instances:

(1) When one gets a glimpse of people at a distance, but on

arrival at the spot finds no trace of them, not even a footprint, they are believed to have been ghosts, the spirits of the departed.

(2) When one sights animals at a distance, but finds no trace whatever of their having been there, it is said that they were *inama yaŵakaaluwe*—that is, that they belonged to the guardian spirit of the herds. Lamba belief in this connexion is fully considered in Chapter XX, where the profession of *uŵupalu*, hunting, is dealt with.

(3) The same term is applied to the ghostly visions seen by a person when 'sickening' for spirit-possession. The sick person about to become a *moŵa* is said to see visions of people travelling in the sky. The wise will say, *Koku, taŵali ŵantu, mipishi waŵona!* "No, they are not people, they are ghosts you have seen!" These are said to be the spirits of the long-departed dead.

(4) The mirage is put into the same category, and is believed to represent a river, swamp forest (*umushitu*), lake, or pool belonging to the long-departed dead.

(5) Mysterious evening heat is also termed *imipishi*. Natives say that sometimes when travelling at night they come upon a spot where there is heat as from a fire. One will call out, "What heat there is here!" His companion will quickly reprove him for speaking like that, and say, "Let us go. It is the fire of the dead. Let them warm themselves at it!"

(6) The *ifinkuwaila*, goblins, and the *ifiŵanda*, demons, are also included under the general term of *imipishi*, because of their invisibility. The beliefs of the Lambas concerning these two classes of beings are an integral part of their conception of the spiritual, and will be dealt with at some length.

The Lambas are diffident about talking of *imipishi*. Should some women, coming back from foraging in the bush, say, "We saw some people coming toward us, but when they were quite near we did not see where they went to," one of the villagers will reply with the proverb, *Taŵalaŵila-mipishi kumushi*, "One does not mention ghosts in the village."

Ifiŵanda—Demons

The *ifiŵanda* are not to be confused in any way with the *imipashi*, spirits of the departed. They constitute a separate creation. The term 'demon' is not an adequate translation of the term, for the *ichiŵanda* is able to act beneficially toward human beings at times. Nevertheless, the *rôle* of the *ichiŵanda* in causing madness seems parallel to our conception of demon-possession.

The *ifiŵanda* are said to wander about in the forest, and old men are said to have seen them as ghosts moving at a distance. They are believed to have long red hair, which stands straight up on their heads, and their eyes are continually turned upward. They are otherwise like *aŵantu*, black people. They do not clothe themselves at all.

Another name for the *ichiŵanda* is *isongwe*, or *ichisongola*, while a praise-name used is *kaŋumba*, a name also applied to the wind because of its invisibility.

These beings favour the darkness, and for that reason, among others, the Lambas dread darkness. They say, *Wemwanichye taŵekala mumutando'mufitile*, "Youngster, one doesn't sit in a dark zareba," lest a demon coming in to get out of the rain should find one there. They also say, *Koshyeni-po umulilo, twikalukulya nefiŵande'nshima, ikashila bwangu!* "Stir up the fire [and brighten the hut], lest we should have demons to share the porridge with us in eating, and it should come to an end quickly!"

Evil Work of Ifiŵanda

Ifiŵanda are said to kill people by beating them. A person on reaching his village may say, "Something struck me while I was in the bush, and I did not see what it was that hit me." The village elders will say, "It was the *ifiŵanda* which struck you." The Lambas say that if an *ichiŵanda* desires to attack a man he comes to him invisibly. The man feels a blow, say, on his eye, and searches round to see whence it has come. He finds nothing. On his return to the village the *umulaye*, doctor, is summoned, and he brings *amaŵula afiŵanda*, leaves efficacious against demons. Burning some of the leaves, he smokes the patient. From others of the leaves he prepares medicine for the patient to drink; others again are soaked in water in a bowl of bark. This receptacle is called *isambwe*, and from it the patient is bathed, that the demon may leave his body. The bark bowl is then covered up, and the patient recovers.

It is said that others, when struck by *ifiŵanda*, are spoken to. They hear the voice only, and do not see anything. The demons say, "Don't say anything at the village! If you say anything, your blood be on your own head. You will die!" The frightened man keeps the matter to himself and says nothing. His life is saved, and he does not fall sick.

243

THE LAMBAS OF NORTHERN RHODESIA

The evil work of *ifiŵanda* is revealed in several ways. When a man suffers from a great persistent ulcer which will not heal it is sometimes said that an *ichiŵanda* has brought the ulcer and is dwelling in it. This is quite a different matter from ulcers caused by witchcraft. Similarly, leprosy, *amanata*, is often attributed to the action of *ifiŵanda*. But by far the most baneful thing attributed to the *ifiŵanda* is demon-possession, shown in. madness. An *ishilu*, a madman, is called *umuntu uwawilwa ichiŵanda*, a person possessed by a demon. There is also in Lamba belief a demon of lesser powers, called *umusako*, which may possess a person and cause morbid dumbness and mild idiocy. They say of an idiot, *Alinemisako*, "He has demons."

Demon-possession

The Lamba account of demon-possession is as follows: A man is ill; maybe it is an ulcer from which he is suffering. The various medicines applied have had no effect whatever; the man gets worse, and begins to speak incoherently. Some of the onlookers will say, "This person is already out of his mind; this is the work of *ifiŵanda*." Then one day he begins to rage, and rushes out of the hut. The people say, "Catch him, he has gone mad; these are demons which have taken possession of the man." When *ifiŵanda* thus take possession of a man they are said to 'eat' him or to 'kill' him, though the result is madness, not death.

Exorcism of a Demon

The *aŵalaye* (diviners) are credited at times with being able to *ŵuka'mashilu*, exorcize the demon from madmen. This is the Lamba account: When a man becomes mad the villagers hasten to fetch the doctor, who diagnoses the case as one of demon-possession. The mother and father of the afflicted man then desire the doctor to procure *umusamu* (medicine) for him. The doctor brings the necessary medicine, which is mixed with water in a calabash cup, *ichyeso*. A small circular hut without any opening, *akaŋanda kambuluŵulu*, is erected around the madman. Some one, holding the *ichyeso* of medicated water, then climbs to the top of the hut, immediately above the place where the madman is seated, and pours the water down upon him. Thereupon the madman shouts out, *Mweŵakalume imfula lelo e!* "Oh, ye slaves, how it is raining to-day!" But the people give him no reply. In the evening they take him out, and he says, "Did you not see how it rained in my house?" Thereupon the doctor spits upon his

back other *umusamu* which he has been holding in his mouth,
and goes on to deceive him by saying, "Wash your face—the
rain has made you very wet." After this the patient is given
gruel mixed with portions of a python. After drinking this
concoction he vomits violently. Then succeeds a period of deep
depression, during which he does not speak at all. He is restored
to the village life, and in place of his madness a quietness comes
over him. He will once more take his part in the work of the
village, but will very seldom be heard to speak.

Attendant Ifiŵanda

According to Lamba belief, every one has his attendant *ichiŵanda*, who looks after his interests, and is able to bring punishment upon anyone wronging his ward. This punishment is
effected by sending sickness to the evildoer or some member of
his family, or by exposing him to the wisdom of the *umulaye*, who
is thus able to 'smell him out' as a wizard. The *ichiŵanda* can
further assist his ward by arranging for *imbiko*, omens of evil, to
appear in his way, and so warn the man against going to his death
or into disaster. This beneficent action of the guardian *ichiŵanda* is also seen in the driving force behind the imposition of
the death-dues which must be paid by a widow or a widower.
When a person dies it is said that his *ichiŵanda* returns to the
forest, whence he has come, to resume his wanderings; no longer
does the *ichiŵanda* have any association with the *umupashi* (spirit)
of his ward. When that *umupashi* is reincarnated it is another
ichiŵanda that comes to act as guardian over the child. If, however, there is a *mukamfwilwe*, widow or widower, left on the death
of the ward, the *ichiŵanda* delays his return to the forest, and
remains to see that the rights of the deceased are observed, that the
death-dues are paid, and that the redemption of the relict is completed. If a woman dies her attendant *ichiŵanda* watches the
husband to see what he does. Should he marry before the death-
due is paid, the demon may cause his new wife to become ill.
When the *umulaye* is called in he will tell the man that it is his
own fault for not having redeemed himself, and that the *ichiŵanda* of his late wife is bringing this trouble upon him. The
man will humble himself, make a present of beads to the sick
person, and beseech the demon, saying, *Nasasa, wechiŵanda, tanje
mbone uŵuŵoni, mbweleshye uko natulile!* "I repent, O demon.
Let me first seek for the goods to restore whence I have come!"
This is called *ukunwo'mufungo*, drinking bitter fruit.[1] The

[1] *Cf.* "eat humble pie."

demon will hear his prayer, and the woman will recover. When the man has carried out his promise the demon will leave him. Death is believed to be the lot of anyone who is persistent in ignoring the claim of the *ichiŵanda* for the payment of the necessary death-dues.

Ifiŵanda are believed to protect their wards from wild beasts. If a person meets a lion out in the veld, and the lion merely stands and looks at him, despite the fact that he is quite close to it, he will say on his return to the village, "My *ichiŵanda* saved me to-day; otherwise I should have been eaten by a lion!"

Ifiŵanda are even said to take the part of *imfwiti*, witches or wizards. It is maintained that during the poison ordeal at a witch-trial, when the *umwafi* poison is being administered to a fowl, the guardian demon of the witch will at times sit in the mouth of the fowl, and take the poison himself, so that the fowl escapes death, the witch consequently being exonerated.

But the guardian *ifiŵanda* do not always remain faithful to their wards. If the demon no longer wants a man whom it has been guarding it will prompt him to commit some foolish action, and then will not save him when he gets into danger. It may lead him to enter a brake after a wounded buffalo or leopard, or make him trust himself on a rotten branch.

Ifiŵanda and Taboo

The *ichiŵanda* is credited with playing a peculiar part when certain taboos have been broken. When a man has committed an anti-social crime, such as rape, incest, copulation outside a hut, soiling of an unredeemed widow, or secret murder, the *ifiŵanda* see to it that the secret is revealed. If, for instance, a man and a woman have intercourse in the bush, not in a hut, it is said that the demons will follow them and catch them; they will fall ill, for they have broken a social taboo. The doctor, when called, will say to the man, "It is an *ichiŵanda* which has caught you. Confess what you have done!" In fear the man will confess, and the doctor will say, "The *ichiŵanda* came to reveal your crime." The sick man will beg of the demon to leave him alone, and his mother and father will come with hand-clapping, and address the demon with the words, *Pano fuma-mo wemukwasu, twakwishiŵa*, "Now go away, our brother. We have recognized you!" And the demon must go, because the case is no longer a hidden one. If the sick man refuses to confess, or if the doctor is called too late, madness is the usual result. Others say that it is the *ifiŵanda* who prompt a man in the first place to commit one of these anti-social crimes.

If the *ichiŵanda* has pursued his vengeance so far as to cause several deaths in the village the *umulaye* is sent for. He carries out the ceremony of *ukuŵuka*, divining, exactly as in a case of witchcraft (Chapter XIX), using his *imiseŵe* (rattles) and pot of water. After this his verdict is, *Chiŵanda echilukumwipayeni*, "It is a demon which is killing you!" He then says to all the relatives of those who have died, "You must be cleansed [*samba*]." The *umulaye* then goes in search of the necessary *umusamu* and a bark trough (*ichikwa*). In this he places a quantity of the medicine when he has set it down at a crossing of the paths (*kumashilampindwe*). Some people are sent to fetch water, which the *umulaye* pours into the trough. When night has fallen all the people gather to the spot. The *umulaye* now takes his zebra tail (*umuchila*) and dips it into the water, shaking it therein (*ŵunshya*); he then takes it out and sprinkles it toward the east, then toward the west, then toward the other two points (*mufiŵafu*). After this he sprinkles the assembled people wherever they are sitting. All then return to the village. The next day the ceremony is performed again in the evening; and it may even be done on the third day. When this is finished all have to sweep their houses, and take all the rubbish—broken pots, old mats, ashes, and even the ant-heap pot supports (*amafwasa*)—and deposit it in a heap at the *amashilampindwe*. The *umulaye* then makes fire for them with his fire-sticks (*ulushiko*). Each woman now comes to obtain fire, and starts her fire in her hut. Then the doctor goes from hut to hut, putting medicinal leaves upon each fire, the smoke from which cleanses the hut. The doctor is now paid for his services, and returns to his home. This whole ceremony is for the purpose of driving the *ichiŵanda* and its polluting influence from the village.

There is a Lamba proverb which says, *Ichiŵanda tachikata-ko*, "A demon does not hold tight"; this is equivalent to our saying, "Do not tempt Providence." A man must not bear his weight upon a hanging object; the *ichiŵanda* which normally protects him may let it go. The *ichiŵanda* is credited with being responsible for accidents due to carelessness. If a youngster points a gun at a friend the demon may cause him to pull the trigger; or if he poises a spear to make a feint with it at some one the demon may cause the spear to slip from his hand.

THE LAMBAS OF NORTHERN RHODESIA

Ifiŵanda and Animals

Ifiŵanda are said to possess wild beasts, especially if they approach human beings, as, for instance, lions, leopards, snakes, and buffalo. It is believed that if one shouts out, *Wechiŵanda! wechiŵanda!* "Thou demon! Thou demon!" the demon will see that it is recognized and make off. No native would throw his spear at one of these beasts without shouting out thus, and he would never shout, *Wenkalamu!* "Thou lion!" or *Wensoka!* "Thou snake!" Wild beasts seen normally are not believed to be thus possessed, and naturally would not attack people. It is the *ichiŵanda* within to which an appeal must be made.

Dogs and lions have attendant *ifiŵanda*. The Lambas say, *Ichiŵanda chyambwa tachilala*, "The dog's demon does not sleep." If a man kills a dog for no real reason its *ichiŵanda* will pester him and kill his children or make them mad. Fowls may be killed without any such risks; so may dogs if they have been killing the village fowls.

During the year 1920, when word had gone out that all native dogs were to be taxed, I visited the village of Kaŵunda-Chiŵele. Word came that the Native Commissioner was approaching, and many who could not afford to pay the tax or did not want to do it caught their dogs, took them out into the bush, and hanged them with bark rope. They did not do this, however, without first bidding them farewell with the words: *Wembwa weŵo nshikwipeye lukoso, ndukukwipayilo'kusonka, nshikwete-ndalama!* "O dog, I am not killing you without cause. I am killing you on account of the tax, for I have no money!" And it was said that the *ifiŵanda* of the dogs heard and understood.

Ukushilike'chiŵanda—Warding off Demons

If a man has recently died, and many people dream about him, they say, *Chiŵanda*, "It is a demon." They believe that 'the *ichiŵanda* (demon) has taken possession of his *umupashi* (spirit), and has come to the village to tell them all. They therefore send for a prominent *umulaye* (diviner). When he comes the *umulaye* divines, and asks, *Muno mumushi tamufwile-po umuntu?* "Has not some one died here in this village?" The people say, "Yes, So-and-so's slave has died." He will say, "That is he. You did not treat him properly!" Then the owner of the slave confesses to the harsh way in which he treated him. The *umulaye* then informs them that if they do not exhume (*shikula*) the body quickly he will cause deaths in the village. The people

248

then beg the *umulaye* to do the exhuming, promising him a gun. In the morning the doctor will call the people who buried the man to show him the way to the grave. Of these one or more then accompany the *umulaye* and his attendants. The guide stops at some distance, points to a certain anthill, and says, "The grave is over there." He then returns to the village. The *umulaye*, carrying his *ulusengo* (horn) and *umuchila* (zebra tail), now advances silently and stealthily to the grave, sticks his horn upright on it, lays down his switch thereon, and says, *Naikata mwefiwanda*, "I have caught you, ye demons!" Then all his attendants come up and begin to dig open the grave with a hoe. The *umulaye* sits still while his men are digging. When the diggers have practically reached the corpse they come out from the grave, and the *umulaye* enters. One other then enters to assist the *umulaye* to take out the body. Some of the assistants now begin to cut up the body (*pampa*), while others collect firewood from *imiwanga*-trees. The pile of firewood is set alight, and when only glowing coals remain the lumps of flesh are thrown on, as in the case of the burning of a witch. When all is consumed the *umulaye* throws on to the embers a stick of the *umwandwalesa* shrub. This blazes up, and is considered potent in stopping (*shilika*) the *ichiwanda*. After this the attendants remain seated round the pyre while the *umulaye* goes ahead alone along the path back to the village. At a little distance he chooses a shrub, a branch of which he strikes with his axe so that it bends over, almost cut through. This is called *uluteeta*. He now seizes the branch, and calls to his companions to come forward without looking behind them. They approach and pass him. He then leaves the *uluteeta*, and follows on after them. When they reach the village they do not enter it, but erect a zareba (*umutanda*) on the outskirts, and sleep there. To this *umutanda* the villagers bring them their payment. On the morrow the *umulaye* returns to his home.

This belief in the action of the *ichiwanda* is behind the necessity for burning ceremonially each witch or wizard (*imfwiti*) that is killed.

Should the corpse have been buried already for a long time, so that it has disintegrated, and mice have taken up their abode in the grave, the *umulaye* will consider, if he catches a mouse (*imbewa*) when digging, that it contains the *ichiwanda* of the dead man who has been disturbing the villagers. He will burn the mouse right on the grave with the same ceremony as in the case of the corpse of the man, believing it to be a reincarnation.

Birds of Ill-omen

In addition to being responsible for *imbiko* (ill-omens) in the ordinary way, *ifiŵanda* are said to be able to warn people by appearing in the *ikwikwi*, the hornless owl, and in another bird, called *lwitaŵila*.

The *ikwikwi* comes to the village if a person is ill, sits in the *uluŵansa*, or courtyard, at night, and calls, *Kwi kwi kwi, putu putu, whe whe whe* (whistling). The people who hear it will say that the sick man cannot recover, "for to-day the *ikwikwi* has cried." If no one is ill, and this bird comes repeatedly, it is believed to presage a death. The hornless owl is a bird of ill-omen.

The *lwitaŵila* lives in the bush, and does not come to the village. It calls *Wo! Wo!* at night in a deep voice, and is heard from afar. It is also regarded as *imbiko*. Little is known about it, but it is said to be a bird with a human voice. Sometimes it calls, *Uŵuta bwanji e . . . !* "Oh, my bow!", or *Nafwa e . . . , nafwa e . . . !* "Oh, I'm done for! Oh, I'm done for!" Some say it is like a big snake, and lives in the clefts of trees, emerging therefrom at night to climb the tree and call. No one has ever seen a *lwitaŵila*.

Ifiŵanda in Folklore

Ifiŵanda (demons) have their place in Lamba folklore, but the Lambas are very careful to distinguish between what they actually believe regarding these beings and what they relegate to the purely fanciful in their folklore. In one story an *ichiŵanda* is depicted as appearing in human form in a village and marrying a young woman who had refused every previous suitor. He would eat none of the food she prepared for him, and when eventually he was followed by the woman's father and mother into the forest it was found that he was in the habit of pulling off his arms and legs to attract the flies to the open flesh, and then gobbling up the flies which constituted his food. The story goes on at length to describe the plan which was necessary to make the *ichiŵanda* leave the village.

A far more common story, however, is the one entitled *Ichishimichishyo chyamuntunshi nechiŵanda*, "The Story of the Man and the Demon." In this story a man is depicted as digging a game-pit by himself. A demon came and offered to help him, on the understanding that each animal caught which pointed its head toward the demon's path should belong to him, the others to belong to the man. The man repeatedly tried to deceive the demon by turning the entrapped animals round, till at length the demon warned him that he would "fear what he would see." The next morning the man's mother-in-law went out gathering sticks, and fell into the covered game-pit. Great was her son-in-law's consternation when he found this, and as he was trying to get the old woman out the demon appeared and claimed her heart as his prize. The protestations of the man were unavailing; the demon sprang in, tore out the old woman's heart, and made off.

But these are mere folk-tales, as all the Lambas recognize. Apart from these ideas, they have a very real conception of demonism, one in which they thoroughly believe.

Ukuwilwa—Spirit-possession

We have already observed the Lamba belief that *ifiẁanda* may possess persons, and in doing so drive them mad; but among the Lambas there are three definite types of spirit-possession, *ukuwilwa*, which confer on those so afflicted a certain status in the tribe, one which generally leads to the acquisition of wealth. First there are the *ẁamoẁa*, who are said to be possessed by the spirits of *ifinkuwaila* (of which we shall treat immediately); then there are the *aẁayambo*, possessed by the spirits of Twa hunters; and lastly the most important, *ẁamukamwami*, possessed by the spirits of Lenje chiefs. All these are foreign spirits. They do not displace the original *imipashi* of the persons possessed; and although they may be of different or of no *umukoka* (clan), they do not change the *imikoka* of the persons possessed. We shall now deal with each of these types of spirit-possession in turn.

Ifinkuwaila

It is impossible to find an English word adequate to translate the Lamba *ichinkuwaila*, so I shall retain the Lamba word in all references to these beings so firmly believed in by the Lambas.

The *ifinkuwaila* are weird denizens of the forests and hills. They are said to resemble a man split down the centre, with one leg, one arm, one ear, one eye, one nostril, and so on. They are taller than human beings, and hop along on the one leg as they travel. Unclothed, they wander about the forests, hills, and *imishitu*, swamp forests, always carrying their *imisengelo*, reed sleeping mats, ready for use when night-time comes. They emerge from their hiding-places when they wish to catch *ẁamu-kamoẁa*, those whom they will possess. Their food is said to be *umufuẁa*, meal mixed with a little water, but not cooked. *Ifinku-waila* are believed to be male and female, old and young. The

251

young ones are said to have been heard in Mulumbwe's garden at Mukolwe's village, calling out, *Mama mpembeni-po*, "Mother, wait for me!" The reply given was, *Kawendeshya ili nalemo' kwita, wekawanda!* "Hurry up, I'm tired of calling you, you little demon!" This calling has been heard at night, early in the morning, and late in the evening.

Elsewhere in the bush in the early morning the *ifinkuwaila* are said to make noises imitating people; they say, *Wele wele wele wele!* At times, when walking through the bush in the late afternoon, one may hear in the distance the sound *ŋaŋwá ŋaŋwá ŋaŋwá*, and think it is a child crying. Then will come the mother's voice, comforting the young one, "*Rr . . . rr . . . rr . . .*" Some one not in the know will feel sure that he has come near to a village of people. He will become tired out with searching, and then he will hear the same sound again behind him. Then will he realize that it is an *ichinkuwaila*, and make off with speed.

The present Mushili stated that his elders recorded the singing of the *ifinkuwaila* as follows:

> *Pumputu, pumputu, ngatuwe,*
> *Fwenkashi shyakubweleshya.*
> *Twalukuchinda newakawa.*
>
> " Trip, trip, let us fall,
> Us sisters who will go back.
> We were dancing with those who will fall."

A Lamba, Paul Kaputula, related that one night, the rest of the people being away sleeping in the gardens (*mututungu*), he and Chiweshya and an old woman were the only ones sleeping in the village of Senkwe. Early in the morning they heard wailing voices approaching the village. They came out from the huts to see what was coming along the road, and heard a tremendous noise of persons passing along and through the village, but saw no one. In fear they went back into the huts, while the wailing passed on through the village and along the road to Kalimbata. When the people returned from their gardens they asked what the wailing had been about, for it was heard afar off. Those in the village said that they were *ifinkuwaila* which had passed.

Kawunda Nkana, an old woman from Mushili's village, related how, long ago in the winter-time (*pamwela*), when she was in Lenjeland, she saw *wamumpilwe* (another name for *ifinkuwaila*) early in the morning in a column passing in the sky from east to west. They were carrying *amasasa* and *imisengelo*. There were little ones, and the big ones were carrying loads and smoking.

One day when, travelling with a number of carriers, I was

passing the Chipese river I heard a lion roaring in a swamp forest about half a mile away. My carriers contradicted my assertion that it was a lion, and assured me that I heard an *ichinkuwaila* imitating a lion.

At the Minshinshye stream, a tributary of the Kafulafuta river, no native will pass the night if he can help it, for his sleep, they say, will be disturbed. He will hear *ifinkuwaila* passing to and fro, and calling, *Palalo'muntunshi pano*, "A human is sleeping here!" and others crying, *Mweŵame tupembeleni-po*, "Mates wait for us!" Men are too scared to sleep through that.

At times, when men are travelling after dark with dogs, the dogs get on the scent of these *ifinkuwaila*, who, it is said, call out, as they drive the dogs away, *Topoke'mbwa shyoŵe nshino wemuntunshi!* "Take away your dogs. Here they are, O human!" Anyone hearing that would run for his life in another direction, calling to his dogs.

Ifinkuwaila are thus invisible to all except the *ŵamoŵa* who are already possessed by one of them. Nevertheless, they like the company of human beings, and will call out to them when travelling, *Pembeni-po*, "Wait a bit!" When, however, a traveller stops, thinking it is his companion, no one will appear. A man may turn at hearing a cough behind him, but will see no one—it was an *ichinkuwaila* wanting his company. The Lambas have this saying of the *ichinkuwaila* making his lament over a deserted village: *Mwali ŵantu, mwali ŵantu, mwamwene muno, shimusachila-milundu, mwali ŵantu*, "There used to be people, there used to be people, here in the chief's village; it is overgrown like the veld; there used to be people."

Ŵamoŵa

It is said that if a man gets into a crowd of *ifinkuwaila* they do not touch him, but just move aside to let him pass. Should one of these beings, however, choose to possess the man, he strikes him in the face with his hand. On his return to the village the man becomes ill, and sees visions of beings in endless march across the heavens, going westward, arrayed in feather headdresses and carrying their sleeping mats. His companions say, *Mipishi waŵona*, "'Tis ghosts you have seen!" With others the visions are even more definite. They see the *ifinkuwaila* travelling in lines, some arrayed in white feather headdresses and some carrying drums. These catch up their quarries, take them off to

253

the hills, and to the beating of their drums dance the night through.

When the sick man describes this his companions will say, "Fetch an initiated *mukamoẁa*!" And one is fetched. He comes carrying his *inkombo shyamusoolo*, calabashes with long, straight handles. In them he has his medicine, a special medicine which the *ifinkuwaila* have told him how to dig and concoct. This medicine he gives to the patient to drink, together with *umufuẁa*, soaked meal, the food of the *ifinkuwaila*. After that there is a dance at night, for which the patient, who is now the initiate, pays the *mukamoẁa* as much as ten shillings. Then a new name is given to the initiate by the initiator, a name which is supposed to be that of the possessing *ichinkuwaila*. Such names are those of Mutoloẁale, a man of Mpokota's village, Kantumoya, another man from Mpokota, Mukalutoẁala, a woman from Mukungu's village, Funkwe, another woman from Mukungu, Kankobwe, a man from Mukungu, Mukankwashi, a man from Chikolwa's village, Lutwika, a man from Chimbalasepa's, and many others.

These spirits generally enter young men and women. It is immaterial of what *umukoka* (clan) the person may be, as the *ifinkuwaila* have no totemic clan distinctions themselves.

Dancing of Ẁamoẁa

When possessed by an *ichinkuwaila* a person is called *moẁa* (plural, *ẁamoẁa*) or, alternatively, *mukamoẁa* (spouse of the *moẁa*—plural, *ẁamukamoẁa*). These *ẁamoẁa* may not eat *imita* (barbel) or *imbishi* (zebra); they are taboo. This taboo lapses when the *ẁamoẁa* grow old and are treated with special medicine. These people have a certain standing in the community on account of their skill in dancing. As their services are much in demand at mourning and initiation ceremonies, and as they are paid for dancing, *ukuwilwa ẁumoẁa*, becoming possessed as a *moẁa*, is a lucrative business. Not only are they known for their dancing, but they are the composers and singers of a special type of song, called *inyimbo shyaẁamoẁa*. Their dances too are called after them, *ishyaẁamoẁa*, though they sometimes dance the *ifimbwasa* dances.

Here are four examples of songs composed by *ẁamoẁa*:

(1) *Inshima ilaẁa yakulya-po, kanshi ngaẁalishyo'lumbeta, nganailya-po neẁo . . . !*

  "Pap for food is to be desired ; if only they would blow the horn I would eat of it . . . !"

SPIRITISM

(2) *Aŵaŵakashi ukuchyenjela ŵapile'misenga, ŵashya kwaŵo, alaye mama !*

   " What a cunning wife this is, who has bailed out sprats, [but] left them at her home [with her mother]. Well, I never, Mother ! "

(3) *Ili yakolele'nsale'chimbayambaya chyalilele !*

   " When the hunger became severe the rejoicing in plenty went to sleep ! "

(4) *Akale panjingo'kwelawila, munshi yachiti nakukungama neŵo; ifyende'shitima nikumungwenyuko, munshi yachiti nakukungama neŵo !*

   " Long ago up and down I bobbed upon a bicycle, under a tree will I lean ; the way the train travels is with a sweep down the incline, under a tree will I lean ! "

Umulenda Waŵamoŵa

When a man becomes possessed as a *moŵa* he procures *insangwa*, rattles for the ankles, and an *uŵuyombo*, a dancing skirt made of a fringe of grass beads; and for the storing of these insignia of his profession he builds a special kind of shrine, called *umulenda waŵamoŵa*, the professional dancer's shrine. This type of *umulenda* is built as an *insama*, a shelter erected for bird-scaring, with open sides. A number of upright poles are planted in a circle, and a thatched conical roof erected above them. Often the trappings of the dance are left exposed to view beneath this shelter [1]

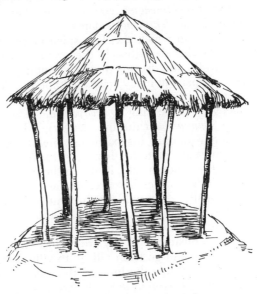

FIG. 75. UMULENDA WAŴAMOŴA

day and night, but no one would think of stealing them, for fear of death at the hands of the *ifinkuwaila*. There are no ceremonies gone through on erecting these *imilenda*, and the

[1] See Fig. 72.

255

whole work is carried out by the *moẁa* himself. The term *umulenda* is used in this connexion because the *ifinkuwaila* are looked upon as *imipashi yaẁamoẁa*, the spirits of the *ẁamoẁa*.

The term *ẁamoẁa* is of recent origin;[1] in older Lamba these people were called *amashyaẁe*, or *ẁamukupe*. The Kaonde people believe in similar possession, and they used to call the persons possessed *ututangu*, but now *aẁayembe*. The Lalas also believe in *ifinkuwaila* possession, and call the possessed *ẁachiwila*.

Ifinkuwaila are found in Lamba folklore, wherein they usually play some ridiculous part in scaring people.

Aẁayambo

The *aẁayambo* are the professional hunting dancers. It is believed that the spirits of dead Twa hunters, from the Ẁatwa or Lukanga Swamp region, take possession of certain Lamba men—never women. These possessed men are not necessarily themselves hunters, but they follow the profession of composing *inyimbo shyachinsengwe*, songs of the chase, and of singing and dancing in the *ichinsengwe* dances.

The way in which the Twa spirit takes possession of a man is much like that described in the case of the *ẁamoẁa*. One day a man falls ill, and dreams that he is singing *inyimbo shyachinsengwe* in the company of many *aẁapalu*, hunters. When morning dawns he actually begins to sing, and all those who hear him recognize his songs as those sung by *aẁayambo*. They send for an acknowledged *umuyambo* (hunting dancer), who comes that evening, bringing with him his particular medicine, *umusamu*, which he gives the sick man to drink. Afterward, that very night, an *ichinsengwe* dance is held, in which the patient takes part. Thereafter he will recover his strength, and be in a position to dance professionally. He will pay his initiator about ten shillings for his services on this occasion. The *aẁayambo* have the same food taboos as the *ẁamoẁa*, and, like the *ẁamoẁa*, make their dancing a lucrative business. They are requisitioned to dance at hunting celebrations, and go from village to village, receiving payment at each place. While the hunters themselves dance the *ichinsengwe* in honour of *mwishyaŋombe*, the *aẁayambo* dance it in honour of the Twa hunters by whose spirits they are possessed. These *aẁayambo* are dressed with rattles (*amansangwa*) on their ankles, a feather headdress (*ichingalangala*), and round the waist a grass-bead skirt, called *uẁuyombo*. The payment (*imfupo*) they receive is in beads, fowls, or money.

[1] It is said to have come into use about the year 1915.

SPIRITISM

Inyimbo shyachinsengwe are very numerous. Two of them were given when dealing with the ceremonies connected with the building of an *umulenda*. Here are two more examples:

(1) *Akale lukoso akale,*
Nali muyinga akale!
Nalukwipaya akale!

" Long, long ago,
I was a hunter long ago!
I used to kill long ago!"

(2) *Bwachya, wo wo ya ya!*
Pano bwachya, bwachyo'ŵushiku!
Aŵapalu ŵanama ŵaliweme, bwachya!
Walepaye'nama, katulya-po,
Bwachyo'ŵushiku!

" 'Tis dawn, *ta ra ra ra*!
Now 'tis dawn, the night has cleared!
Hunters of game are fine, 'tis dawn!
They kill game, and we eat of it.
The night has cleared!"

Isambwe

The *aŵayambo* are said to be able to give to hunters medicine to give them success in hunting, especially to favour them with finding the game out grazing, not lying in concealment. A bowl of this medicine is called *isambwe*. The *umuyambo* procures a certain root, and gives the hunter the following instructions: "Prepare a bark plate [*umukwa*], and put this powdered medicine upon it; then pour water over the medicine. Next tie together a bunch of leaves of the *umusamba*-tree, and make this resemble the tail of an animal. Then dip the bunch of leaves into the *isambwe*, and sprinkle your body all over with the medicine by continually flicking the bunch." One cannot help noticing the element of sympathetic magic which comes into this prescription. The bunch of leaves resembling an animal's tail is flicked or 'swished' in applying the medicine. This is the normal action of the tail of a grazing animal. Then there is a remarkable connexion between the terms used The whole operation is called *ukusamba*, to bathe. This same root is found in the word *isambwe*, indicating the particular bowl of medicine, and it is leaves from the *umusamba*-tree that are needed to make the switch. *Aŵalaye* (doctors) and *ŵamukamwami* (mediums) are also able to supply this medicine to hunters requiring it.

Like the term *moŵa*, the term *umuyambo* is of recent origin;[1]

[1] It is said to have been first used about 1910.

257

the older Lamba term was *uŵutwa*. The Lambas think it likely that both terms, *moŵa* and *umuyambo*, will eventually give place to new terms, according to the whim of the time.

Possession by the spirits of Twa hunters has nothing whatever to do with the *umukoka* (clan). The original hunters may have belonged to any of the clans, and Lamba men of any clan may become possessed. *Aŵayambo* take the names of the spirits which possess them, and it is significant that all the new names of *aŵayambo* are in the Twa language or are Twa names prefaced by the Lamba prefix *muka*, "the spouse of." Such names are Chinkunta (a village headman of commoner's clan), Tampila (a man at Luntantwe's village), Mukandoso (a man at Lupumpaula), Mukachyeso (a man of Kaŋonde), and Mukalyuni (a man of Malakata). All these men are *aŵayambo*.

Aŵami and Ŵamukamwami

The most influential of the spirit-possessed people in Lambaland are the *ŵamukamwami* (literally, the spouses of the chief). In Lenje and in Ila *mwami* is the term for 'chief,' and the *ŵamukamwami* of the Lambas are said to be possessed by the spirits of Lenje chiefs. Lamba chiefs are not known to *wila* (possess a person), not even in another tribe. The clan of the Lenje chiefs is that of the *aŵenatembo*, the wasp clan, but the same clan among the Lambas is a clan of commoners, and has no connexion with the *aŵami*. The Lambas say that they know that the *aŵami* are Lenje spirits, because the *mukamwami* gives the name of the deceased chief; *e.g.*, one will say, *Neŵo ninechitanda naisa*, "I, Chitanda, have come!" Chitanda was a prominent Lenje chief.

Ukuwilwa Kwaŵamukamwami

This is how the possession is said to come about. A person falls ill, and his illness gets worse and worse, no remedy giving any relief. He then begins to speak in a weird way, using the most extravagant language, telling of wonderful things he says he has seen. On hearing these things the villagers send for a prominent *mukamwami* to come and see the patient and prescribe the necessary medicine, for they have recognized that this is not an ordinary sickness, but probably possession by an *umwami*. When the *mukamwami* comes, and finds the patient singing, he says, *Ŵami aŵa!* "This is a Lenje chief!" He then orders the drums to be brought for the dancing. That night a great concourse of people comes together in order to greet "the chief," as the initiate is called, and to hear the matters he has to tell them. Then that man who had been so ill begins to speak with a loud voice. Sometimes he will climb on to the *ichitupa* (loft) of the house to speak. He says, "I have come from Chitanda's village; I am Chitanda himself. I am moving my residence from that country ; I have come here to my relatives; so I have caught this my servant [indicating himself]. Furthermore, behind me I have left many pestilences—they are coming. Behind are small-pox and locusts. All of these [latter] are coming to eat your food-stuffs; they are my soldiers, with which I travel." On hearing that fear takes hold upon the people, and they all bring offerings (*imilambu*) to the chief, to prevent those disasters from coming upon them. Then the chief says, " It is well, my children. I have warded off the locusts, and the smallpox too I have warded off; I shall cause them to pass round you to your neighbours; maybe they will go to the Luapula river and destroy the people there."

In the morning the new *mukamwami* will go out and travel through the gardens, accompanied by many people, who keep up a chorus of *lululu*-ing, calling out, "*Aẇami* are going through the gardens, warding off the locusts." In this fashion the *muka-mwami* goes from village to village through the country; he pro-vides medicine for drinking and for washing lest the people should contract smallpox.

It is one of the most lucrative practices of the *ẇamukamwami* to foretell the coming of evils, which they claim to be able to control, in order that the people may bring them offerings to induce them to exert their power. It can readily be understood that these practitioners are generally held in awe by the people, and that they are in great demand when any real calamity threatens.

The old *mukamwami* who pronounced the new initiate as pos-sessed of an *umwami* is the one who instructs him in the herbal lore necessary to his trade, and initiates him into the mysteries of prophecy. The initiate will pay his initiator as much as the value of a gun for his services.

Appearance of a Mukamwami

The *mukamwami* does not cut his hair; he plaits it so that it hangs down in tassels all round his head, freely anointed with castor-oil and red ochre (*ulushila*). He also wears *impande*, as a symbol of chieftainship. These are generally discs carved from elephant tusk, and attached to a string encircling the head. The genuine *impande*, cut from the huge shell, used to be obtained by trade from the Mbundu traders, but are becoming increasingly rare now among the Lambas. A circlet of threaded cowrie-shells (*imiŵela*) is also worn on the head, and ivory bracelets (*amakoosa*) on both arms. A woman *mukamwami* may also wear *insambo*, bracelets of twisted wire. Calico is worn round the waist and over the shoulders. The *mukamwami* observes the same food taboos as the *moŵa* and the *umuyambo*. In addition he may not eat *inshima* prepared by *aŵanichye*, young people, but only that made by *aŵakulu*, elders. When travelling the *mukamwami* carries over his shoulder a small knob-headed ornamental axe, called *impompwe*, *imbafi*, or *ichiŵanga*, and also his *akasako*, a long staff with beads wound round the centre. This is his sign of office. His sleeping mat, blankets, and other belongings are carried by his *chipyaila*, or by others who are acting as his servants.

Chipyaila

The *chipyaila* is a youth who enters the employ of a *mukamwami*. He shares a proportion of the 'spoils' gained by his master when a journey is undertaken. His work consists in looking after the *akapeshi*, to protect it from the termites, in sweeping the house of the *umulenda*, or, as it is called in Lenje, *ichyonde*, and in carrying the *akapeshi* on journeys. The *ichyonde* is a small lean-to house (*inkunka*), in which are kept the *akapeshi* and other paraphernalia of the *mukamwami*, and in which sleeps the *chipyaila*. The term *chipyaila* is derived from *ukupyaila*, to sweep. A *chipyaila* never becomes a *mukamwami*.

Akapeshi Kaŵami

The *akapeshi* is a small grass basket (*ichilukwa*) with a support beneath it (*ishyula*), like that of a beer-basket (*intumbe*). This basket, *akapeshi kaŵami*, is the receptacle for the offerings (*imilambu*) of the people. These gifts, whether of beads or money, are placed in the basket, which is wrapped up in a piece of red calico (*ichimbushi*) such as used to be obtained from the Mbundu traders, and carried on the head of the *chipyaila* as the *mukamwami*, accompanied by a concourse of people, goes from village to village. This *akapeshi* is reverenced by the people as though it contained the spirit of the *umwami*, or, as the Lambas express it, *Ŵalachichindika'ti ŵami*, "They reverence it, believing it to be the *umwami*."

Consultation

Occasionally, at the time of the new moon, a *mukamwami* is heard to scold to himself or to his wife in the house at night.

SPIRITISM

The people say, *W̱amukamwami pano w̱alukubwa muŋanda*, "The *mukamwami* is now 'popping' in the house." *Ukubwa* is the term used of fish 'popping' in a still river, and is used in this connexion and in that of the 'popping' out of ejaculatory information at intervals by the *mukamwami*. Sometimes he will imitate the roar of a lion. Then they will hear him say, "This year you will see no harvest, and the rain will not fall, because you do not humble yourselves [*lambila*] before the *aw̱ami*. And here I have in my hand smallpox and disease, birds and locusts. I shall let them out." On hearing that many of the people leave their huts and assemble at the prophet's hut to beg for pardon (*ukusaasa*).

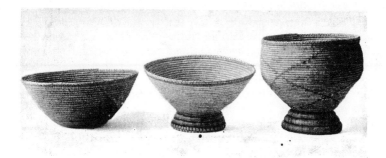

FIG. 76. ICHILUKWA, AKAPESHI, AND INTUMBE
Photo by W. Paff

Then, when they have satisfied him with offerings, the *mukamwami* takes out some *umusamu* and gives it to them, saying, "Take and pound this medicine, and mix it with your seed corn [*amasaka*]; then sow, and you will see an abundant harvest." And this rejoices the hearts of the people.

The *mukamwami* claims power over the elements. It is said that when a great storm of wind and rain comes, if there is an *umwami* in the village he rushes out of his hut, scolding (*pata*), disregarding the fact that he is getting drenched through, and shouts out, *Tamubwene, mwew̱ashya, mwe mulukupichishya, w̱oneni ifi w̱alukuchita'w̱ami!* "Don't you see, ye slaves, ye who are arguing, see what the *aw̱ami* are doing?" Every one on hearing these boastful words is afraid, and all rush out from their huts, uttering the shrill *impundu*, praising the *umwami* and uttering his name. "Ward off this wind, *shikulu* [lord]," they plead, "that it kill us not." Again they all utter the *impundu*. Then, when they see that the hurricane has passed, they say, "Indeed our

261

umwami has helped us to-day; he has saved us. Were it not for him all our huts would have been blown down!"

Rain-prophet

When the rain is long delayed, or when that which falls is insufficient, the people say, *Aŵami ŵakana kwiulu*, "The *aŵami* have refused in heaven!" When consulted the *mukamwami* says, "First build an *umulenda*, and let us put therein the *akapeshi kaŵami*; then you will see the rain." They set to work and build the *umulenda*, and the prophet says, "Now, my children, the rain is near!" If still the rain holds off, the *mukamwami* says, *Iseni mulukuŵomba!* "Come and humble yourselves!" *Ŵomba* is a term used in much the same way as *lambila* and *saasa*. It indicates grovelling servility, and is what is done by a defeated enemy. *Ukuŵomba kuŵami* can, then, hardly be taken as equivalent to worshipping the *aŵami*, but rather as humbling oneself before the *aŵami*. When thus called by the prophet many go and humble themselves ; but the rain still holds off. Then one day the rain comes, and far and near it is heard that rain has fallen at such and such a village, where the *mukamwami* lives; and people flock there with their gifts to beg for rain from the *aŵami*.

Sometimes the *mukamwami* travels from village to village prophesying rain. He may do this for as long as two months at a time, going all through Mushili's country and as far as the Congo, everywhere collecting offerings of money and kind. All of this goes to increase the wealth he amasses.

Hunting-prophet

Sometimes the *mukamwami* will reach a certain village and say, "Don't you eat meat here in this village?" The answer may be, "No, *shikulu*, we get no meat here." Thereupon the *mukamwami* tells them all to bring their guns. The guns are all brought, and the *mukamwami* stacks them together near to a fire. He then goes and picks a quantity of leaves, which are his special *umusamu*, throws them on to the fire, and blows the smoke produced over the pile of weapons. He then asks, "Who is there here who wants to kill an eland ?" Some one answers, "I want to kill an eland!" He asks again, "How many eland do you want to kill?" The reply may be, "Three, *shikulu*!" Then the *mukamwami* gives him three leaves, and says, "Smoke them! When you have smoked these three leaves you will kill three eland!"

SPIRITISM

In the same way he distributes leaves sufficient for everybody. The people in return hand over money to him. When he has finished distributing the leaves he moves on elsewhere. Those who remain, however, have no success in hunting; their money has been thrown away. By such methods of deceit the ŵamukamwami amass their wealth, playing on the credulity of the people, and then returning home to enjoy their ill-gotten gains.

Ukuŵomba

The ŵamukamwami have established themselves in the country as prophets, oracles, and mediums for the spirits of the aŵami to such an extent that people come often from a great distance to consult them. These consultations are carried out with certain formalities, and are called ukuŵomba, the term already discussed as indicating a servile submission to the spirit of the deceased Lenje chief. On these occasions the mukamwami remains silent in his house, but his assistants, aŵantu ŵamilimo, and his chipyaila keep up a continual shouting (ukuwela) during the night, and lishye'mpundu, utter that shrill sound which resembles lululululu! Meanwhile, the people are gathered in the court (uluŵansa) outside the house of the oracle. The mukamwami does not appear outside. From time to time his assistants sing. There seems to be but one definite ulwimbo lwakuŵomba, song of the consultations; it is this:

> Nalaŵila lukoso,
> Nikaseŵa, aŵene ŵankanga,
> Yo!
> " I have merely spoken,
> I, Kaseŵa, Nkanga herself,
> Yo!"

When they have finished singing the mukamwami will begin his business. For a time he will consider the cases brought before him; then there will be singing again, and after that more cases. Sometimes the aid of the mukamwami is sought because the birds are eating the corn. The people will gather at the door, and beg him to forbid the birds to eat the corn. If this is done, on the next morning they go through the gardens, as has been already described, carrying the akapeshi, and forbidding the birds. In some cases the mukamwami enters his ichyonde for consultation. The chipyaila acts as his mouthpiece outside the door to communicate to the people what he says, and to give him the people's reply.

263

At times there is no singing, only the consultation and the *impundu*. But all is invariably carried out at night.

Birth-prophet

Quite commonly people come to ask for children, and the *mukamwami*, who has ready-prepared medicines of every kind in his house, gives them *umusamu* to drink, with the promise that they will have a child. For this ample payment is made, and if perchance (though this seldom occurs) a child is born additional money is claimed by the *mukamwami*. The child is called *katungu*, and the *mukamwami* will address him as *umwana wabwanga* (child of the charm). The same is done by the *aŵalaye*.

Sometimes the *mukamwami* calls or sends out his *chipyaila* to call the people, saying, "I know that you people have matters; come and ask me!" Then a woman and her husband will come and sit in the doorway of his hut, and say, "As for us, our children die as soon as they are born." The *mukamwami* says, "I shall give you some *umusamu*, of which you are both to drink, and then your children which will be born will be strong." They move away for the next to come, maybe a woman who says, "I have some internal trouble [*ndi mulwele mumala*] and do not give birth." To her he gives some *umusamu*. The *umusamu* of the *aŵami* is called *ichitondo*. All of these supplicants place money, beads, or calico on the floor of the hut for the *mukamwami* to take.

They will pay as much as five shillings for childbirth medicine; for success in hunting, for the driving off of birds from the corn, or for the prevention of locusts each person may pay a shilling. For the bringing of rain much more is collected. In any one village the chief will pay as much as five shillings, each adult a shilling, and each child the equivalent of sixpence.

A Lucrative Profession

It is only too well known in Lambaland that the *ŵamukamwami* 'get fat' on the credulity of the people. Some ten years ago I knew a lazy young man of the name of Lumina, who used to act as mail-carrier for the mission, and who worked so badly that his services had to be dispensed with. On one occasion he was one of a squad of natives carrying boxes of bricks from a kiln to a new building. He was found to have but three half-bricks in his box, and when detected dropped the box and went home. I think that was the last stroke of 'work' he did, for shortly afterward he fell ill, visited by the spirit of a Lenje chief, and recovered to find himself a *mukamwami*. For ten years he has never done any real work, yet I hear he has bought a bicycle now for £7 10s., and that is no little wealth for a Lamba.

After a tour round the country the *mukamwami* often settles in his own village. Sometimes he is accompanied by a number of people who have come to hoe his gardens for him, as they had been unable to give any donation in money or kind to his funds. These *ẃamukamwami* may be of either sex. Some are the owners of their own villages, as, for instance, Mukamwami, a Ŵulima chief on the Mpongwe river, Mukamwami Umwanakashi, a Lenje chieftainess on the Chisangwa river, near Lwamala, Mukachintu, a Lenje chieftainess on the Kasu river, Chiẃatata, a Lamba chieftainess who died in 1922, near Kachyeya, the mother of Stephen Lutongamina, and Mukaluẃumba, a Lamba chieftainess from the Kafuẃu river, near Old Ndola. Others are commoners, as, for instance, Lumina, an *umwinanguni*, a man from Chibweshya, Kanuŋuna, an *umwinatembo*, a man from Katanga's village who died in 1924, and Mwanamashyaẃe, an *umwinansofu*, a man from Kachyule.

The Spouse of the Spirit

Male *ẃamukamwami* usually marry but one wife. Many female mediums do not marry at all, as they consider the *umwami* to be their husband. It is significant that only male *aẃami* take possession of female *ẃamukamwami*, while both male and female *aẃami* enter male *ẃamukamwami*, and the men are permitted to marry in the ordinary way. Sometimes a married woman becomes possessed, and then her marriage is dissolved. Here is an instance. Chiẃatata was married to a man named Chipotela, and gave birth to Lutongamina (male), Mutakula (male), Kalendu (female), and Chyembo (female). Then she became possessed (*ukuwilwa*), and the marriage was dissolved, for, she said, "Now I am married to the *aẃami*." So she lived alone. Her husband went elsewhere, and married again. The children remained in the village with their mother. In such a case it is said that a woman could not refuse the *umwami*, lest she should die. Some women, who are not respected as true *ẃamukamwami*, do marry.

A Lenje chief, named Musaka, died, and his spirit was said to have entered a youth named Kaẃunda, who became a *mukamwami*, and was called Mukamusaka (the spouse of Musaka). Kaẃunda feared the chaffing of his old companions, who had come under Christian influence, and his power waned through *insoni*, a feeling of bashfulness. He practised less and less, then took the name of Jim. His friends called him Longwani ("Long One"), but in self-depreciation he dubbed himself Jimu Half, because of his small stature. He married a woman named Sula, of Katanga's village, but failed to have any children, and this caused him considerable embarrassment. He has now become a Christian, and has abandoned all his previous practices.

Some *aŵami* are reputed to enter persons *mukutushishya-mo*, in order to rest therein, and then to pass on. There are thus some who are *ŵamukamwami* only temporarily. It has also been known that one *umwami* has taken possession of more than one person at the same time. This is akin to the spiritual influence which we noticed to be an essential element in the Lamba belief in reincarnation, not the whole spirit, but a kind of afflatus taking possession of the person. The spirit of the Lenje chief Chitanda is said to possess a man at Mwefyeni, on the Lufuŵu river, and also a woman at Kalumbwe, in the Lala country.

From time to time the *mukamwami*, whether man or woman, brews beer (*kumbo'bwalwa*) in honour of the *umwami* which is possessing him. He calls together the people to the beer-drink; and after the drinking is over the *mukamwami* dons his *uŵuyombo* (dancing skirt) and the *insangwa* (rattles). The *insangwa* are fastened round the calves of his legs; on each leg are four sticks, on each of which are threaded four rattles, making a total of thirty-two. Holding his ornamental dancing axe (*impompwe*), the *mukamwami* now commences to dance the *ichimbwasa*. In the middle of the court (*uluŵansa*) is a grass mat (*isasa*); on this is placed the *akapeshi*, on top of which is the *akasako*, or wand of office. The people bring offerings of beads. This is called *taila*. They do not give the beads into the hand of the *mukamwami*, but place them in the *akapeshi*.

Female *ŵamukamwami* sometimes dance for payment at initiation ceremonies, *ifisungu*; the dance in which they take the leading part is the *ichimbwasa*.

In addition to the medical prescriptions of the type already described, the *ŵamukamwami* are able to prepare *ubwanga bwashiŵuwungu*, the charm for protecting the gardens, as are the *aŵalaye*. This is dealt with under the subject of "Ubwanga" in Chapter XVIII.

There is an important rule which must be observed when with a *mukamwami*—no one must step on or over his shadow, for it is reckoned to be the shadow of the *umwami*, who is a chief, and such action would be insulting to a chief.

Prophecies

Though generally using the Lamba term itself when referring to the *ŵamukamwami*, I have sometimes used the terms 'prophet' and 'medium.' Such a man without doubt acts the part of a medium in conveying to people the wishes of the spirit possessing him, but I think the term 'prophet' is perhaps the more significant of the two. There are several well-known prophecies of the *ŵamukamwami* which are said to have been fulfilled. Long, long ago it is said that they predicted, *Mukanwo'mukalo'mo,* "You will all drink in one well!" meaning that race-distinction would be lost. Now that the white men have come into the country, and inter-tribal fighting has ceased, this prophecy has come true. Another has it, *Nangaŵa'ti tulikele fino, kulukutulila kumbonshi aŵantu ŵamutongola ukupinta ŵonse sela!* "Although we are living thus now, there are coming from the west loadsmen all fully loaded!" Many, many people have entered Lambaland with the opening up of the mines, but not from the west. And now they prophesy that the time will come when the white men will 'roll up' again their railway-line, and take their departure with it back to the sea from whence they came!

Ifimpelampela

It is not out of place, in a consideration of the Lamba beliefs concerning the spiritual world, to close with a short account of the belief in the possibility of transmutation. We shall see how this is connected with their conception of the workings of witch-craft; but they relate as historical certainties some of these trans-mutations, and treat them all as *ifimpelampela*, miracles. There are four of which I have heard: (1) a man turning into a stamp-block or mortar, (2) people turning into long grass, (3) people turning into trees, and (4) a man turning into a pheasant.

(1) The Chikunda raiders came to a certain village early one morning, while it was still dark. All the young men rushed out and made off, shouting that the enemy was upon them. But the old chief of the village could not run. He came out of his hut, stood in the centre of the village, and turned into an *ichinu*, a hollowed log, stood upright, in which mealies are stamped. When the raiders arrived they knocked over the stamp-block and stamped on its side, shouting, "The demons have gone off with haste and left a stamp-block!" and passed on. The chief resumed his own form, re-entered his hut, and began to smoke. Only his back was sore, where they had trodden on him. In the evening

his 'children' all returned, and he recounted to them what had happened. They all marvelled at him.

(2) Swahili raiders came to the village of Lumina, near Nsakanya, but the chief Lumina was forewarned, and with all his people rose very early in the morning and left the village. Shortly afterward the raiders reached the village, and, seeing that the people had gone, followed hot-foot on their tracks. Presently they espied their quarry crossing a plain, and doubled their speed to catch them. Lumina looked up and saw them coming, and called together his people. They came together, each with a heavy load of goods, and they changed into clumps of long grass. The raiders arrived and searched everywhere, without avail; they found no traces of them. Then they gave up the search and returned, saying, "Lumina is too clever for us!" Then the grass clumps (*imisanse*) changed back into people, and all returned to their village. Lumina died about 1900.

(3) There is a story of people turning into trees when pursued by their enemies, but I have not been able to ascertain the locality or occasion of this 'miracle.'

(4) A man named Lyongoli, from near Lesa's village, was once entrapped by the enemy in his own fenced garden. He saw no other way of escape, and so turned himself into a pheasant, flew up with a whirr, and went and settled in the plain. All who saw it were amazed. His own people who were with him said, *Walyongoli ŵaaluka musokoshi, fweŵaŵyaŵo ŵatushila!* "Lyongoli has changed into a pheasant, and left us, his companions, behind." Lyongoli died about 1924.

CHAPTER XVI

UŴULAYE—THE RÔLE OF THE DOCTOR

Professions

In the previous chapter we dealt with three distinct professions, those of the *moŵa*, the *umuyambo*, and the *mukamwami*, professions of considerable status in the tribe, professions which carry with them considerable authority and no little opportunity of acquiring wealth. These professions are the result of spirit-possession, *ukuwilwa* ; those concerned have no choice—at least, they are believed to have no choice—in the taking up of their profession. But involved in the social structure of the Lamba people are certain other professions which are entered upon by deliberate choice. Four of these are of such importance as to demand special individual treatment. Of the four, three carry with them very considerable social standing in the tribe, and one considerable social degradation and abhorrence. They are the professions of (1) *umulaye*, the doctor or diviner, (2) *imfwiti*, the witch or wizard, (3) *umupalu*, the hunter, and (4) *umufushi*, the blacksmith. There are many minor professions of necessity carried on in village and tribal life, but none of these commands any special respect from the people. These four professions, which will now be considered in turn, may be learnt by anyone desiring to enter them and willing to pay the price for initiation into the mysteries. For mysteries there are in each one of these, mysteries which touch upon the realm of spiritism in some cases, but principally upon that other realm which plays so large a part in Bantu religion, the realm of dynamism, that hidden power in nature which only the initiated may tap with impunity.

Umulaye

In the discussion of the character and work of the *umulaye*, or, as he is also called by the Lambas, the *iŋanga*, the assurance was given that there is no *umupashi waŵulaye*, spirit of divination or doctorship, but that *aŵene ŵalasalulula*, men choose for themselves, and learn the profession. It is difficult to find a satisfactory derivation for the term *umulaye*, though it has been given as fróm the word *laya*, promise, summon, for in Lambaland the doctor never looks for his patients, nor practises his healing arts until sent for; he answers the summons, he promises to come when called. In a Lamba village a man could break his leg next door to the doctor's house, but the doctor would not move a finger to apply any remedy until he was called by the patient or by his relatives. Another significance of the term *laya* is 'make an appointment,' and the Lamba explains the connexion of this with *umulaye* by saying that when anyone goes to fetch the doctor *mukuŵuka* (in order to smell out a witch), the doctor remains to make ready his things, and does not come till the next day, so as to divert suspicion from the one who called him. The other term, *iŋanga*, is clearly connected with the terms *ubwanga* and *ichyanga*, which, as we shall see presently, indicate charms variously used to ensure good fortune, protection, or guidance, and may even be used of poisons for detecting witchcraft or charms to kill thieves. The *iŋanga*, then, is one who has the knowledge and power of preparing and administering these charms, bound up as they are with dynamic belief.

Learning the Profession

If a young man desires to enter the profession of a doctor he will come to some well-known *umulaye* and say, *Naisa mweŵachiŵinda, ndukwenda nenu, munsambishye uŵulaye*, "I have come, O great doctor. I would travel with you, that you may teach me the art of divining!" If the doctor agrees the young man becomes his disciple. The first thing he is taught is *ukuŵuka kumupini*, to divine by means of an axe-handle. Should the *umulaye* be called in to prescribe for some one suffering from chronic headache, he will send his new pupil, saying, "Go and divine, but, remember, do not diagnose the case as one of demon interference; you must say it is his *umupashi* [spirit], which is angry because light beer [*ifisunga*] has not been brewed in his honour." Such are the instructions the pupil gets continually. The Lambas say, *Ichiŵanda tachikatwa kumulaye umwanichye*, "A demon is not caught by a young doctor!"

Ukuŵuka Kumupini

When the young doctor reaches the village he finds that the interested friends and relatives of the sick man have already congregated in his hut. The patient is lying on his bed, and they squat on the floor around, some sitting on his bed. The *umulaye* sits down just within the doorway, and places his axe on the floor in front of him, the axe-head toward himself and the handle (*umupini*) pointing toward the patient. Then those who have summoned him, the chief one of whom may be the sick man's mother, begin to put forward the usual questions for the doctor's divination. This is called *ukusanshila*. The first question may be, "Is it an *ichiŵanda* which has come to this young man?" On hearing the question, the doctor repeatedly strikes the axe-handle with the under-side of his closed fist, as though to hammer it firmly into the ground; he then rubs the axe-handle backward and forward. It has not stuck tight to the ground, and he says, "It is not a demon; *ubwanga bwakana* [the charm has replied in the negative]." With the Lamba *umulaye* divining seems to be dependent upon the efficiency of the *ubwanga* of which he has control. As will be seen presently, *ubwanga*, though often referred to by the term 'charm,' really signifies much more; it is inseparably connected with the belief in dynamism.

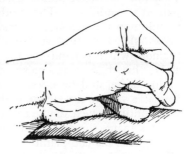

FIG. 77. DIVINING BY MEANS OF THE AXE-HANDLE

The freedom of movement of the *umupini* having demonstrated that the *ubwanga* "has not caught," the questioner puts forward another question (*ukusanshila*). "Is it perchance his *umupashi* which is angry?" The doctor says, "Just listen whether his *umupashi* is angry or not." He then proceeds to knock with his knuckles on the axe-head, making as though to pull the axe up; again he strikes the axe with the under-side of his clenched fist, this time upon the flat of the blade. Then he pretends to try to tear up the axe-head by catching it with his fingers, wrenching at it unsuccessfully. In the eyes of the credulous audience the axe is no longer loose; it is held tightly to the ground by the power of the *ubwanga*. *Ubwanga bwaikata*, "The charm has caught!" Clearly it is the *umupashi* who is offended, and who has caused the illness of the young man. The wrath of the *umupashi* must be appeased. There is no need for medicines or medical treatment, so the doctor says, "Brew *ifisunga* [light beer], and make your peace with the spirit to-day, and the young man will recover. *Epo chyambule'chyanga popele apa!* It is just here that the charm has caught on!" He warns the people, however, that if they do not brew the *ifisunga* quickly the man will die. Again he pretends to wrench with all his might at the axe, but it will not come away. Then he says, "Give me *ichyakulambulo' bwanga* [an offering for the charm], that I may go." The people thereupon make an offering for his services. Immediately the *ubwanga* lets go the axe—it is loose; and the doctor takes it up and goes his way.

Ukuŵuka Kumiseŵe

It very often happens that the patient gets no better for all these instructions. The light beer has been brewed and the *umupashi* has been honoured, but there is no difference in the patient's condition. The mother of the sick man then goes off to summon the *umulaye umukulu*, the fully qualified doctor, that he should come and ascertain if perchance it is an *ichiŵanda* (demon) which is troubling her son. He does not come immediately; his dignity and position do not permit him to exercise undue haste, and he does not want the villagers to connect the woman's visit to his village with his own visit to her village. He waits until the next day. Even then he does not go to the hut of the sick man; the doctor does not need to see his patient in order to diagnose his complaint. When he reaches the village he goes off to a spot in the bush a little distance away. He takes with him his pupil, and maybe the father and mother of the patient, but no one else. He is going to *ŵuka kumiseŵe*, divine by means of the rattles, and to *sanshile'miseŵe*, put the questions to the rattles; this he will do by himself. His pupil makes a small clearing (*uluŵansa*), scuffling away the grass and small bushes with a hoe borrowed from the village; he next brings a little water in a small pot, puts some *umusamu* in the water, and sets the pot on an *inkoshyanya*, a ring of grass set on their heads by the natives to assist them in carrying water-pots, firewood, and loads of all kinds. He then sets on end one horn. Meanwhile, the *umulaye* himself is sitting on the ground, and begins to rattle one *umuseŵe*. The mother of the sick man begins to *sanshila*, and says, "My child is dying, and will not recover." Thereupon the *umulaye* says, "Just listen; she is telling you!" He shakes his rattle, and listens to it with his head on one side. "She says her child is dying!" And he bends over the pot of water and gazes into it. Then he says, "No, he is not going to die; but it is witches that I see sporting in the water!" and adds, "It is all right, I shall speak with them at night, lest they should kill him."

After this he searches for the appropriate *umusamu*, a portion of which he administers to the patient as a draught, using another portion to foment his body (*china*). This medical treatment is not intended to cure the patient, but to strengthen the weakened body. The doctor depends on other means for the cure; he simply uses herbs in order to keep the patient alive until the effect of the witchcraft has been removed. Without doubt, however, in many cases these *aŵalaye* use really effective remedies, which directly contribute to the patient's recovery.

When night has fallen the *umulaye* climbs an *ichyulu*, a great anthill, and shouts out, "You, O witch, who are in this village, I see you! It is my demand that you loosen the grip [*sunsulula*] which you have on this young man. If you kill him, I too shall not go away. I am waiting to kill you! I saw you last night walking about this village; it was you I saw." On hearing that everybody is afraid, believing that the *umulaye* has seen the witch.

In the morning the doctor goes back home to his village, and his pupil, the young doctor, goes from time to time to visit the sick man. When he is recovered a handsome offering (*ichilambu*) is made. Should the patient die, however, the doctor is summoned to catch the witch or wizard whom he saw in the first instance. The procedure in this case will be fully dealt with when we consider the whole subject of witchcraft. For attention to the sick man the doctor is paid anything from two to ten shillings in cash or in kind. As we have said, the *umulaye* has considerable real knowledge of herbal remedies, but it is important to realize that these are dispensed with a view to strengthening the man who has become weakened by sickness; the doctor holds out no hope of recovery unless the offended spirit is appeased, or the evil-working witch or wizard is frightened enough to remove the power of his evil charms, or some other power for ill is countered.

During his period of learning and probation the pupil is taught by the older *umulaye* the different types of herbs, their preparation, and their uses; and his daily association with his master teaches him all the arts of the diviner. When he has completed his training, he pays his teacher as much as £2 or a gun, and then leaves him, to set up on his own.

Ukufishya Kuŵulaye

Before leaving his master, however, there is one important rite which has to be performed. This is called *ukufishya kuŵulaye*, bringing into the profession of doctor, and is gone through by all who aspire to the title of *umulaye wachishyala*, doctor of the instrument bag, *ichishyala* being the name applied to the bag containing the doctor's paraphernalia. Such a doctor must have the sign of having killed a man, for he will be called for the detection of witches. Doctors who do not aspire to this eminence are called *aẇalaye ẇakankwese*, doctors of the circling of the axe-handle, for they divine by means of the *umupini*, or with one *umuseẇe* only.

When the old *umulaye* is summoned to another village in order to *ẇuka* (divine) he takes with him the younger man, and maybe diagnoses the case as one of an *ichiẇanda* (demon). In the morning they, with their attendants, go to the grave of the person whose *ichiẇanda* has been causing the trouble. The older man will give his *ulusengo* (horn) into the right hand of the younger man and his *umuchila* (zebra-tail switch) into his left. The younger man now goes ahead and sticks the *ulusengo* into the grave, saying, *Naikata mweẇakalume*, "I have caught you, ye slaves!" The attendants now come and dig up the grave in the way described already for 'settling' an *ichiẇanda*. When the body is reached the workers come out from the grave; the two *aẇalaye* enter, and take out the body to give it to the assistants. The assistants now cut up the body, the two *aẇalaye* sitting and looking on. When the head is cut off the old *umulaye* takes it, cuts off the back of the skull (*akabwangala*) with his axe, and cleans out any of the brain still adhering, leaving a clean bowl. This he gives to the younger *umulaye*, saying, *Lelo wafika*, "To-day you have arrived." After this the younger man superintends the work of burning the remains of the body in the approved fashion, while the older man watches him. In this way he is fully initiated. The *akabwangala* he will carry in his *ichisoko* (bag), and from it cut off bits to make the *umutaḥu* (medicine for exorcizing) when it is needed.

During his time of probation a learner will gradually amass sufficient money to make the necessary payment to his teacher, as it is an understood thing that he keeps the offerings made to him when he is sent by the master-doctor to divine.

Cause of Sickness

Among the Lambas there is no natural death, and no illness due to natural causes. All illness, apart from that which results in the *ukuwilwa* (spirit-possession) of the *ẇamukamwami*, the *ẇamoẇa*, and the *aẇayambo*, is attributed to one of four causes:

(1) the anger of the *imipashi*, (2) bewitching by *imfwiti*, (3) capture by *ifiŵanda*, and (4) the direct dealing of Lesa.

(1) As we have already noticed, the resentment of the *umupashi* (spirit of the departed) is roused if the owner does not erect the *umulenda* (spirit hut), but allows the *inkombo* (gourds) representing the spirit to lie outside, for the spirit argues, "It is we who are then sleeping outside." The cure of a person suffering as a result of this negligence depends upon the carrying out of the necessary duties. Beer has to be brewed, people summoned to honour the *umupashi*, the *umulenda* built, and the *inkombo* placed therein. The result anticipated is the recovery of the sick person. The resentment of the *umupashi* is also roused if the periodical brewing of *ifisunga* (light beer) is not carried out. The spirit must not be neglected.

(2) If the sickness is persistent the evil machinations of a witch or wizard are suspected. Jealousy or enmity or the desire for revenge may be the cause behind the practice of witchcraft. We have already described how the *umulaye* shouts from the anthill to frighten the witch into undoing the spell she has cast. The sickness is but the outward manifestation of the hidden power; it is useless to depend upon medicines; the root cause must be sought and eradicated.

(3) The illness may be caused by an *ichiŵanda* (demon) punishing a man who has secretly indulged in unnatural vice, anti-social evil. If the man does not confess when confronted by the accusation of the *umulaye*, madness is the expected result. This matter was dealt with when the whole question of the *ichiŵanda* was considered. It is significant that this belief in interference by a demon is a strong incentive to the confession of rape, incest, or murder.

(4) Such scourges as smallpox, Kafir pox, leprosy, and 'Spanish influenza' are often said to be sent by Lesa. For the Lambas there is no way of pleading with Lesa for a cessation of these evils; the *umulaye* can prescribe no remedy; they must have their way.

Medical Treatment

In a few cases only the doctor does not divine (*ŵuka*), but uses some type of medicinal treatment. For instance, some *aŵalaye* are said to treat persons struck by lightning, giving them medicine to drink (*ukupuupulula'ŵantu*) even when they are unconscious. In cases of barrenness in women (*iŋumba*) the doctor prepares certain roots and gives a potion to the woman to drink. This medicine is usually composed of stamped roots mixed with meal and then heated to the consistency of *uŵusunga*; it is taken every day. This medicinal gruel is placed in a calabash (*insungo*) and hung above the doorway. Should she after such treatment bear a son, she would have to make a substantial payment to the doctor, perhaps as much as a gun. Such a child is called *katungu*, or *lukamfi*, and is addressed by the *umulaye* as *umwana wabwanga*. If the treatment had no satisfactory result no payment at all would be made. Generally if a mother loses each child in infancy the doctor will divine for possible witchcraft, but sometimes it is found that the woman is suffering from some internal disease, in which case the *umulaye* prescribes a medicine.

Though medicine is usually administered in the form of a drink (*nwinshya*), certain ailments are treated by hot fomentation (*china*). Various medicinal leaves are placed in a pot of water, which is heated, but not to boiling-point. The wet leaves are taken out and repeatedly pressed against the affected part, being dipped in the water again and again when they have become dry. This type of treatment is not confined to *aŵalaye*; numbers of ordinary folk know how to foment.

Detection of a Thief

When some article of value is missing the village headman says, "Bring the *chimulonda*. Let it come and help us!" Thereupon the *umulaye* is summoned to come with the *chimulonda*,[1] a long sable antelope horn filled with a certain powerful medicine. When he arrives one of the villagers takes hold of the horn, while the *umulaye* shakes his rattle (*akaseŵe*). The person who holds the horn does so with both hands, keeping it near the ground. It is said that the horn draws its holder on and on, wavering from side to side, and causing him to move forward in the right direction. When they come to the houses the holder passes near the doorways with the horn, while the *umulaye* follows behind, shaking his *akaseŵe* and saying, as they come to each house, "If the thief is in here, *ukose* [harden]!" After a while, when they reach a certain house, the horn commences to bob violently up and down. This is called *ukukosa*, hardening. The holder has to grip it more tightly to prevent its slipping from his hands. Then the people know that the thief is in that house. If it is a case of maize-stealing the culprit will confess that he broke off the cobs. At the confession the *chimulonda* will stop its violent movements,

[1] See the illustration on p. 176 of Melland's *In Witch-bound Africa*.

and lie passive in the villager's hands.   Having served its purpose, it will be restored to the *umulaye*.

Ichisoko

Unlike the doctors in many other Bantu tribes, the *aŵalaye* of the Lambas perform no bone-throwing or divining by means of bones or similar counters.   Nevertheless, the Lamba doctor of renown has his bag of instruments, and this is called *ichisoko*, or, in old Lamba, *ichishyala*.   This bag con-
tains his *imisamu*, medicines made from leaves, bark, roots, twigs, etc. (but never from stones), sometimes in the form of powder made up in packets, and the *umutalu*, medicine for exorciz-ing spirits, demons, etc.   Sometimes the various medicines are put up in horns (*insengo*); they are then called *ifishimba*, and comprise nail-parings, hair, rags which have been discarded, python-skin, lion-skin, elephant-hide and rhino-hide, human skull-bones, roots, herbs, etc.   The

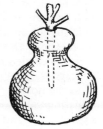

FIG. 78. UMUSASHI
WITH INSHINKO

doctor is never without *ulushila*, the red ochre so necessary to certain forms of divination.   Then in his bag he carries the *imiseŵe*, those rattles which play so large a part in his divining, the *impindo*, the pieces of stick used in divination, and an *umusashi*, a double calabash used as a container for castor-

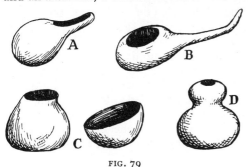

FIG. 79
A, *ichinkuli*; B, *ulukombo*; C, *ifitele*; D, *umusashi*.

oil and for certain medicines.   This is closed by a small stick chosen and cut because of protrud-ing twigs which can act as a grip for pull-ing out this 'stopper.' The whole stopper is about six inches in length, with about one inch of twigs pro-truding.   His bag also contains a zebra's tail (*umuchila wambishi*), two horns (*insengo*), and some small sticks for drawing lots (*ututi twafipa*).   He also usually has the *akabwangala*, part of the skull of a man whom he has had to disinter and burn for being an *ichiŵanda*. Some *aŵalaye* also carry *inkusu*.   The kernel of the fruit of the *inkusu*-tree is taken and whittled down until it is about three-quarters of an inch in diameter, and oblong in shape. Sometimes the *inkusu* is smeared with medicine which has been pounded up. A hole is pierced through the centre for a string, and the 'charm' is often worn by the *umulaye* himself on his ankle. When he enters a hut where there is death he takes it off. Others carry *imbilichila*, another kernel treated in the same way. Neither of these is of Lamba origin, and they are seldom met with. Most *aŵalaye* carry portions of armadillo shell (*inkaka*) or bones of this animal, and put them into horns or shells of tortoises; the whole charm resulting is also termed *inkaka*, and is used for rendering an opponent helpless.

Sometimes the doctor carries his *ichisoko* himself, but very often it is carried by a boy who acts as his attendant. The doctor also carries spear and axe. His attendant (*mulonda*) carries his big sable horn. The *umulaye* does not have any special dress to distinguish him, as does the *mukamwami*, for the doctor's name is sufficiently known everywhere.

The duties of the *umulaye* in the community are varied. He will be summoned at times of sickness, as we have already seen, to divine the cause and prescribe the remedy, which in very few cases is medicinal. He will be called at death to 'smell out' the witch or wizard, or after a theft to detect the thief. He will prescribe for barrenness, and prepare charms (*ubwanga*) for many contingencies. The part the *umulaye* plays in the detection of witchcraft will be considered in Chapter XIX, and the whole subject of dynamism, lots, and charms is dealt with in Chapters XVII and XVIII.

The *umulaye*, principally on account of his powers of divination, is a person of very considerable standing in the community. Especially owing to his powers of witch-detection, his influence and sway over the people are unbounded. He is feared, and people fear to provoke his anger, for, with all their belief in genuine witchcraft, they know well enough that the cry of "Witch!" can be raised only too readily if they offend those in authority.

Inferior Doctors

Among the Lambas there are other doctors whose status is much inferior to that of the *umulaye* proper. Two of these are called *aŵalomweshi*—the *aŵalomweshi ŵansoka*, snake-bite doctors, and the *aŵalomweshi ŵabwanga*, charm doctors. The third type of inferior doctor is called *umulaye watuluŵi*, the ventriloquist doctor.

UŴULAYE—THE RÔLE OF THE DOCTOR

Umulomweshi Wansoka

The Lambas have a strange belief regarding the *lukungwe*, a long, thin tree snake. They say that its bite is not poisonous, but that it often attacks in quite another way. Holding in its mouth a stick, twig, grass-stalk, or stone, it throws the stone at its victim or strikes him with the twig, causing him to fall immediately. If two natives are travelling together and one suddenly falls, his companion, should he see a *lukungwe* making off, travelling with head erect and body bent backward, will know that it has struck his companion. If the village is near he runs to call assistance, shouting, "My companion has been struck!" He dare not mention by what he has been hurt, for it is taboo to mention the *lukungwe* in the village, lest the victim should die. In practically every village are to be found *aŵalomweshi*, and one, hearing the man's shout, quickly fetches some *uŵusunga bwamawo* (gruel made from the small red millet), which is always kept in his hut, adds to it some *umusamu*, and carries it to the stricken man, who is made to swallow it. The sick man vomits violently, throwing up a black bile. When the fit of vomiting is over it will be seen that he opens his eyes a little; then he is given some other liquid *umusamu* to drink. After that he quickly recovers, and the people conduct him to the village. For such services a patient may pay the *umulomweshi* from five to ten shillings, according to the seriousness of his case.

If a man is bitten by an *umuswema* (a dun-coloured snake) or an *akapinisansa* (a small species of adder) he is quickly brought to the village. The *umulomweshi* goes and collects a quantity of medicinal leaves and piles them in a heap. They are set on fire, and the affected limb, arm or leg, is held in the smoke. Further *umusamu* is chewed by the doctor and smeared on the wound. Then a sharpened stick, resembling a knife, is taken and the wound scraped, in the belief that thus the teeth of the snake will come out of the wound, where they are believed to have been left. After the scraping further *umusamu* is bound over the wound, and another oily medicine supplied for rubbing on. Recovery is assured to the patient. Kalimanama, a village headman on the Kafulafuta, is an *umulomweshi wansoka*.

Umulomweshi Wabwanga

An *umulomweshi* of another type will treat a patient suffering, for instance, from a swollen leg. The doctor, when summoned, addresses the swelling with the words, *Kani uli bwanga ufume-mo;*

kani toli bwanga koikele! "If you are a charm, come out of it; if you are not a charm, stay there!" Then he cuts incisions (*inembo*) in the leg, and rubs in certain *umusamu*. After that he takes a stick with a sharp edge like a knife and begins to scrape, saying, "Don't you see what quantities of *ubwanga* are coming out [this when the white scrapings of the skin appear]? Witches have badly bewitched you!" On hearing that the patient's heart is greatly cheered. When he has finished this treatment the doctor says, "Now pay me, that I may go home!" Payment up to ten shillings will be given to him. Sometimes such a swelling goes on year after year without relief, and the sufferer throws away all his money on doctor after doctor. Kapumba, of Nsensenta's village, and Nswana Nkashyafiputa, of the same village, are *aŵalomweshi ŵabwanga*.

The *aŵalomweshi* are a very inferior type of doctor. They are never honoured with the name of *aŵalaye* or *iŋanga*, and travel about with their bag of medicines looking for patients. When asked for tobacco they say, "No, this is *umusamu wakulomona* [medicine for treatment]." In this way they advertise their trade. The *aŵalaye*, on the contrary, are renowned for their skill, and never go to a sick person unless summoned.

Aŵalaye Watuluŵi

The doctor who practises by means of ventriloquism also commands but little respect among the Lambas. The term *akaluŵi* (plural, *utuluŵi*) is applied to any imitation of a person, such as a doll or figure. The doll is the centre of the work of the *umulaye watuluŵi*. In some cases it is made out of a small *umusashi* (type of double calabash), into which is put certain *umusamu* called *umutalu*. In other cases the doll is carved out of a piece of wood, with legs, arms, and head like those of a man; bee's-wax is stuck to the head, and holes made in it so that castor-oil beans may be inserted into the huge nostrils of the *akaluŵi*. People come to this image to consult it. The image is called *mukolo*, the principal wife, and is considered as such in relationship to the *umulaye*. The people say, "We have come to the *mukolo*, that she should give us information." The doctor sits at the back of the hut, with the image near him. Those who come to *ŵuka* (consult) sit in the doorway. The *umulaye* proceeds to address the *akaluŵi*, saying, "People have come, O *mukolo*, to see you!" The people say, "Let the *mukolo* tell us!" Then in a small piping voice the *akaluŵi* says, *Mbacisa'ceŵo?* "What is the matter?" They reply, "Our child, O *mukolo*, is sick. We are wearied with getting *umusamu*, O *mukolo*, but he shows no improvement!" She replies, *Mipashi yakwe!* "It is his spirit!" On hearing that the people go away, saying, "We shall pay our respects to the spirit, and brew some *ifisunga.*" They leave an offering in the hut for the doctor.

One of these doctors was Chifunshya, of Nkambo's village. One day a certain woman found that her meat had been eaten by some one. She made up her mind to consult the *mukolo* in order to find the thief. The woman arrived and said, "Tell me, O *mukolo*, for my meat has been eaten by somebody!" The answer came, "It is your husband who ate it, while you were away at the river!" The woman went home, and her husband immediately asked her what was the result of the divination. She replied, "The *mukolo* says it is you who ate the meat!" The husband was furious. He caught up an axe-handle, and went straight to the person who had made the *akaluŵi.* He vigorously belaboured the *umulaye*, shouting, "Where did you see me stealing the meat out of my own house?" People came and separated the men, rescuing the much-battered doctor. The *akaluŵi* was not seen; it had been hidden.

CHAPTER XVII

IFIPA—LOTS

Ukuŵuka and Ifipa

In the previous chapter we considered the art of divination as practised by the *umulaye* in order to discover what had happened in the past and to ascertain the cause of illness, theft, etc. All of this is covered by the term *ukuŵuka*. We shall in this chapter consider the art of divination when directed to discover what the result of sickness, a journey, etc., will be. In order to probe into the future *ifipa* (lots) are used; in Lamba the term used for casting or drawing lots is *ukuteye'fipa*. The use of the term *ichipa* (lot) is not, however, confined to ascertaining what is going to take place. As we shall see, *ifipa* are used even in detecting the cause of illness; and there is one use of this term closely akin to that of *ubwanga*, a charm designed to bring about some definite result. This is discussed in the next chapter. As with *ubwanga*, or *ifyanga*, the use of *ifipa* is not entirely restricted to *aŵalaye* ; certain *ifipa* are cast by ordinary people.

Ifipa in Illness

When a person falls ill the *umulaye* is often summoned to cast lots in order to ascertain whether the sick man is going to die or to recover. The doctor brings with him his three *ifipa*. These are little sticks, the length and size of a finger, scraped

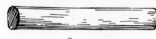

FIG. 80. ICHIPA

evenly, so that they have the shape of a cigarette when finished. A special tree is chosen from which to carve out the *ifipa*, but I have not been able to discover the name of the tree. The people say to the doctor, "Set [*teya*, the same word as is used for the setting of a trap] the *ifipa*, for the man is very ill, and we want to know whether he is going to die." Thereupon the doctor takes his *ifipa* and goes into the bush beyond the village, sometimes alone, sometimes accompanied by his assistant. There he clears a small *uluŵansa* of rubbish and bushes, and in the centre digs a little hole. To one side of the hole he places meal, making a white strip several inches in length. Then he takes some leaves, mixes them with a certain *umusamu*, and chews the mixture. Next, holding the three *ifipa* in his hand, he spits the chewed mixture upon them, squeezing them together in the same way as a man works putty. The three *ifipa* stick together, and the doctor takes them and sets them up on end at the edge of the hole he has dug, between it and the line of meal. The *umulaye* then addresses his *ifipa* as follows : *Utuŵule wefipa*[1] *fyanji; kani uyumuntu wakufwa uponene mukalindi; kani akuŵuuka uponene*

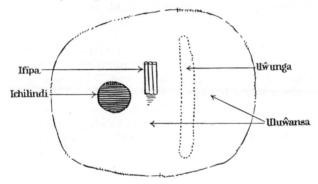

FIG. 81. HOW THE IFIPA ARE SET

muŵunga, "Tell us, O *ifipa* of mine. If this man is going to die, fall into the hole; if he is going to live, fall into the meal."

As is only to be expected, the various elements in this performance are symbolical. The meal (*uŵunga*) invariably represents life, as is seen when considering its ceremonial use after the payment of the death-dues. The hole (*ichilindi*, or its diminutive, *akalindi*) symbolizes the grave, and hence death. The *ifipa* in this instance represent the sick man, and the fact that they are three in one may be due to the Lamba conception of man's being made up of body (*umuŵili*), spirit (*umupashi*), and person, or soul (*umuntu umwine*). The test is to see whether the *ifipa* (the sick man) will go into the *akalindi* (into death) or into the *uŵunga* (into life).

When the *umulaye* has thus arranged his symbols he leaves them and returns to the village. After a considerable time he goes back and finds the *ifipa* still standing. He returns to the village, and later once again visits his symbols. They are still standing.

---

[1] *Ifipa*, though a plural, is here treated as singular, since the three have become one ; the concords for ' thou ' are used.

He therefore goes back to the village, and says, "He is merely ill; he will recover." But in order to make quite sure he will go in the evening and set the *ifipa* again, and address them, saying, "If he is merely ill, and is going to recover, tell us." That night maybe the *ifipa* fall into the meal. The *umulaye* will then say to those who are caring for the sick man, "Don't be anxious; he is going to recover." After that the same *umulaye* will find the necessary medicine for strengthening the patient; and, says the Lamba, "The man will recover if Lesa tells him to."

If, however, the *umulaye* finds that the *ifipa* have fallen into the hole (*akalongelo*, or *akalindi*) he is afraid, seeing in this the sign that the man is going to die. Very early in the morning he takes up his *ichisoko* (bag) and leaves the village. He has been paid in advance for his services, and he leaves before anyone is about. When his host carries to his hut his morning food he finds the hut empty, and the villagers say at once, "The man is going to die, for the *umulaye* has run away secretly."

The people, however, are seldom satisfied with such a verdict, and send for another doctor, who comes with his bag and his lots. He sets the *ifipa* in the same way, and addresses them, saying, "Tell me if he is going to die!" When he next visits the place maybe he finds the *ifipa* still standing. He takes them up, puts more *umusamu* upon them, and says, "If it is an *ichiŵanda* [demon], tell me!" Having set them again, he returns to the village. When he goes back in the evening he finds, perhaps, that the *ifipa* have fallen into the hole; from this he divines that his last question has been answered, and that an *ichiŵanda* has knocked them in, showing that he is concerned in the man's illness. The *umulaye* then goes to the village, and says, "No, it is an *ichiŵanda*, and the man will recover." It is now his business to discover what it is that has caused the anger of the *ichiŵanda*. Fear of death or of madness now seizes the patient, and he confesses to some unnatural sin which he has committed. When he has confessed the demon can no longer hold him. The *umulaye* now procures for him the necessary medicine, and he begins to recover. When he is fully recovered he gives to this second doctor a handsome gift of goods. This type of *ichipa* is sometimes called *ichipa chyabwanga* or *ichipa chyafiŵanda*.

Ichipa Chyakasuŵa

There is another way in which an *umulaye* may *teye'fipa* (cast lots) when summoned to divine whether a patient will recover or not. He goes out early in the morning, and chews certain leaves just as the sun is emerging red in the east. He then spits out the chewed leaves (*pala*) in the direction of the sun, and begins his divination by questioning (*sanshila*), saying, *Kani pali ichyeŵo ichyakufwo'muntu, ŵekasuŵa, ulukuŵilaka! Kani teshi afwe, teku-lukuŵilaka!* "If this is a matter involving the death of the person, O sun, boil! If he is not to die, don't boil!" Then, as the doctor stands and gazes, he seems to see the sun whirling round as though it is boiling. Again he puts a question : *Kani uŵulwele bwakukula, kani akutenda-po lukoso, ŵekasuŵa utuŵuule!* "Whether the sickness will get worse, or whether the man is merely unwell, tell us!" Again he sees that the sun is boiling. He goes back to the village and says, "Whether he will recover one cannot tell!"

Ichipa Chyaminyeŋu

When the time for the return of a man from a long journey—maybe one of three or four months' duration—has passed his mother or his wife will go to the *umulaye* and say, "Set an *ichipa*, that we may see whether the traveller is ill or whether he is dead." Thereupon the *umulaye* goes and begs some salt. He chews this with certain medicinal leaves. He finds a nest of large black biting ants, *iminyeŋu*, and spits the chewed leaves into the mouth of their hole, saying, *Kani alifwile mutuŵuule mushinchile, kani epwali mufumishye posonde umusamu napala mubwina bwenu!* "If he is dead, tell us and shut it in; if he is alive, bring outside the medicine I have spat into your hole." Then he leaves the place and goes back to the village. After a little while he calls the mother of the man, and says, "Let us go and see!" Perhaps they find that the ants have brought all the leaves outside, in which case the *umulaye* says, "Look, your child is living!" The woman will go home contented. If, however, they find that the ants have taken all the leaves into the hole, and closed up the hole with mud, the doctor will say, "Your son has no life!" and the mother will go away to wail, fully believing her son to be dead.

In this type of *ichipa* we again see that what happens is symbolic. The hole of the *iminyeŋu* represents the grave. The taking in of the chewed leaves and the closing up of the hole is symbolic of burial, the pushing of the leaves outside symbolic of escape from the grave. It may also have further significance. *Pesonde* (outside) is the term used of mortal life. The phrase, *Walale' myaka inga pano pesonde?* "How many years have you slept here outside?" indicates "How old are you?" The outside, then, like the meal, indicates life.

Ichipa Chyakwe Sumba

There is another type of *ichipa* used in cases such as the above, and also in the detection of adultery. This is called *ichipa chyakwe sumba*, testing of the green lizard, or *ichipa chyapawuchyende*, testing for adultery. It may be carried out by an *umulaye*, but is more commonly performed by an ordinary person.

If a man has been away from his home for several months, and now the last day of his journey home has come, he will set an *ichipa* in order to find out whether his wife has been faithful to him or not. He gets a number of leaves of any kind and chews them, making from the pulp (*ulukamfi*) a small round ball the size of a marble. Then as he walks along he keeps a look-out for a *sumba*, a large green lizard with a very long tail, and watches where it goes into its hole at his approach. These lizards are very commonly seen along the path. The man then puts the *ulukamfi* at the mouth of the hole, and says, *Wechipa chyanji, kani umukashi alichitile uwuchyende winjishye mubwina ulukamfi; kani tachitile wiinjishya, yo!* "O my *ichipa*, if my wife has committed adultery, take the *ulukamfi* into your hole; if she has not done so, don't take it in!" He then goes away to a little distance and sits down by himself. He allows a considerable time to elapse, and then returns to the hole of the *sumba*. If he finds that the *ulukamfi* has not been taken in he accepts it as a sign that his wife has been faithful, and goes on to the village happy in mind.

If, however, he finds that the lizard has taken the *ulukamfi* into his hole there is hate in his heart, and that night he will tie up his wife, and demand that she give him the name of the man who has injured him. Often the woman will have no answer, and will just cry with fright at her husband's violence. But sometimes, owing to the pain of the cords, the distracted woman will name some man. When the accused man is caught in the morning he will demand that the woman explain her accusation, and she will say it was untrue, but that she spoke in order that her husband might loosen her quickly. In such a case the husband would have to compensate the wrongly accused man. The Lambas, despite such happenings, pin great faith to the accuracy of this type of *ichipa*. Without any doubt here too we have a test which is symbolic. The taking into its hole of the *ulukamfi* by the lizard is symbolic of the action of an adulterous woman.

286

Tossing-up

The term *ifipa* is also used in cases equivalent to those in which a coin is tossed by Europeans. When travellers are not certain which of two paths they should take they decide to *teye'fipa* (cast lots). They pluck two leaves of any kind, and throw them into the air to see if they *pawama*, come down right side up, or, as the Lambas put it, *akapafu peulu*, stomach upward; for with them each leaf has an *akapafu*, a stomach, and an *inuma*, a back. If only one leaf descends *akapafu peulu* the travellers will take it as an endorsement of their choice of the path over which they are 'tossing' the leaves. This type of test is sometimes called *ichipa chyeshyamo* (trial of ill-luck).

Something similar is done when honey is being sought. If the men have found honey they put it on a dish made of bark and then eat it. The chief man among them will then take the bark dish (*umukwa*), point in a certain direction, and say, "If we go that way, shall we eat honey?" He will thereupon throw the *umukwa* into the air. If it comes down bottom upward (*ifunama*) he says, "It has refused over there." Again he will say, "Shall we go that way?" and will again throw the *umukwa* into the air. If it comes down face upward (*pawama*) he says, "It has consented. Let us go this way."

Ichipa Chyamalya

When natives set out to visit friends at a neighbouring village they very often decide to *teye'fipa* in order to see whether they will get *inshima* (thick porridge) given to them. They look for a certain bush called *ulupaapi*. Taking a small branch, they tear it down between forked pieces, dividing it as is done with withies (*imango*). If it snaps quickly it is understood that they will not get anything to eat, but if it splits right down (*lendewuka*) they expect to find food provided. If the latter happens they will go on to the village fully expectant. Then when their friends begin at once to prepare food for them they will say, *Ichipa chyesu chyachita bwino*, "Our *ichipa* has done well." This is called *ichipa chyamalya*.

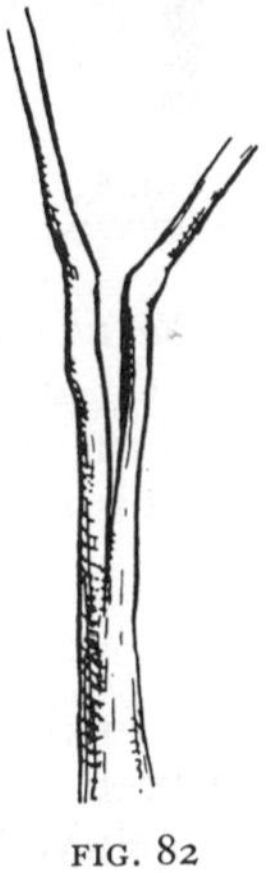

FIG. 82
UKUKWAMU-
NO'LUPAAPI

Ifipa fyamalya are also used to settle a quarrel over the ownership of food or even of any article and to find the direction in which honey may be found. The term *amalya* is derived from the verb *lya*, eat, and has to do primarily with food.

287

Ichipa Chyawukulu

Children indulge in a game of lots, also called *ukuteye'chipa*. When arguing as to who is the biggest in their company they often appeal to the *ichipa* to settle their dispute. They plait a piece of string from old cloth and set fire to it half-way up. Standing round, they pass it quickly from hand to hand, and the person in whose hand the string eventually burns through and breaks is called the biggest. "Yes," he says, "I'm the biggest!" The others all laugh and say, "You are the child of a witch, because the *ichipa* has told us."

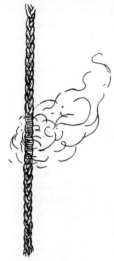

FIG. 83. ICHIPA
CHYAWUKULU

The Delaying of Sunset

Under the heading of *ichipa* the Lambas include a peculiar practice which they have for the purpose of 'delaying' the sunset. When a man on a journey sees that the sun is about to set while he is still some distance from his objective, he knocks off the top of a small ant-heap (*ifwasa*) and sets it up on a stick, saying, *Wekasuŵa ukuwa ili nakuya kufika uko ndukuya epakuwa!* "O sun, in setting, when I arrive where I am going, that is when to set!" It is then believed that the man will reach his destination before dark. This use of *ichipa* is much akin to that of *ubwanga*.

Ichipa in Folklore

In folklore *ifipa* of various kinds are recorded, but they are regarded by the natives as being merely fanciful, and hence are not believed in as genuine tests. One such is recorded in the *Ichishimichishyo ichyaŵamwana-nkalamu naŵamwana-ŋombe*, "The Story of Mr Lion-child and Mr Cow-child." [1] When the two heroes were about to part company the one who was going away, Cow-child, conjured (*chite'chipa*) with porridge in a cooking-pot, covered it over with leaves, and gave it to his brother's wife, saying, "Now I am going far, five nights and five days; so if my *ichipa* dries up you will know that Cow-child is dead!"

[1] See *Lamba Folk-lore*, by C. M. Doke, p. 19.

IFIPA—LOTS

In the story of *Ŵakalulu neyaliile Ŵulambe*, "Mr Little-hare
and what ate Ŵulambe," [1] the term *ichipa* is used to indicate a
trick, a feat of strength or unusual cleverness. The Little-hare
lures the lion into his big sack by saying, "Sir, I have a splendid
trick [*ichipa*]! If you were to see it you would just love it at
once!"

[1] See *Lamba Folk-lore*, p. 37.

CHAPTER XVIII

UBWANGA—THE CULT OF DYNAMISM

Ubwanga

WE have already dealt with two aspects of the Lambas' religious beliefs, that of the existence of Lesa, the Creator, a monotheistic belief, and that of a spiritual world of disembodied spirits, demons, and other spiritual beings, a spiritistic belief; and now we come to consider their belief in a power quite separate from that of Lesa or of the *imipashi* or the *ifiŵanda*—what has been termed a dynamistic [1] belief.

Dynamism with the Lambas indicates a belief in the inherent potentiality of certain preparations, charms, medicines, actions, and even words to bring about certain definite results. The operation of this dynamic power is, generally speaking, automatic, but in many cases it is seen to be controlled by the *umulaye* (doctor). Most of the preparations used in this connexion are made by the *umulaye*, though we shall see that the *aŵapalu* (professional hunters), the *aŵami* (mediums), and even ordinary people may make these preparations in particular cases. This dynamic power generally is covered by the terms *ubwanga*, or *ichyanga*, and a practically synonymous term, *umusamu*. In derivation *ubwanga* has the same root as the Lamba word *iŋanga*, synonymous with *umulaye*. It is the power behind the *umulaye*, a power which the uninitiated may well fear to dabble with. The word *umusamu* is the Ila equivalent of the Lamba *umuti* (tree), which is generally translated as medicine. *Umusamu* is the visible form which the unseen *ubwanga* takes when it is being manipulated by the *umulaye*. It matters not whether the doctor has prescribed a herbal remedy which we should recognize as a genuine medicine or whether he has prepared a duiker's horn of some special concoction which has to be hung in a specified place; both are called *umusamu*, and both represent the *ubwanga*, the power for healing or for destroying, for protecting or for hurting. One of the most sinister things in this dynamistic belief is the

[1] See Smith and Dale, *The Ila-speaking Peoples of Northern Rhodesia*, vol. ii, chapter xx.

conviction that *imfwiti*, witches or wizards, can also tap this
hidden source of power, and use it for their nefarious purposes.
The *umulaye* is always trusted to exercise the powerful *ubwanga*
in a way beneficial to the whole society, but the *imfwiti* is invariably credited with using it for the hurt of the society.
The *imfwiti* is therefore a danger to the community; his or her
presence is regarded as a cancer which must be cut out at all
costs.

Ubwanga is of many kinds, for many purposes, and prepared
and administered by several types of people. In this chapter we
shall consider those manifestations of it controlled by the *aŵalaye*,
by the *aŵami*, by the *aŵapalu*, and those which may be controlled
by anyone. The *ubwanga bwakulowa*, that of the *imfwiti*, will be
considered in the next chapter.

It must further be pointed out that the term *ubwanga* is also
used synonymously with *uŵulembe*, the poison which the Lambas
put on their arrows. The *uŵulembe* is a type of creeper, with
long trailers the thickness of one's finger, found hanging in the
trees. It has a sausage-shaped fruit about seven inches in length.
These are picked, and broken open. The seeds are then extracted,
dried, and pounded; the fatty pulp resulting is pasted on to the
arrows behind the head.

Ubwanga for Protection

We have already observed that the *aŵalaye* do not offer their
services for the diagnosing of diseases, divining of causes, or the
healing of the sick—they wait to be summoned. There is, however, one thing which they do advertise, and that is the *ubwanga*
which they stock for the prevention of certain evils. On his
arrival at a village an *umulaye* may announce, *Neŵo ndikwete
amano, ndi nemusamu wakuŵulo'kwikatwa kunkalamu; nebwanga
bwansoka ndikwete naŵo!* "I am wise, I have medicine to prevent
one's being caught by a lion; and a snake charm I also have!"
This will attract customers, and in the morning he will go into
the bush to dig about for the necessary roots, bring them to the
village, skin them, and pound them. He then calls all the people,
old and young, to bring duiker horns (*insengo shyanshya*). Everybody has to take the horns by night to the *umulaye* in the bush,
and there he fills them with the potent *umusamu*. This process
is called *ukupando'bwanga*. The doctor also prepares *impindo*,
small sticks with dynamic power, to be worn on arm or leg to
prevent snake-bite. These *impindo* are about an inch long, and

THE LAMBAS OF NORTHERN RHODESIA

the thickness of a pencil; through one end is a hole for inserting a string. All of these charms, whether *insengo* or *impindo*, are hung up in the trees in the bush, and thus left during the night. In the early morning the owners come to take them down, and the *umulaye* instructs them in some of the needful prohibitions (*imishiliko*) to be observed by the holders of these charms. He says, *Tekupiniko' lukuni uŵushiku neli kutwo'ŵushiku. Kani mukatwe, inkalamu ikamwikateni; nelukuni kani mukapiniko' ŵushiku ikamwikateni*, "Do not chop any firewood at night, or stamp food at night. If you do stamp, a lion will catch you ; and if you cut a piece of firewood by night it will catch you!" These prohibitions are carefully observed; they are called *imishiliko yaŵalaye*, prohibitions of the doctor.

Ubwanga Bwankalamu

To secure protection from lions certain pounded roots, known only to the *umulaye*, are placed in a duiker horn and two *impindo* cut by the *umulaye* from various roots, one of which is that of the *umumpulumpumpi* shrub. The *impindo* are strapped one on either wrist. When travellers are going to sleep in the bush, they build a zareba (*umutanda*), and hang their *insengo* on trees outside, believing that these will drive away any lion that may approach, and so protect them.

Ubwanga Bwansoka

As a protection against snake-bite one *ulupindo* (singular of *impindo*) is worn above the ankle. This type of charm is called *ulupinga*. It is said that a snake will sense this charm and make off at speed when the wearer approaches. It is further said to prevent a snake from biting the wearer even when he treads on it.

Ubwanga Bwangwena

There is a type of protection, *ubwanga*, prepared by the layman to give him safety from crocodiles when crossing rivers. Incisions (*inembo*) are made on the legs below the calf and over the shoulder-blade. The roots of the *intetele*, a kind of wild snapdragon, are dug up and burnt, and the powder rubbed into the incisions. Then two *impindo* are worn on the leg below the calf when a river is to be crossed in the rainy season. A man so protected is believed to be immune from attack by a crocodile.

UBWANGA—THE CULT OF DYNAMISM

Ubwanga Bwamfwiti

Ubwanga bwamfwiti (charm against witches) is prepared by the *umulaye*, and placed in a duiker or grysbok horn. Usually the horn is secreted in the side of one of the doorposts. It is said that the horn has the power to leave its place and pursue the witch, driving her away. Others say that when the witch or wizard approaches the horn causes the hut to become invisible, so that the visitor is baffled in his attempt to do evil. If the owner of the hut goes away for any length of time he leaves the horn at the village to protect his home. Sometimes a man will have more than one of these potent horns, and will place one at the back of the hut as an added protection.

Ubwanga Bwalwela

There are two types of *ubwanga* prepared by the *awalaye* to give assistance in warfare, the *ubwanga bwalwela*, for protection in the fight, and the *ubwanga bwachimbwembwe*, for putting fear into the enemies' hearts. The day before a party sets off to fight the *umulaye* procures a certain *umusamu*. He then brings a little child (*ichinjishi*), one who has not yet commenced to talk. The *ichinjishi* urinates, and the urine is mixed with the *umusamu*, the resulting concoction being placed in little horns (*utusengo*). The intention of this is that the enemy, on meeting the fighters with these little horns on their persons, will all become like *ifinjishi*, and be overcome by fear.

When such a party of fighting men, having spent a night on the road within striking distance of their objective, set off to the attack, with their officer behind, they all wear these *utusengo* attached to a circlet round the head. When they reach the village they are to raid they take another *ubwanga*, *ubwanga bwachimbwembwe*, intended to give their enemies such fear that they will be unable even to get up. This particular *umusamu* is mixed with gunpowder (*imfundanga*), and with it one of the guns is loaded. In this way the men reach the village early in the morning, and surround it. Then the gun with the medicated powder is fired, and is believed to ensure complete victory. The men issue terror-stricken from their huts, and are quickly dispatched. The women and children fall a prey to the raiders, and are carried off into slavery.

If the raid is unsuccessful, and the enemy is found to be on the watch for them, the men will throw the blame upon the child chosen for the preparation of the *ubwanga bwalwela*. "This

293

child," they will say, "did not arrange the preparation properly." Or maybe they will look for an offender among their number. It is an *umushiliko* that no brave may lie with his wife on the day before going to war. Maybe one has offended in this respect.

Ubwanga Bwalukawo

A bundle of special leaves is tied up and attached to a pole set

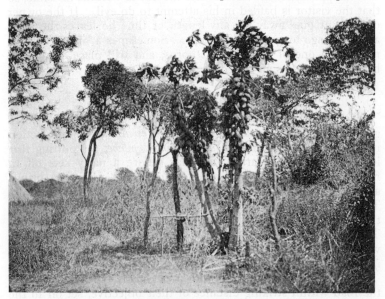

FIG. 84. PAWPAW-TREES PROTECTED BY UBWANGA BWAYAMBA
Photo by C. M. Doke

in the midst of a garden of foodstuffs, such as ripening maize, pumpkins, potatoes, or nuts. It is said that if a thief comes and touches any of the foodstuffs his hand is caught fast, so that he cannot let go the thing he is trying to steal. When the owner of the charm comes the thief is secured.

Ubwanga Bwayamba

Ubwanga bwayamba is also a potent charm for the protection of foodstuffs and the harm of any would-be thief. A man who has a special crop, such as some fruit-trees or a patch of tobacco, which he wishes to protect from thieves will go to the *umulaye* to procure *ubwanga bwayamba*. This may consist of certain

294

pounded leaves, which he puts into a duiker horn. The horn is tied on to a cross-pole (*umutembo*) supported by two upright forked sticks (*impanda*), which are planted in the ground near the foot of the tree. There is sympathetic magic in the preparation of this charm, for it is said that the person who now plucks

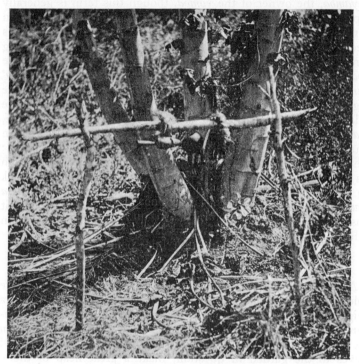

FIG. 85. UBWANGA BWAYAMBA, SUPPORTED LIKE A DEAD BODY ON A
CARRYING-POLE, TO PROTECT PAWPAW-TREES FROM THIEVES
Photo by C. M. Doke

this fruit will to-morrow be carried *pamutembo*, by means of a carrying-pole, as is a corpse, the supported duiker's horn representing the dead body of the offender. Some believe that the death of one ignoring the *ubwanga* will be by lightning. They say, at all events, that such a one commits suicide; the onus of his death is upon himself.

Yamba Wamulukombo

There is another type of *yamba*, called the *yamba* in the calabash, which is used for prevention of rain. At the time of the early rains people will go to an *umulaye* and say, "We want to drink *yamba*." The doctor prepares a mixture of water with flakes of mica (*amamba akwe Lesa*) and certain pounded roots and leaves in it. This he puts into a drinking calabash (*ulukombo*), and gives it to his client to drink. The doctor may be called *umwine wayamba*, the owner of the *yamba*, though this term is generally applied to the person who has drunk the potion. Such a person is more commonly called *uwayamba* (plural, *aŵayamba*), and is credited with special powers in the prevention of rain. During a rain-storm, if much thunder is heard (*Lesa alukupata*), the *uwayamba* rushes out shouting, *Kopata bwino, ulukutiinishya' ŵantu mumfulo'mo!* "Steady with the thundering. You are frightening the people in this rain!" He then shouts in the village, *Kani pali uwalya-po umusale, kani kwiŵa aiŵa fimbi, ngalaŵile, yamba wafiitwa!* "If there is anyone who has eaten young maize-stalks, if some of them he has stolen, let him speak; the rain-charm is angry!" Some one in fear will come out from his hut and say, "It is I who ate So-and-so's maize-stalks. I took no one else's!" And the *uwayamba* replies, *A'a, naŵona Lesa ukufiitwa, kanshi niwe!* "Aha, I saw that God was angry, and it was you who were to blame!" Other types of rain-prevention will be considered under *ubwanga bwamfula*.

Ubwanga Bwashiŵuwungu

As it is believed that certain persons, called *ŵashiŵuwungu*, are able to practise witchcraft in order to transfer the strength of a neighbour's crop to their own, *ubwanga bwashiŵuwungu* is prepared to thwart their designs. Both *aŵalaye* and *ŵamukamwami* are able to prepare this *ubwanga*. They bring certain roots and leaves to the garden in question, make a great heap of them, and set fire to the heap, so that dense clouds of smoke are given off. This smoke they try to drive to all parts of the garden. It is then believed that if any *ŵashiŵuwungu* come to take the 'virtue' from the crops this *umusamu* will drive them away before they have accomplished their purpose.

Ubwanga Bwanama

It will be seen when we consider the hunting profession, *uŵupalu*, that the whole of the hunter's success depends upon the efficacy of the *ubwanga* which is at his command. *Ubwanga* is necessary to ensure straight shooting; it is necessary to ensure coming upon game in the first place; and it is necessary to ensure the safety of the hunters. Here we shall consider but one instance of its use. In order to ensure that he will quickly find and kill an animal the professional hunter, *ichiŵinda*, digs up the roots of a shrub called *umumpulumpumpi*. He then prepares a bark dish, *umukwa*, and places in it the roots and some water. The roots are not pounded, but are placed in the water as they are. He next takes a sprig of the *umusamba*-tree with leaves on it—this to represent the tail of an animal, an instance of sympathetic magic— dips it into the *umukwa* of medicated water, and sprinkles his weapon as though to wash it. Then he is ready to set out for the hunt. The *umusamba* is usually the tree used in connexion with washing (*ukusamba*) ceremonials. The connexion of the roots of these words is obvious.

Ubwanga Bwaŵulwele

Ubwanga is employed for both the prevention and the cure of sickness. For certain ailments ordinary people may prepare the *ubwanga*, or they may obtain it from a doctor.

Ubwanga Bwamutwi

As a cure for headache the Lambas carve *impinga shyandale*, charm-sticks from the *ndale*-tree, and tie them round the head of the patient with a string of beads. They further pick *ndale* leaves, chew them, and rub them on to the patient's head. It is possible that the *ndale*-tree is used because of the connexion of its name with *lala* (to sleep)—for example, *Ndale* means "Let me sleep!"

Ubwanga Bwakalwani

For chest troubles, such as pneumonia and pleurisy, they carve four *impindo shyamulemu*, charm-sticks of the red protea, pierce them, thread them on a piece of string, and carry them on the person. If a woman or an old man has one, it is worn round the waist. When some one is taken ill this charm is taken and tied round the affected part. A medicinal drink made from the root of the *mukona*-tree is given to the patient, and some is put into his gruel. All this is practised by people who are not necessarily doctors. The 'pneumonia string' is consistently worn round the chest by old men to keep away pneumonia and other chest complaints. The term *ubwanga* may thus be applied to preventive medicine, which in cases of sickness is identical with the curative. It may also be applied to the sickness itself, or, rather, to the dynamic force behind the sickness. Such phrases as these are heard: *Ubwanga bwanjikata mukuulu*, "*Ubwanga* has caught me in the leg," *Ŵandowo'bwanga mukuulu*, "They have bewitched me with *ubwanga* in the leg."

Ubwanga Bwamfula

Charms for the prevention of rain are very common. We have already noticed the use of *yamba* in this connexion. When a person is starting on a journey early in the morning during the rainy season he comes out of his hut at dawn, plucks a handful of fresh green grass (*umwefu*), heats it over the fire, and sets it on the end of his spear. As he starts along the path he says, *Wemfula ukalochye uko natulila, kuntanjile nyendele-ko bwino*, "O rain, you may rain where I have come from, but ahead of me let me have a comfortable journey!"

Aŵakoleshi Ŵamfula

Certain individuals are credited with further power over the rain. They are ordinary people themselves, but it is not every one who has this ability. They are called *aŵakoleshi ŵamfula*. When rain is threatening these people pluck leaves of the *akapota-*, *umwenje-*, or *umusafwa*-trees, and throw them toward the clouds. It is believed that just as the storm travels in the direction in which the wind carries the leaves from the trees, so this will have the effect of driving the storm in the direction in which the leaves have been thrown. This is another case of sympathetic magic.

Another type of *umukoleshi wamfula* does not drink any water on the road. In the early morning he goes out and picks some leaves of the *akapota*-tree, and enters the house chewing them. He then spits some of the *inkamfi* (chewed leaves) about the house; the rest he rolls in the ashes, until they become white, and then puts them on a stump of wood outside. Other *akapota* leaves are stuck up above the doorway, and the people are instructed that when evening comes they must take them down and burn them, so that it may rain. The same is done with the ash-covered *inkamfi* on the stump. They are thrown on to the fire, lest they should keep the rain away indefinitely.

When travelling the *umukoleshi wamfula* ties a bunch of *umusuku* leaves to the end of his spear and carries it over his shoulder. This is called *ichipeela*, for it swings from side to side as he walks (*peela*, to swing to and fro). When he wants to rest by the way he hangs up the *ichipeela*, sits down, and makes his meal. When

UBWANGA—THE CULT OF DYNAMISM

he resumes his journey he takes the *ichipeela* down again. On his arrival at the village to which he is going he undoes the spell by throwing the *ichipeela* into the fire. If he wants to bring rain he puts the *ichipeela* on the ground and pours water over it. This charm is always hung up if there is no desire for rain.

The principle of sympathetic magic is seen in all this. Abstention from drinking on the road is designed to minimize the likelihood of rain. The ash-covered *akapota* leaves are probably symbolic of the dry winter-time (*umwela*), when no rain falls. The constant swinging of the *ichipeela* denotes the moving onward of the clouds; its being hung up indicates that the clouds will remain high; while when it is put on the ground and drenched with water we see a picture of the lowering clouds discharging their moisture.

The *awakoleshi wamfula* believe that they have the ability to ward off lightning. If they are inside a hut and see that there is much lightning about they go outside, spit into the air (*shipila' mate mwiulu*), and say, *Koloka bwino, nindo twachita, fwewana wowe?* "Rain carefully. What is it that we, your children, have done?" This is addressed to Lesa. The women, meanwhile clapping their hands, utter the shrill *impundu*, a sign of humbling themselves (*saasa*) before Lesa, lest he should throw down their houses. At other times the *awakoleshi wamfula* snap their fingers (*lishyo'lusota*), and address Lesa, saying, *Koloka bwino, fwewantu wowe twakuwomba!* "Rain carefully. We, your people, have paid homage to you!" At other times they scatter ashes into the air and address the deity.

Ubwanga Bwankatulo

A special process of *ubwanga* is gone through to prevent the *utuyewela*, those peculiar creatures employed in witchcraft, from stealing foodstuffs. This is called *ubwanga bwankatulo*. The day before seed is sown, roots of the *umukokolo*-tree are dug up, peeled, and pounded. The seed, whether maize, sorghum, or pumpkin, is mixed with these ground roots, and on the next day it is sown. It is believed that the *utuyewela* would know that the *umusamu* was there, and that, should they steal, they would no longer be invisible.

Ubwanga Bwawusuko

Ubwanga bwawusuko is used if the pumpkins begin to rot. Leaves of the *uwukumbwayombe* bush are picked and placed on

299

a small bark dish (*akakwa*), and then sprinkled on the runners of the pumpkins. When the sprinkling has been completed the dish of medicine is covered over.

Ubwanga Bwakufyala

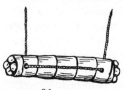

To ensure successful and easy birth a pregnant woman obtains from an *umulaye* what is called *katungu*, or *ubwanga bwakufyala*, a charm for giving birth. A small horn is cut through at both ends, *umusamu* inserted, and the ends closed each with four beads. Holes are pierced near both ends for the insertion of

FIG. 86. KATUNGU

a string. The charm is worn suspended from the neck.

Various Uses of Ubwanga

It must be observed here that *ubwanga*, this mysterious power, is said to be behind the work of the *aẁalomweshi* (see Chapter XVI), and to be at the root of the *ifimpelampela*, or miracles of transformation practised by certain individuals (see Chapter XV). *Imfwiti*, witches and wizards, are believed to tap its sources for their nefarious work, and even thieves bring it to their aid. One day I was visited by a man named Malisope, who had taken a violent fancy to the skin of a long-haired hyena which adorned my floor. I would not part with it. Recently I found that he wanted to use the skin as *umusamu* to procure for himself invisibility while carrying out a theft he was planning.

Ukushilika

In Chapter XIII the term *umushiliko* was noted as indicating a taboo of the strongest kind. The word is derived from the verb *ukushilika*, which means to prohibit, forbid, prevent, or ward off. In connexion with hunting it will be noticed that there are numerous *imishiliko* to be observed to ensure successful hunting. Kaaluwe, the sprite of the animals, has to be propitiated and guarded against. The observances necessary for this are termed *ukushilika Kaaluwe*. The same term is used in connexion with certain preventive observances carried out for the protection of the crops. Here are three such:

(1) *Ukushilike'ngulu ẁe*, warding off wild pigs. If wild pigs are worrying the crops certain *umusamu* is procured, together with the snout-bone of a wild pig. At night the people go to the

300

gardens, sit down on the west side, light a fire, and place on it the snout-bone and the *umusamu*. The owner of the gardens then fans (*pekawila*) the smoke over them. When the medicinal leaves (*umusamu*) are all burnt the people retire silently and return to the village. The next day no one goes near the gardens, but the day following that they may go.

(2) *Ukushilika ŵakolwe*, warding off monkeys. Medicinal leaves and an old monkey's skull are brought. The people then dig up *umumbu* marsh roots, which are carried by little children. When they reach the gardens a fire is made. The skull is broken to pieces, and it and the leaves are thrown on to the fire. Then the children climb up on to tree-stumps and eat the *umumbu* roots, imitating monkeys. When this is done all return to the village. The children are now warned by their elders, *Teku-lukuninina pafishinga, ŵalishilichile aŵene ŵeŵala*, "Don't climb on to the stumps any more, for the owner of the garden has forbidden them!"

(3) *Ukushilike'fyuni*, warding off birds. As in the other cases, smoke is produced in the gardens by medicated leaves, and while this is being done the people shout out, *Wa! Kalyeni kumulyashi ekuli ifyakulya fyenu twamupeleni. Tekwisa kulya kuno yo!* "*Wa!* Go and eat at the burial-ground—that is where the food we have given you is. Don't come to eat here again!"

CHAPTER XIX

UŴUFWITI—WITCHCRAFT

Witchcraft among the Lambas

THE existence of the spirit world around is a very real thing to the Lambas. We have noticed the respect they show for the *imipashi* of their departed relatives and the fear they have of the *ifiŵanda* which watch their actions. Their belief in the dynamic power which may be tapped by the man versed in *ubwanga* is equally strong. But perhaps even stronger than these is their belief in and their dread of witchcraft. The belief in witchcraft is a necessary corollary to their acceptance of the existence of dynamistic powers. If the doctor can tap these powers for the good of the community, is it not likely that there are those who can tap the same powers for their own selfish ends and for the harm of the community?

We have seen that, to the Lamba mind, sickness is attributable to one of several causes—the displeasure of the *imipashi*, a warning from the *ifiŵanda*, the hand of Lesa, or the work of *imfwiti* (witches or wizards). Now it is further said that the *imipashi* never kill—they only cause illness. The *ifiŵanda* too seldom, if ever, kill—they cause madness if they are not satisfied. Certainly Lesa does at times kill, but Lesa has so little to do with mankind that in the matter of death he is seldom considered as the cause. With what are we left? There must be a cause for every death. Natural causes of sickness and death, except in the cases of new-born babies or very old people, are not accepted. Hence practically every death among the Lambas used to be put down to the baneful work of the *imfwiti*. Does not this explain what a tremendous place in the life of the people witchcraft occupies? It is not only useless, it is incorrect, for Europeans to tell the natives that "there is no such thing as witchcraft." In the following description of the beliefs and practices of the Lambas we shall see how real a thing, and how pernicious a belief, this is.

In Lamba witchcraft is denoted by the term *uŵufwiti*; to practise witchcraft is *ukulowa*; while the witch, wizard, or warlock is termed *imfwiti*, a term which is used of a person of either sex.

302

UŴUFWITI—WITCHCRAFT
Ŵemba Creation of Lions

The Lambas give credit to the Kaonde people for superiority in the practice of witchcraft. It will later be seen that the Lambas sometimes obtain means for practising witchcraft from the Kaondes. They also maintain that, along certain lines, the Ŵembas are far superior. They say that the Ŵembas dig a certain *umusamu* and place it on a small potsherd in the bush, together with two *impindo* (sticks); one of these they call the lioness, the other the lion. When they visit the place in the morning they find that the *impindo* have actually changed into lions. To begin with they are very small, no bigger than mice. The owner of the *umusamu* feeds these little creatures, and they gradually grow up. When they are full grown he sends them whither he desires them to go, to kill some one against whom he has a grudge. Supposing a man has taken his wife away and married her, he sends these lions, which are under his control, to eat the offending man, and his wife who has left him, and his mother-in-law who connived at the desertion and subsequent marriage. The lions obey him. They remain in hiding until they see their victims, then destroy and eat them, returning afterward to their master.

The Lambas say that they are not able to do this. It is seen that a man does not have to *wilwa*, become possessed by a spirit of witchcraft or by a demon, to become an *imfwiti*; the profession is one of choice. A man becomes an *imfwiti* merely by buying from some *imfwiti* whom he gets to know the necessary *ubwanga bwakulowa* (witchcraft medicine). Should a Lamba desire to make lions as described above, he would have to procure the *ubwanga* from a Ŵemba.

Transmutation

One of the *ifimpelampela* attributed to *imfwiti* is the power of transmutation, the ability to change themselves into some animal, and in that shape to carry out their sinister work. An *imfwiti* may accost his victim as he travels along a lonely section of the path, and ask him if he is travelling alone or whether others are behind. If he gets the answer, "I am alone," he quickly goes behind an anthill and keeps quiet. When the man has gone on a little the *imfwiti* changes himself into a lion, pursues his victim, and eats him. After eating him he changes back once more into human form, picks up his axe and spear from behind the anthill, and goes his way. The Ŵemba and Ŵulima people are said to have been able to do this, and recently I came across an instance of firm belief in it among the Lambas.

A few years ago a man, Mwansa by name, was the regular mail-runner from the Kafulafuta Mission to Ndola. It was a time of lion-scare, for a man-eater had accounted for a number of natives in the vicinity of Ndola. Mwansa came with the mail one day, very agitated about what had happened on the road. He said that when he was about twelve miles from Ndola he was accosted by a man whom he did not know. The man asked him if he were alone. Mwansa, awake to the possibilities, replied, "No, my companions are a little way behind me!" The man vanished ; but a mile farther on he appeared again, and put the same question. "My companions," replied Mwansa, "have just stopped to light their pipes!" (A rather laborious business this, necessitating the lighting of a roadside fire from which to take hot embers to place on the top of the tobacco.) Again the man vanished; and this time Mwansa, thoroughly scared, ran for his life, not stopping until he was within sight of Ndola. "Had I given any other answer," he averred, "the visitor would have changed into that man-eater and devoured me."

There is much in Lamba folklore of lions becoming men, marrying women, and then attempting to devour them. Though this is generally accepted as purely fanciful by the Lambas, they have a saying regarding a stranger who comes to a village to marry one of the girls: "Ask him concerning his home and his ancestry; if you don't you may find yourself marrying a lion, that will eventually devour you!"

Witchcraft Practices

Imfwiti, whether men or women, generally carry out their work at night. They are able to render themselves invisible to ordinary eyes, but are said to go about stark naked. Possibly this is because their *ubwanga* for invisibility applies to their bodies only. It is significant, however, that, among the Lambas, should a man go about naked, he would be called an *imfwiti*.

In their night prowling they are said to enter the houses of their victims. This they do either through the closed door or through the roof without disturbing the thatch. Once they are in the hut so deep a sleep comes upon the inmates that nothing will waken them. One *imfwiti* takes off the head of the victim, and, going outside with it, with his or her companion tosses the head backward and forward. Before dawn they re-enter the

hut and restore the head. The victim, on waking, feels severe
pains in the neck, and soon dies. If in the tossing the head should
be dropped the victim complains of severe aching and swelling
on his head before death.

If an *imfwiti* has a grudge against a person, and notices that he
has a large sore (*ichilonda*) on his leg or arm, he will approach
him when he is asleep at night with his potent *umusamu*, and put
some of it on the wound. This will prevent the wound from
healing, and it will become a chronic swelling ulcer (*soŵongo*).

Imfwiti often carry their potent *umusamu* in a large snail-shell
(*inkofwa*). It is said that the power of this medicine is increased
by the admixture of portions of human flesh. They are said to
exhume a body, cut off portions of the flesh, dry it, and grind it to
powder, which is then mixed as one of the ingredients. The
belief goes even further : that they take the earth from graves,
and, by sprinkling it on a person's face, cause him to cough
(*ichifuŵa*). The *inkofwa* must of necessity be kept carefully
hidden.

At times an *imfwiti* acts in quite a different way. He takes a
horn filled with *ubwanga* and sets it in the path along which he
expects his victim to travel. Generally the horn is buried in the
path, with only the tip poking out. When his victim comes
along he trips at the spot where the horn is and cuts or scratches
his foot. The sore thus made becomes septic and spreads. The
victim says, "I tripped and knocked myself along the path," but
the people who see his spreading sore say, "No, it is an *imfwiti*
who has trapped you with his *ubwanga*." A woman of the name
of Malasa came for treatment to the Mission dispensary in 1920.
She had a terribly ulcerated foot, almost half of which was
already eaten away. Asked how it happened, she gave her
story. For a long time her husband had been treating her badly,
until she finally said she was going to the *boma* (magistracy) at
Ndola to obtain a divorce. The husband threatened her that, if
she persisted in going, he would bewitch (*lowa*) her on the road.
She persisted, went to Ndola, and obtained the divorce. On the
return journey to her home village she tripped and cut her toe.
From that wound the whole foot became ulcerated. Nothing
would alter her firm belief that her husband was an *imfwiti*, and
was the cause of this. Under British law she could do nothing
to him, but such a case would have been taken up very quickly if
it had happened a few years before. Then, in all probability, a
husband would have been more careful about uttering such a
threat.

Poison

Imfwiti also use poison to secure their ends. They prepare the *umusamu*—for poison when used by an *imfwiti* is *ubwanga*—and secretly put it in their victim's food. On the death of the victim people will say, *Nimfwiti shyamulowa!* "It is witches who have bewitched him!"

In other cases it is said that the *imfwiti* administers the poison during a night visit to his victim's hut. On waking in the morning the man will say, *Nafwe'fintu kumutimo' kwenda,* "I have a feeling of nausea!" Again people say, *Nimfwiti shyakulowo'ŵushiku!* "It is witches who have bewitched you at night!" A man may recover from this after a brief illness.

The poison may even be administered more openly; but, provided it is done without the victim's knowledge, it is still *ubwanga*, and the one who administers it *imfwiti*. There is to the Lamba mind a distinct difference between *akapondo*, a murderer, and *imfwiti*, a warlock. The former does his work openly, using weapons, stabbing, shooting, or beating, but the *imfwiti* kills with *ubwanga* and acts secretly. In the ordinary way poison would not be called *ubwanga* or *uŵufwiti*, but when it is secretly administered, with intent to kill, then it is so regarded. If, for instance. a man and his wife both eat of a certain fruit, and the wife dies, while the man becomes ill, then there will be no witchcraft charge against him when he recovers ; but witchcraft would be imputed to him if, in such circumstances, the wife died, while the man did not even sicken.

It is said that an *imfwiti* need only point the index finger at a child for him to sicken and die. Though it is recognized that the power of the *ubwanga* must be behind the pointing, it is considered very unlucky for anyone to point thus at a child; should the child sicken, the person who had pointed would be accused of witchcraft.

Wild beasts can be brought into the service of *imfwiti* in order to kill their victims. The death of a man bitten by a snake may be divined by the *umulaye* as being due to witchcraft. A man named Kuulu was badly mauled by a lion in 1916. He was successfully treated at the Mission for about two months. His friends said, "Some one has prepared *umusamu* in order that the lion should catch him!"

When a man undertakes a long journey, from which he never returns, it is said, *Imfwiti eyasweseshyo'mutima wakwe ati eme*

306

alukuya akafwile-ko! " A witch cleansed his heart that he should get up and go to his death!"

Witchcraft is even attributed to a woman with an insulting tongue. She is called *imfwiti*; but if no death or sickness occurs in the village she is not molested, but will get the title of *imfwiti yankumbu*, the merciful witch. Should such a woman be married, her husband would divorce her.

The wives of elephant-hunters are in constant dread when their husbands are out hunting; for should a hunter be killed by an elephant, it will be assumed that his wife has broken one of the elephant taboos (see Chapter XX), and she will be branded as *imfwiti*, and put to death.

When a man commits suicide it is commonly said, *Imfwiti shyamusomwena ati afwe*, "Witches have made him rush headlong to his death!" Elephantiasis of the leg is always attributed to witchcraft ; the Lambas say, *Ŵalimulowele umusantu*, "They have bewitched him with a swelling like a bundle of grass!" Similarly, regarding dropsy of the stomach they say, *Ŵalimulowele uŵutumbefumo*, "They have bewitched him with a swelling of the stomach!"

Treatment of Imfwiti

From the preceding account of what the Lamba people sincerely believe to be accomplished by witchcraft it is not difficult to realize that the *imfwiti* is feared, dreaded, and hated beyond measure. He (or she) is a menace to society, and when convicted —nay, when accused—is generally rushed off to death, a death by the spear. So great is the detestation in which an *imfwiti* is held that the body is invariably burnt in a special way, so that the death of the contaminated *umupashi* may be also secured and the community be rid of the possibility of a reincarnation of such a spirit. If, however, the *imfwiti* has many and powerful relations, the people would fear to kill him. They would drive him out from their community, and he would lead an exile's life. Such treatment, however, is rare.

Ukuŵuka

The *imfwiti* taps the hidden forces of dynamism for the power to carry out his designs. Naturally the only way to attack the *imfwiti* is through those who also are able to tap those same sources of power. We have seen that the *umulaye* has this ability. He can utilize the forces of dynamism expressed in *ubwanga* for the curing of the sick, for success in hunting, or for protection from accident, and those expressed in *ifipa* for looking into the future; but by far his greatest use of these forces is in the detection of witches and wizards. For this reason the *umulaye* is very commonly called a witch-doctor, and unfortunately many people confuse the work of the witch-doctor with that of the witch. From the Bantu point of view the witch is a person who is a curse to society, while the witch-doctor is a blessing, in that he eradicates

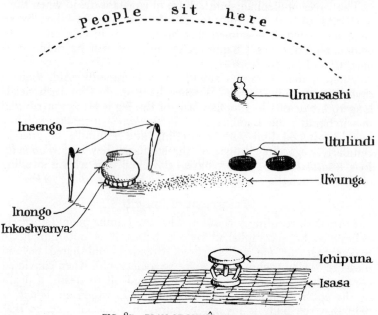

FIG. 87. PLAN OF ICHIŴANSA CHYAMFWA

this curse. We shall see presently how in practice the *umulaye* may really be a danger to the community.

Let us now consider what the *umulaye* does in order to detect, *ŵuka* (*nuka*, 'smell out,' as the Zulus have it), an *imfwiti*, and how he disposes of such a person.

When a person dies his relatives send a gift of two shillings to the *umulaye*, to summon him. In the old days beads were sent, or sometimes a fowl. He responds, and comes to their village with one or more of his assistants (*aŵantu*). The next morning early he goes to the bush and begins to divine (*ŵuka*), alone with his rattle (*umuseŵe*). First his assistants clear a large space, hoeing aside the grass and bushes. This space is called *ichiŵansa*, the great courtyard, or *ichiŵansa chyamfwa*, the court of death.

308

UŴUFWITI—WITCHCRAFT

The people who summoned him bring a supply of water. The *umulaye* now digs two holes with the 'paddle' (*chyochyo*) of his spear. The holes are about a foot apart, round, big enough for the insertion of the hand, and about nine inches in depth. He makes these holes in the middle of the *ichiŵansa*. To one side of these holes he places on the ground his *inkoshyanya yachisansa*. This is a rolled ring of twisted dark cloth, very carefully made, which the *umulaye* always carries. The *inkoshyanya* is used by the natives of Central Africa for balancing more easily pots or loads on their heads. On the *inkoshyanya* he places a medium-sized pot of water. The pot has been supplied from the village which summoned him. On either side of the pot he plants in the ground, point downward, a large bush-buck horn. These two horns contain his potent *ubwanga bwamfwiti*, charm for detecting witches. Next he lays down a line of meal (*uŵunga*) from the pot to the vicinity of the two holes he has dug. The meal has been brought from the near-by village in a small basket (*akalukwa*), which is laid aside, as it plays no part in the divining. A little distance from the holes he places an *umusashi* (a double calabash) of powerful *umusamu*. The mouth of this *umusashi* is closed by a wooden stopper. When these preparations are complete the *umulaye* fills the two holes with water and proceeds to smear the sides with mud in order to prevent drainage.

The *umulaye* now sits on a stool (*ichipuna*) set on a grass mat (*isasa*). Both the stool and the mat have been supplied by the villagers who summoned him. He commences to shake his rattle and to sing.

Here are two specimens of the type of song sung by an *umulaye* on such an occasion:

Ŵakalulu amatuntashi newaswe, kwani wabwene'chipini chyamalombe?

  " Little-hare, I'll have none of your playful bobbing about. Where did you see the nose-stud of the fine young men ? "

Nemulaye nshilya-mukungu, sombi ichikuuku chansumbi chilinkonwene!

  " I, the doctor, I don't eat relish of *kungu* leaves, but the hind-quarters of a fowl have broken me ! "

When he has finished singing he questions the symbols which he has arranged, asking, *Kani chiŵanda ichili umu ichilukwipaya' ŵantu, kani nimfwiti imbi ili-mo?* " Is it a demon which is killing people here, or is it some witch?" It is said that if it is a case of witchcraft the symbols answer, "There are witches!" Again he asks, "Are there two of them?" And the answer comes, "They are two!" Then he leaves off questioning. For this interrogation the *umulaye* has rubbed soot (*imishyangalala*) on the left side of his face and flour (*uẁunga*) on the right side. On his forehead he has rubbed red ochre (*ulushila*), and he wears on his head his feather headdress (*ichingalangala*), which he has carried in his large bag of grysbok skin. All this preparation, as well as the setting up of the symbols, is intended to impress the people and to put fear into their hearts.

It is time now for the people to gather to the *ichiẁansa*; but before they come the *umulaye* goes a little distance away to micturate, because, once he has started to *ẁuka*, he may not leave the *ichiẁansa*, where he sits from early morning to sunset. He returns to his stool, and sits down to await the people. This is a very momentous occasion, and the people gather in large numbers, for an absentee by his very absence may be suspected of being the guilty *imfwiti*. The people have a proverb, *Ichipuswa pachiẁansa nimfwiti*, "What is missed in the courtyard is the witch." The children too are brought, but there must be no crying among them. If the babies cry they must instantly be comforted. All the people sit down in a semicircle, facing the *umulaye*, with the symbols between him and them. They keep silence.

The *umulaye* now addresses the assembled people with the words, *Ichyeẁo chyaluẁa*, "The matter is a lost thing!" All maintain silence. He now takes two little black stones (*utubwenje*), the size and shape of marbles, and puts them both into one of the holes. Sometimes *inkamfi*, chewed leaves hardened into little balls, are used. They both sink to the bottom of the water. The headman of the village is now summoned, and the *umulaye* says to him, *Aẁulo'to'tubwe toẁilo!* "Take out both of those stones!" The man puts his hand into the hole and finds nothing but water therein. Then the *umulaye* says, *Tamubwene'chyeẁo ichi? Epo chili ichyeẁo, mulukukana, mulukufisa lukoso!* "Don't you see this matter? There is matter enough, you deny, you are just hiding the thing!" This is all said in an angry tone, in order to instil fear into the hearts of those present. The *umulaye* himself puts in his hand, takes out the stones from the hole, and says, *Tefifi?* "Aren't these they?" In this he evidently practises some sleight of hand. Then he adds, *Umuntu'yu nimfwiti yamwipeye!* "It is an *imfwiti* who killed this person!" All the people respond to this by saying, *Chipale koku tali nimfwiti!* "Maybe it is not an *imfwiti*!" He says, *Koku!* "No!"

The *umulaye* rises now and says, *Tanje mwense chyelele!* "Silence, every one of you!" He then proceeds to select one of the young men present, gives him a certain *ubwanga* in the

UŴUFWITI—WITCHCRAFT

form of small stones, called *utumwengwemwengwe*, and tells him
to go and throw them away in the bush at a distance. The
young man goes and throws them away. When he has returned
the *umulaye* gets up and goes over to one of the old people, and
says, *Tanje ima-po apo!* "Just stand up here!" When the
old man gets up, behold, that very packet of *ubwanga* is found
in the place where he had been sitting, or maybe among his
clothing. Fear immediately catches hold of every one, for they
think that the *imfwiti* has now been caught. Then it is that the
umulaye begins to dance with his *imiseŵe* (rattles), and asks the
old man, *Mwalimŵipailendo uyomuŵyenu?* "For what reason
did you kill your fellow?" But the old man can only tremble with
fear, and say nothing.

The *umulaye* now sings his song of triumph:

> *Mushyana-chinselawila, nikwilala mfumine,*
> *Ili afwile ŵanangwa, nkalala nensengo!*

> " [I] the dancer of the dance of abandonment,[1]
> It is from the Lala country I have come,[2]
> When [I] the great doctor die,
> I shall lie with the horns [in my hands][3]! "

At this the crowd scatters in haste, every one making for the
village in fear of the *umulaye*. Meanwhile, the assistants of the
umulaye, together with some of the stouter-hearted villagers,
seize the unfortunate accused man and carry him off to the
village. There they say to him, "Name your companion in
this witchcraft and we shall set you free!" In fear he answers,
Ŵanangwa ŵalya eŵo tulowa fweŵilo! "So-and-so over there—
the two of us practise witchcraft together!" They catch the
second man, and both are put to death. The promise of release
is only a blind to make the accused implicate some one else, and
a man or woman once caught in this way is never let off.

Trial by Ordeal

Usually the second person will expostulate and protest his
innocence. He will say, "This man is just lying about me,
because he does not want to die alone!" Sometimes the
people will say, "Very well. Let us first try [*peeshya*] a fowl!
If the fowl survives[4] we shall let them go, and if the fowl

---

[1] The people are so relieved that their fear is removed that they can now
dance in abandonment.
[2] *I.e.*, " I have come from far—a prophet from another country."
[3] *I.e.*, " People will bury me with my powerful medicines."
[4] Here they use the word *bwela*, return, meaning " return from the bush to the
village."

THE LAMBAS OF NORTHERN RHODESIA

dies we shall kill them both!" Meanwhile, both men are bound.

Now the *umulaye* sings a song which is borrowed from the *ichisungu* initiation ceremonies:

> *Nkunkulula'kaŵondwe-mushi;*
> *Ŵamame'li ŵafwile tamwali-mano;*
> *Ŵonsa'ŵa ndaŵaŵuula,*
> *Muŋomba walila!*
>> "Let me fully harvest the spinach in the village;
>> When my mother died there was no wisdom [in me] [1];
>> All of these I tell them,
>> The ground-hornbill has cried!"

The next morning they catch a fowl for the trial by ordeal. This trial is held in the bush. A potsherd (*akayinga*) of water is set over a fire to warm; it must not get too hot. A portion of outside bark is taken from an *umwafi*-tree, and either sliced (*kwesa*) or ground on a stone to powder. The slices or the powder are then mixed with the warm water, which takes on a reddish tinge; this mixture is, with the help of a funnel made from a leaf (*akansokolwa*), given to the fowl. The *umulaye* then says to the fowl, *Kani ulyamuntu nimfwiti ufwe!* "If yonder man is a wizard, die!" The opposite formula is then repeated, *Tekufwa lukoso kani taili nimfwiti!* "Don't die if he is not a wizard!"

As soon as it has been given the poison the fowl is allowed to go into the bush so that it may be seen whether it will eat. If the fowl begins to eat the people say, "It is just lies that have been told about these people," and they catch the fowl and take it back to the village. "The fowl has come back," they say, "these people are not *imfwiti*!" And they release them.

Many people, however, would not be satisfied by this, and some would say, "It is an *ichiŵanda* [demon] that has saved these *imfwiti* by drinking the *umwafi* [poison] before the fowl could get it." They therefore catch another fowl and have another trial. If in this case the fowl dies the accused men are carried off to their death.

Sometimes a different fowl is used to represent each of the accused. One may die and the other may survive.

An *imfwiti* is generally put to death by the spear. A large stack of firewood cut from *imiŵanga*-trees is made. The body is then cut up into small pieces, and when the fire is raging the pieces are thrown into it. With long poles the people now poke the fire to make sure that all is properly burnt. When they have

[1] *I.e.*, "I was still young."

ascertained that every vestige of the body is destroyed the *umulaye* brings a handful of leaves of a special tree and throws them on to the fire. The leaves burn and the smoke goes up. In this way the body and the spirit (*umupashi*) are both completely destroyed.

Another Method

At times the *umulaye* employs a different method. After the headman has put his hand into the hole of water and brought it out empty the *umulaye* says, *Yo, taili nimfwiti imfumu!* "No, the headman is not the wizard!" Then one by one the people are called out to go through the same test; and as each passes it successfully he is glad, knowing that he will not be accused of the witchcraft. Now there is one man left, and he trembles when he sees that he is the last, for he knows that the *umulaye* has so arranged it. When he comes forward the *umulaye* asks him, *Mpeni-po kafwaka!* "Give me a little tobacco!" The man says, "I have none, sir!" Then the *umulaye* says, *Ifipa fyaluŵa, ulenda shyani?* "The counters are lost. How do you behave?" He replies, "No, sir, I don't behave myself ill!" But the *umulaye* says, *Ikala bwino, utuŵuule bwino!* "Steady now. Tell us carefully!" Now the man is really afraid. At this point the headman of the village, who has summoned the doctor, may break in with, "Men, catch the enemy!" They catch him. Cases have been known of one thus threatened making a dash into the bush, and getting away successfully to the care of some other chief. The *umulaye* on these occasions has his axe or spear. Some of the distant onlookers come with spears, but the people who are gathered together must be unarmed.

Confession

In a great many of these cases the confession of witchcraft is made because the accused knows that all protestations of innocence are useless, so that he often admits having done what he never committed. He can then implicate some one else against whom he has a grudge by saying, "It is not only I; So-and-so was in the plot as well." Nevertheless, in many cases confession is made because the accused has actually been employing *ubwanga* with the object of causing the deceased person's death. He has tried and tried, and at last the person has died; this may be a mere coincidence, but he is convinced that his *ubwanga* has been successful. Sometimes it is actual poison he has administered in the deceased's food, and the cause is real. At times, if such

313

a person fears the outcome of the trial, when he hears that an *umulaye* is being called he will visit the *umulaye* secretly, confess his guilt, and offer him a child as a slave in order to bribe him. If the doctor agrees, after divining he will say to the people, *Ichiŵanda chilukumwipayeni!* "A demon is killing you!" This will stop any witch-hunt. Later on the culprit will send along the child, making out that the *umulaye* is a relative of his; in reality, however, the child will become a slave to the *umulaye*, the price of the father's life.

Funeral Detection of Imfwiti

Sometimes the detection of the witch or wizard is carried out at the time of the funeral, without the calling of any *umulaye*. In the morning, when they are about to bury the dead man, the people bring out the bier with the body, set it down in the court-yard (*uluŵansa*), and throw meal (*uŵunga*) upon it, saying, *Kani muno mumushi pali uwakwipeye, wiya-po, ubwele, umwikate wemwine!* "If the person who killed you is here in the village, do not go away. Come back and catch him yourself!" Then the undertakers take up the bier (*imiseeŵa*) and start off. When they have gone but a little distance from the village the body begins to get very heavy. On feeling this they turn round and return with it to the village. When they reach the village their burden forces them on and on until they reach a certain hut; they are driven right into the doorway of the hut, until the bier sticks there. Here the bearers set down the bier. The brother of the dead man comes, and throws some more meal on the corpse, and says, *Twamuŵono'wakwipaya, pano wime lukoso ulukuya*, "We have seen your murderer. Now just get up and go!" Then the bearers take up their burden, and go to the burial without any more delay. The owner of the hut where the corpse came to rest is seized as the *imfwiti*.

Sometimes, when the corpse is thus brought back to the village, it is to find the mourning villagers still assembled. On seeing the funeral returning the people scatter in fright, shouting, *Imfwa yabwela*, "The dead has come back!" But the bearers call out, *Mwitiina iyine'mfwa ikate imfwiti!* "Do not fear. Let the dead himself catch the wizard!" Then they go on, and set down the bier near some old man. Every one in relief shouts out, *Emfwiti iyi!* "This is the wizard!" and drag him off to his death.

All this merely shows that the relatives of the deceased have made up their minds to fasten the blame upon some one who is a burden upon the community owing to old age or who has for some reason become unpopular ; they are thus able easily and with popular acclamation to rid themselves of the unwanted person.

Utuyeŵela

In witchcraft the Lambas look upon the Aŵenambonshi, people living to the west, Kaonde and border peoples, as their superiors. It is said that a person will go to those western districts with money or goods and say that, as many of his relatives have died as a result of witchcraft, he wants to buy powerful *ubwanga* to compass the destruction of the *imfwiti*. A Kaonde man skilled in this trade will receive his offering, and provide him with two *utuyeŵela*,[1] a male and a female. These *utuyeŵela* are curious little creatures said to resemble, in size and appearance, a genet, but to be able to converse with people. Mr Melland's description of them, based on that of the Kaondes themselves, is that they are like tiny men. The man returns to his home with the *utuyeŵela*, and prepares for them a place to sleep in in the bush not far from his house. His wife grinds meal, and he takes it to them every day. The man then tells them that they can kill people in the village. The *utuyeŵela* are said to come invisibly to the village at night, carrying stones. They watch for the person whom they are to kill, and when they see him they throw a stone at him and strike him. The man re-enters his hut, and says that something struck him as he stood outside. After that he falls sick, complains of pains all over his body, and dies. This the *utuyeŵela* do day by day, killing such persons as their master instructs them to kill.

When their victims have been buried the *utuyeŵela* go to the graves and in a miraculous way change the bodies into other *utuyeŵela*. This interference with the dead affects their bodies only ; the *utuyeŵela* cannot touch the *imipashi* of their victims. In this way the number of *utuyeŵela* goes on increasing, each person killed adding one. They all assist their master in cultivating his gardens. His gardens are naturally larger than those of anyone else, and when such beliefs are held the charge of witchcraft made against the progressive and prosperous villager can be understood.

When the master's food comes to an end he will say to his *utuyeŵela*, "The food which you have been eating has come to an end. Go to So-and-so's place and steal food!" The little

---

[1] See Mr Melland's description in *In Witch-bound Africa*, pp. 204–206.

creatures go by night and steal food, bringing it and putting it into their master's grain-store. The owner of the corn will be amazed in the morning at the state of his bins, and say, "My corn has been stolen by *utuyeŵela* here in this village."

One day the whole crowd of *utuyeŵela* come to their master and say, "Give us a person to kill!" Their master will say, "Go and kill So-and-so!" But they refuse. They say, "We want your wife. If you do not want to kill your wife, we shall kill you yourself." Thus he has to consent to the death of his wife. The *utuyeŵela* kill her and change her into an *akayeŵela*. After some time they will come again and say, "We want a person." The man will say, "I have no one!" If this is true he will be able to take them all up, and carry them back to the west country, and restore them to the man from whom he obtained the first ones. "Here," he says, "are your little things. The people are all finished!" The Kaonde man will then take them all, and their temporary master will go back home. Should the man have any brothers or children left the *utuyeŵela* will not consent to go back home until they have killed them, and he is the only one left.

Detection of Utuyeŵela

Now when the villagers see that many people in the village are getting ill, this one and that one complaining of bad headache, they send and call a *mukamwami*. When the *mukamwami* arrives the people come to *ŵomba* at night, and the *mukamwami* says, "Where you are sitting I see five little creatures, all of them with stones in their hands, and I see the owner of the little creatures." On hearing this every one is afraid. That night the village elders question the *mukamwami*. He says, "Is there not some one who recently went to the west country?" The headman says, "There is!" Then the *mukamwami* says, "It is that very man who brought the little creatures, and it is he who is stealing your food!" Then they all believe that that is the man who has by witchcraft brought the *utuyeŵela*. The offender is caught and burnt as an *imfwiti*. The *utuyeŵela* are then believed to go back home.

The only persons who are able to see *utuyeŵela* are the *ŵamukamwami* (spirit mediums), the *aŵalaye* (doctors), their master, and the man from whom he bought them. Even the wife of their master, though she knows that her husband has them, is unable to see them. Hence if the *mukamwami*, when called, is unable to detect them the *umulaye* is sent for, that he may divine. When he has ascertained who is responsible he tells the village

316

UŴUFWITI—WITCHCRAFT

headman, and then goes back home. That night the headman climbs an anthill and calls out, "We know you who are bewitching by means of *utuyeŵela*; it is you who are transferring our food; for while the food of your fellows has come to an end, you still have some to eat. If you don't make restoration to us, leave our village and go back home!" All who hear this are amazed, and some headstrong ones at once fix the blame for the *utuyeŵela* upon some recent arrival. In the old days they would seize on him and burn him without further proof of his guilt.

Umulombe

Another instance of witchcraft attributed to the Kaonde people is the *umulombe*. A man whose relatives have been dying will go to the western territories, and, taking with him the equivalent of £1 in goods, will buy *umusamu wamulombe*, the charm for *umulombe*. He obtains a small house lizard (*malenganya*), which he carries in a calabash partly filled with meal. When he reaches his home he puts the lizard in the hollow (*ulupako*) of a tree on the outskirts of the village. Every night he visits the place and pours water on the lizard. It grows to an immense size, and eventually changes into an enormous snake, still living in the hollow tree. When it has thus grown it begins to beg of its master, saying, *Mpele*, "Give to me!" meaning that it wants people to kill. Then one morning its master says, *Nakupela liŵe*, "I have given you So-and-so!" The *umulombe*, however, refuses the offer. The man next says, *Nakupa liŵe!* "I have given you So-and-so," mentioning the name of some one else. This time maybe the *umulombe* accepts, and that night the man mentioned is taken suddenly ill and dies. Every day the same thing is done, the *umulombe* saying, *Mpele!* This fabulous snake lives on meal (*uŵunga*) in the hollow tree; its owner brings this meal day by day, and it does not leave its lair. When all the people in the village are finished off the *umulombe* changes its place of abode and goes to its owner's hut. Here it gradually kills off all his children, begging for them one by one, saying, *Mpele umwana woŵe!* "Give me your child!" Then one day it says, "Give me your wife!" Eventually only the master and the snake remain.

Long before this, however, the people might have called in a *mukamwami* (spirit medium), who will say, *Muno mumushi muli umuchyekulu upandile umulombe*, "Here in this village is an old man who has brought an *umulombe* by witchcraft." It is only the old who are thus accused. This accusation is sufficient for the old man to be killed and burnt.

When persistent ulcers refuse to heal it is often said, *Umulombe eulukumyanga-po pafilonda*, "An *umulombe* is licking the wounds!" Witchcraft through *utuyewela* and *imilombe* is said to be carried out by men, seldom by women.

Insanguni

Again, the great wizards of the west are credited with the ability to prepare the *insanguni*, a fabulous monster with the body and tail of a fish and the head of a man. Men go to buy them, saying, "I want an *insanguni* to protect me, so that I shall not die quickly." When a man has bought one he brings it home and puts it into a well which he has specially dug in a secret place. Around the well he plants *iwamba*, a species of cutting grass with spiky points, and reeds (*amatete*), and then returns to the village. When the *insanguni* desires to kill a person it watches for a comely woman or a handsome man, for it desires only the good-looking; as soon as it sees one such going to the river to draw water it steals that person's shadow (*ichinshingwa*) and takes it into its hole beneath the water. When that person returns to the village he dies. In the same way the *insanguni* treats young and old. Only the dead have no shadow.

One day the river will be found to have dried up, but the next day it will again be full. When the people see this they will say, *Muno mumushi muli upandile insanguni!* "Here in this village is a man who has brought an *insanguni* by witchcraft!" They will connect with this the frequent deaths which have taken place. The *insanguni*, when it has killed all the other beautiful women of the village, will eventually steal the shadow of its master's own wife if she is handsome, and the man will be left alone.

Further, the *insanguni* is believed to lick its master all over while he is asleep, and thus to add length of life to him.

If the suspicions of the people are fully aroused they will send for an *umulaye*, who will smell out the person who has brought the *insanguni*. When he is caught the *umulaye* will command him to lead the way to the well. The *umulaye*, with a crowd of people, will follow him there, and spit out (*pala*) a certain *umusamu* into the water in the well. This will bring out the *insanguni*, which will be immediately dispatched. After that its master is killed, and the bodies of both burnt in the fire. The *wamukamwami* are also able to detect the presence of an *insanguni*, but an *umulaye* has to be called in to kill it. It is said that no ordinary person can see the creature until the *umusamu* of the *umulaye* has been spat into the water.

The *insanguni* is also believed to be able to pour forth water, and envelop people and drown them. It is said to cause water trouble in mines.

The Wife of Munyonshi

About the year 1904, in the village of Chyushi, near the Lwamala river, there was an epidemic of deaths. An *umulaye* was summoned, and when he had divined he accused of witchcraft the wife of a man called Munyonshi. Munyonshi's brothers went to him secretly and said, "Your wife is a witch!" Munyonshi was thunderstruck, but at the time he agreed to their suggestion, and said, "All right, you kill her!" So they came by night and caught her, the attendants of the *umulaye* dragging her away into the bush and killing her with their spears, and the *umulaye* himself burning her. Munyonshi was left with two little children,[1] and their continual crying for their mother drove him nearly mad. He took up the two children and went to the old *boma* at Manda, near the Akashiŵa Kaŵena-mofya, where Mr Johnston was stationed, and told the whole case concerning his wife. The result was the arrest of one of his brothers among others. They were sent to Livingstone, where Munyonshi's brother died while serving a sentence of five years. Munyonshi could not return to live at his home near his sisters and other relatives as they were much embittered against him. He therefore moved to the village of Mukumbi, on the Kafulafuta river.

Kalongoŵila

Another interesting case occurred about the year 1909. There was living in Katanga's village an old Lenje man called Kalongoŵila. One day he said he was going out to pick mushrooms, and lost himself in the bush. Search-parties were out for four days, but found no trace of him. Then they sent messengers (*inkombe*) from village to village to inquire for him, but he could not be found. After considerable time relatives of the old man's, hearing of his disappearance, came to Katanga's village and demanded from Katanga a gun, on the charge that he had killed Kalongoŵila as an *imfwiti*. Katanga gave them the gun,

[1] One of these children, Meleki, was a schoolboy at the Kafulafuta Mission a few years ago.

acknowledging that since Kalongoŵila had lived in his village for a considerable time he was really responsible for his welfare.

After the foregoing consideration of the witchcraft practices of the Lambas we cannot deny the existence of definite occult practices, carried through with the intent of bringing about a death—real witchcraft. We have seen in what detestation a witch is held; and yet we have also seen that, although looked upon as a benefactor to the community, the *umulaye*, the witch-doctor, is regarded almost with terror. His power is enormous, and the abuse of that power is only too obvious. He can be bribed to let off a man whose conscience is guilty, and he can be paid, by those who are influential, to condemn some unfortunate innocent man or woman to death. He becomes the instrument of jealousy, envy, hatred, and revenge. His hand is definitely against progress or prosperity of the individual, and his influence cannot be described as other than baneful to the community as a whole.

CHAPTER XX

UŴUPALU—THE PROFESSION OF HUNTER [1]

The Profession

Uŵupalu, the profession of hunting, is held in very considerable esteem among the Lambas, and is akin to that of the blacksmith, *uŵufushi*. Like the two professions, those of the *umulaye* and the *imfwiti*, which we have just considered, this profession is one of choice and initiation, and is inseparably connected with the use of *ubwanga* (charm) and the derivation of dynamistic power. We shall also see that the spiritual world has to be reckoned with, and account taken of that sprite of the herds, Mwishyaŋombe. The Lamba makes an absolute distinction between the professional hunter, *umupalu*, and the trapper or fisher, who gets probably as big results, but has no status in the community. After considering the *rôle* of the professional hunter we shall give some details regarding the trappers and fishers of Lambaland.

The Initiation

When a young man desires to take up the profession of hunting he first tries his hand with the gun—in the old days with the bow and arrow—to see if he has any aptitude. He may repeatedly wound animals, but let them escape. He needs to go to one of the well-known hunters, *aŵapalu*, to procure the necessary *ubwanga*. Even should his first attempts be thoroughly

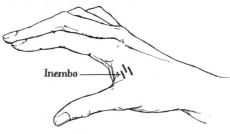

FIG. 88.   UBWANGA BWANAMA

successful, he will go to be tattooed with the charm (*lembo'bwanga*) in order that he may in future kill many animals.   More faith is

---

[1] The substance of much of this chapter appeared in the *Rand Daily Mail* (Johannesburg) some years ago.

placed in the charm than in the huntsman's skill, and an initiate will pay as much as £1 for the necessary initiation.

The professional hunter goes into the bush for a piece of root of a particular kind, slices this up, and puts it out to dry. He then grinds this *umusamu* on a grindstone, together with the head of a

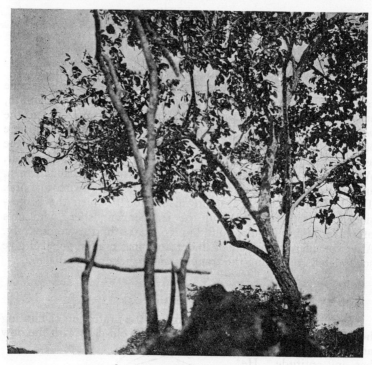

FIG. 89. AN ICHIPANDA ON AN ANTHILL
Photo by C. M. Doke

tree-snake called *lukungwe*. This provides the powerful *ubwanga*. The hunter and the initiate then proceed to the *ichipanda*, the hunter's shrine. Here the young man grips one of the poles comprising the *ichipanda*, in order, it is said, to steady himself, and the old hunter cuts with a sharp blade (*ichimo*) incisions (*inembo*) between the thumb and the forefinger on the back of the right hand, on the biceps of the upper right arm (where vaccination marks usually are), and behind the right shoulder-blade. Three short lines are cut in each of these three places, and into these incisions is rubbed the medicine which the hunter has

322

prepared. The initiate is then instructed as follows: *Tekupama neli nimbwa neli kuteŵe'nkuni lelo, yo!* "Strike nothing, not even a dog, and cut no firewood to-day!" After resting for the one day the initiate will be ready to undertake his hunting. Until he makes a name for himself he is called *umwana wabwanga*, child of the charm, and the professional hunter who has initiated him is called *nyina wabwanga*, mother of the charm.

Ukushilika

As soon as the initiate is successful and he has killed his first animal he must go and fetch his *nyina wabwanga* to perform the ceremony of warding off (*shilika*) the evil effects of his having killed an animal. Unless this ceremony is performed the *umupashi* (spirit) of the animals, called Kaaluwe, will use his power to prevent any other animals from being killed by this hunter.

The *nyina wabwanga* brings certain leaves, and with them flicks (*kupala*) the dead animal all over its body; this is said to be a sign of driving away the *ifiŵanda* (demons) sent by Kaaluwe to prevent the young man from killing other animals; by some it is said to get rid of Kaaluwe himself. The *nyina wabwanga* then inserts a stick into the animal's nose—this in order to block the way of Kaaluwe and prevent him from entering there. Kaaluwe is believed to ride on the backs of live animals, but to enter dead ones through the nostrils and thus steal all the meat. When the animal has been cut up (*pampa*), and the meat removed from the death-place (*ilambo*), the *nyina wabwanga* cuts a wooden peg from the *ulupaapi* bush, and hammers it into the ground on the spot where the meat was cut up. The *uŵufulu*, chyme or contents of the stomach which have been turned out, is deposited on top of the peg to cover it over. It is said that the peg is hammered into the ground in order to ward off the mates of the dead animal (*chichile'shiŵyakwe*). It is believed that there is a type of spiritual connexion between one animal and another, though it is not thought that animals have *imipashi* (spirits) in the way that people have. The *uŵufulu* in this ceremony is the symbol of earth (*iloŵa*) beneath which the death-place is buried. When this ceremony is over the *umupalu* and his initiate return to the village.

Ichinsengwe

At the time of the eating of the meat the vitals (*imitima*, plural of 'heart') and the ears (*amatwi*) are taken to be specially cooked for the *ichinsengwe* dance in honour of Kaaluwe or, as he is also called, Mwishyaŋombe. Men only dance this hunting dance, for which the assistance of the aŵayambo (professional hunting dancers) is often procured. We have already given several examples of the songs used at the *ichinsengwe*; [1] here we include two typical ones sung in honour of Kaaluwe:

> *Chyofwe malimba, walala muchyaŵu, watandaŵala !*
> *Mbe'chyakuŵe'fi, waipaya shyani, wemukombola ?*
> " The hippo bull is a great piano,
> He lies in the ford, his legs stretched out !
> What of a thing like this ?
> How have you killed it,
> O beater of the bark-cloth ? "

The hunter, who spends most of his time in the bush, sings boastingly:

> *Ninechyende-ende,*
> *Wakambwena kumoni !*
> " I am a wanderer in the bush.
> People will find me by the vultures [which
> gather to my corpse] ! "

In the evening, after the dancing is over, *inshima* porridge is cooked, and partaken of by men, women, and children, who also each have a mere taste (*akeshiŵilo kaŵuleme*, a sign of honour) of the vitals and ears. This meat is called *inama shyabwanga*, meat of the charm, and is designed to be eaten by aŵapalu only. Ordinary people may partake of this only when the *nyina wabwanga* has boiled it. It may not be roasted, nor may any salt be added to it. The *nyina wabwanga* digs up certain roots— the *umumpulumpumpi* is sometimes used—and puts them in the bottom of the pot before boiling the *imitima nematwi* (vitals and ears) together. When the mixture is cooked he distributes it to the people.

Kaaluwe

It has commonly been said that the Lamba people " worship the spirits" to ensure good hunting and in giving thanks for success in the chase. This is quite erroneous. Their *ifipanda*, or hunting shrines, which we shall consider presently, have no connexion with the 'worship' (*pupa*) of the *imipashi* (spirits of the departed). They are erected in honour (*chindika*) of "the guardian spirit of the herds." This little creature, who, though never seen, is believed to be like a little baby, *akanichye akamukoa* (a youngster with a navel string), is called by various names, the commonest

[1] *Cf.* Chapter XV.

being Kaaluwe, Mwishyaŋombe, Mwenshyaŋombe (the herd of the cattle), and Mwelaishyaŋombe. He is said to carry two *ifinsonta* (sharp wooden lances), and to travel on the backs of the animals in the herds of big game, such as eland, roan, sable, hartebeest, buffalo, zebra, and black water-buck. It is said that he does not frequent the herds of puku or elephant or the schools of hippo. When a young hunter has been unsuccessful in stalking a herd of game the old hunters say, "We saw Kaaluwe there, taking care of the animals." Kaaluwe watches over them, and if he sees any people coming he utters a hissing sound, "*Ffyu*" (*lishya'kakoŵe*), and off race the animals. Great hunters have *ubwanga* for removing Kaaluwe and for making him bring the animals. When such hunters leave the village they cut down a branch of an *umusaalya*-tree and plant it in the ground; they then carve from it two *ifinsonta* and say, *Chipanda chyaŵakaaluwe, tulukufwaya'ti ŵatupele-po inama ŵakaaluwe!* "It is a shrine to Kaaluwe. We want Kaaluwe to give us meat!" Then they go on their way.

Ichipanda

As Kaaluwe is regarded as the guardian of the animals, and as the greatest hunter himself (*umupalu umukulu*), one who can give game to the hunters, he is held in very great esteem by all *aŵapalu* (hunters). In his honour they erect the *ichipanda*, which may be regarded as his *umulenda* (shrine). There are many Ŵakaaluwe in all the different herds of animals. In Lamba conception they are looked upon as *aŵantu*, people, but not *aŵantunshi*, human beings.[1]

Each hunter has his *ichipanda*, which is not necessarily devoted to any one particular Kaaluwe. He cuts down an *umusaalya*-tree with many branches (*uwamampandakanya*), and sets it up in his *uluŵansa*, or behind his hut, or on a near-by anthill. Then he prepares a drinking calabash (*ulukombo*), and hangs it on the *ichipanda* thus erected. This *ulukombo* is dedicated to Kaaluwe. It is usual for the professional hunter and the novice to erect the *ichipanda* together. On the day on which the young man desires to hunt he goes to his *ichipanda*, as though to bid farewell to it, and grovels on the ground (*lambila*) before it, saying, *Mungofwe-ko ndukuya mumpanga, mumpele bwangu inama!* "Help me, I am going hunting. Quickly give me meat!" This is a prayer offered to Kaaluwe.

When he has killed an animal, and it is brought in from the

[1] *Cf.* Chapter XIV.

bush, all the meat is put down before the *ichipanda*, and the people gather there to get their portions. When the meat is divided out the head is cleaned of flesh, and the skull, with the horns and the vertebræ of the neck (*inkoti*), is stuck up on the *ichipanda*. The *ichinsengwe* is danced in front of the shrine.

If continual ill-success attends his hunting the hunter suspects that Kaaluwe is angry, and sends for the *umulaye* (doctor). The *umulaye*, when he has divined, will probably say, "It is Kaaluwe. He is angry because you have not brewed any beer for him. If you brew beer for him you will be able to kill game!" The

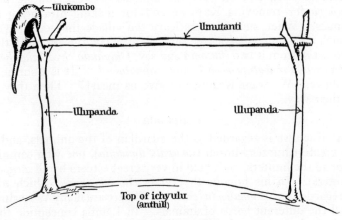

FIG. 90. ICHIPANDA

hunter then beseeches Kaaluwe, saying, "Have mercy on me. First let me get beer; I shall brew it for you!" So beer is brewed, and men dance the *ichinsengwe* while the beer-drink is on. The hunter pays the dancers in beads. No beer is ever put into the calabash of Kaaluwe.

At times an *ichipanda* of quite another type is constructed. Two upright forked poles (*impanda*) are planted in the ground, with a cross-piece connecting them. On this structure are hung the *ulukombo* and trophies of the hunt. There is something of sympathetic magic in this structure, as it is said to resemble the *umutembo*, or carrying-pole, on which the dead animal is carried to the village.

In many cases the *ifipanda* become quite an accumulation of many-branched tree-stems, especially if a village has been using one site for a number of years. Sometimes the dead stump of a tree is used for the same purpose, *inkombo* being hung on it, while around are stacked the skulls and horns. In one case I saw included in the collection an elephant's tail and the dancing

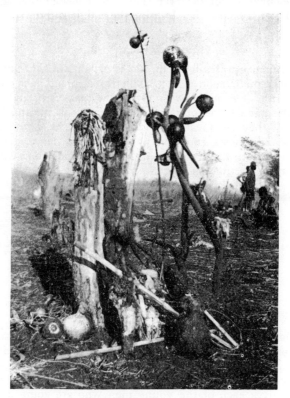

FIG. 91. A TWA ICHIPANDA, OR HUNTING SHRINE,
AT MUẂALA'S VILLAGE
Photo by C. M. Doke

rattles (*insangwa*) and dancing skirt (*uẁuyombo*) of the *aẁayambo* (professional dancers).

Ubwanga Bwaẁupalu

In Chapter XVIII we noticed to some extent the part played by charms in hunting, *ubwanga bwanama* being used to ensure the quick finding and killing of an animal. We have noticed also [1] that the *aẁayambo* (hunting dancers) provided a similar *isambwe* (bowl of medicine) to be given to the hunter that he might find

[1] Chapter XV.

the animals out grazing. In addition to all this there is a great deal more of hunting magic, *ubwanga bwaŵupalu*, practised especially by elephant-hunters. We shall now consider this, and also the *ubwanga* necessary when hunting the buffalo and the rhinoceros.

Ubwanga Bwansofu

The ordinary professional hunter is called *umupalu, umuyinga*, or *ichiŵinda*, but as soon as he has killed an elephant he is honoured with the title of *nkombalume*. When the meat is brought to the village the people do not *ipike'chinsengwe*, cook for the hunting dance, but they cut meat from the heart and head of the beast and *ipike'limbalakata*, cook for the *ilimbalakata* dance. This is a dance learnt from the Kaonde and Mbwela people, and with it go special songs, as, for instance:

(1) *Walindekele,*
   Kanokanama katema'mashyashya [1] *wo:*
   Kanokanama katema'mashyashya.

   " You left me alone.
   This little animal was cutting down branchlets, *wo:*
   This little animal was cutting down branchlets ! "

(2) *Twaŵasanga mumalalo wo:*
   Ŵankalawe ngaŵashyale wo.

   " We have found them in their sleeping-places, *wo.*
   Let the great hunters remain behind, *wo.*"

The hunting of elephants is, then, considered to be so much apart from even the ordinary professional hunting that it is not surprising to find special precautions necessary, special *ubwanga*, and special taboos observed. On the day before the hunt the *umupalu* gives each of the young men who are going a cowrie-shell (*ichilundu* or *umuŵela*). That night some special roots are pounded; these constitute the *ubwanga* (charm), which is put into the *imiŵela* shells at night. All now leave their *imiŵela* on a pot-sherd (*ichiyinga*) at the spot where the *ubwanga* was prepared. The next morning at dawn the hunters go to the place with their guns, their loads of meal, and cooking-pots. They take out the cowrie-shells, and in the potsherd they place the remains of the pounded roots, and fill it up with water. With this medicated water they all sprinkle their weapons and their loads; then they cover over the potsherd.
   The wives of the hunters are then warned regarding the following taboos.

   [1] *Amashyashya* is the Mbwela equivalent of the Lamba *ifisako.*

Tekupamo'mwano'lupi! "Don't strike a child with the hand, to punish him."

Tekusangano'mwalalume nekumupamo'lupi! "Don't meet a man and strike him with the hand, to sport with him."

Tekupyange'toi akasuŵa muŋanda! "Don't sweep the ashes from the house by day."

Tekupatike'chintu pachitupa peulu wemwine! "Don't put anything up on the upper loft yourself."

Tekulomba fwaka kumwalalume! "Don't beg tobacco from a man."

It is firmly believed that if one of these taboos (*imishiliko*) is broken by a woman at the village the elephants will 'tell' the hunter when he meets him; and, say the Lambas, *Insofu taiŵepa*, "An elephant never tells a lie!" Should a hunter see two elephants in the act of connexion he would immediately stop, and say to his younger companions, "Let us go back home. My wife has committed adultery!" Should the younger hunters be obstinate and want to fire on the elephants, the older man would refuse, saying, "No, if we attack it will kill us!" They would then return to the village. On his arrival at the village the hunter would call his wives and accuse them of adultery. In the olden days the word of the elephant was taken against that of the woman, and one of these would suffer the death of the adulteress.

Should a woman break taboo and strike a child in anger, the hunter would know of this by finding when he reached the elephants that one had pulled down a branch and struck another with it.

If a person dies at the village while the elephant-hunters are away they will find the whole herd of elephants lying down. The hunters will return immediately to the village for the mourning.

If a male elephant is found sporting with a female elephant the hunter knows that his wife is 'playing' with the men at the village.

If an elephant is found digging up the earth the hunter knows that his wife has broken taboo and has swept out the hut in the daytime.

If an elephant is seen to raise his trunk to the top of a tree it is known that the wife has stretched up her arm to put something on the loft (*ichitupa*).

If a male elephant is seen to touch the teats of a female, then it is known that irregularities are going on at the village dances.

If an elephant is seen to be plastering mud on his face it is a sign of death, for the women put mud on their faces when wailing.

If the elephant takes a clod of earth in his trunk and gives it to a female it is known that the wife at home has broken the tobacco taboo.

It is noticeable that if any of the taboos are broken by the wife at home the hunter will find the elephants in a roused and angry state, difficult and dangerous to approach, but it is believed that, should all the commands be rigorously observed, the animals will be found *ishitumpile*, foolish and easy to attack.

If the elephants are vicious, and a wounded one charges the hunters in fury, they all put their *imiwela* in their mouths, in order to render themselves invisible, and take them out again only when the beast is dead.

Ubwanga Bwamboo

Buffalo (*imboo*) and rhinoceros (*kakwele*) are dangerous animals to hunt, and there is special *ubwanga* to assist the hunters against them. The hunter carries a *chikasole*, a large reed-buck horn filled with special *ubwanga*. When he leaves the *umutanda* (zareba) in the morning he hangs up the *chikasole*, and goes to the hunt convinced that when he meets these animals he will kill them.

The Omens

However skilful a hunter may be, and however potent the *ubwanga* he has secured, he dare not ignore the signs and omens which he may encounter if he is to be successful and avoid danger and disaster. The Lambas, as we have already seen, have a proverb, *Kumbonshi takuya ubwela*, "To the west he does not go who would return again." And so some hunters, if they desire to hunt in the bush to the west of their village, will start out eastward and then work round to the west. They believe that misfortune would befall them if they started out westward. There are many ill-omens, *imbiko*,[1] which will turn a hunter or a traveller back if he meets them when setting out. If a hare runs away and then stops to look back at him, if a lurie flies toward the west, if a chameleon climbs *down* a stick, or if one of many other unlucky things is encountered, the hunter dare not proceed on his way. He will turn back, and postpone his hunt until the next day.

Should, however, all the omens be favourable, the chameleon be climbing *up* the stick, the hare racing straight off without stopping, and the lurie flying eastward, he will expect a kill, and

[1] See Chapter XIII.

continue along the path with light heart and swift step. When he has reached the point in the path where he considers it wise to turn off into the bush, in order to stalk some glade of which he knows, he utters the following 'prayer' to his *umupashi* (spirit): *Ulumpasumpasu ulwakupasuchila pakana kanama*, "Turning off the path, to turn and meet a young animal." This should give him the necessary success in meeting the animal. The success in killing is already provided for by the doctoring of himself and his weapon. So little does the Lamba hunter consider that his own personal skill counts for anything in the hunt.

When all these precautions fail the hunter is not without an excuse for his comfort. *Mwishyaŋombe alenda petanga lyanama*— "Mwishyaŋombe travels with the herd of animals," he says, "and I have not taken the precaution to win his favour." A hunter, too, may be tempted to kill a guinea-fowl early in his expedition; he will kill nothing else, for is not the name of the guinea-fowl, *ikanga*, derived from the verb *kanga*, to baffle? And will not this prevent his meeting anything else? *Waipaye' kanga, lwakanga*, "You have killed a guinea-fowl, and the journey is baulked!" is a saying they have. The hunter may kill guinea-fowl on the homeward journey, but not when starting out. Like the European huntsman, the native hunter can see the irony of circumstances pictured in this saying : *Inama shilaw̃oneka kuwakuw̃ulo'w̃uta*, "Game appears to the one without a bow."

So bound up with superstition is the hunting of Lambaland that when the success desired has been achieved the huntsman has still numerous taboos to observe. Should he kill a zebra, he must never bring the hoofs to the village; they must be left in the veld. Should an ant-bear be killed, its head must never be brought to the village. If these precautions are not observed misfortune will quickly follow.

Weapons

A few years ago the Lamba hunter depended almost entirely upon his bow and arrows, but to-day very few bows are found in Lambaland, and old guns of the muzzle-loading type are all the vogue. The bow is called *uw̃uta*, and indeed this term may be applied to almost any weapon, the gun, *imfuti*, being often so styled.

The Lamba bow is a very well-made, well-finished weapon, unlike the 'ready-made' inferior bow of the Bushman. When strung it is just five feet in length, and is made of very strong, yet springy wood, smoothly and beautifully shaped. The bowstring is very strong, and is made from well-twisted sinew of stembok or sable antelope, the sinew of these animals being the strongest for the purpose. The string passes through a hole at each end of the bow, and is then wound round the wood for a certain distance, the tightening being accomplished by clever turning of the string. In some cases the string is twined round the whole length of the wood, adding strength and weight thereto.

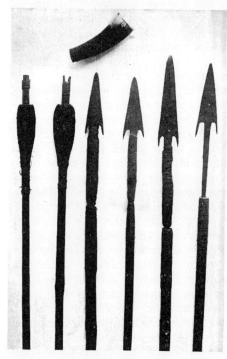

FIG. 92. ARROWHEADS (WITH AND WITHOUT POISON WAD), FEATHERED ENDS OF ARROWS, AND DUIKER PIPE

Photo by W. Paff

Lamba arrows (*imifwi*) are usually very carefully made, the hafts being of smoothed and polished wood, though sometimes stout reed is used instead. The feathering of the arrows is a work of art, and must take considerable time and perseverance. There are two types of arrowheads, each of iron, the *uluŵeshi*, or spear-headed arrow, being not so commonly used as the *umufwi wamatwi*, with its long, delicate barbs.

In the majority of cases the barbed arrows are poisoned; the poison, *uŵulembe*, is fixed behind the barbs in a thick pad, which is sometimes composed of gum mixed with poison, or of bits of soft bark soaked in the poison and wound round. As a rule the seeds are extracted from the sausage-like fruit of the *uŵulembe* creeper, dried, and then pounded. The fatty pulp is then pasted on to the arrows behind the head.

A hunter will seldom own more than half a dozen arrows; he takes great care of them, for they are not easily made. His shooting is remarkably accurate at twenty-five or thirty yards, but seldom will he venture at longer range. Should he miss, he will pick up his arrow again. Should the arrow strike the animal, the poison will be sure to work in an hour or two; the hunter will track the animal till he finds it dead, when he will recover at least the head of the arrow, embedded in the flesh. It is seldom that arrows are lost.

The guns which are widely used by the natives to-day are very primitive weapons, many of them bearing dates from 1850 to 1860. They vary in local value from twenty-five shillings to £5, and are used as exchange commodity for paying death-dues and settling fines almost as much as they are for hunting. The powder used has hitherto been procured from native traders in the Congo and in Angola. Any bits of iron or brass are used as the charge, and when the buck is hit a ghastly wound is usually the result.

No hunter is completely armed without his spear and axe, and to these is sometimes added a hunting-knife. The spear, *ifumo*, varies in length from about 4 feet 6 inches to 5 feet, the metal blade being anything from 1 foot to 1 foot 6 inches in length. In some cases the iron used in the spear-heads is quite pliable, and the weight of the wooden haft will often bend the blade at right angles when it sticks into an animal. Another type of spear, the *impula*, is made of solid metal throughout, much better tempered than in the common spear, is about 4 feet in length, and has a hand-grip of gummed gut tightly wound round the centre. Each type of spear has a 'paddle' on the lower end, which is used for sticking the weapon upright in the ground, for digging up roots, or even, when an axe is lacking, for cutting down small trees to get at the bark.

The Lamba spear has a use intermediate between that of the short stabbing assegai of the Zulus and the 8-foot hurling javelin of the Ilas. It is usually thrown at close range—anything up to ten or twelve paces—and is used for finishing off a wounded animal brought to bay. The spear blade also takes the place of a huntsman's knife, for very few Lambas carry any knife at all. The blade can be loosened from the haft and used to skin the animal and to cut up the meat. The people have a phrase regarding the buffalo which calls him *impulumbi yakatemo nemwele*, "the buffalo of the axe and the hunting-knife," for his skin is so tough (and the same applies to the hippo, the elephant, and the rhino) that the spear is not sufficiently tempered to cut it through; hence the axe and the knife are essential.

The Lamba axe, *akatemo*, is made of the hardest and best-

333

THE LAMBAS OF NORTHERN RHODESIA

tempered iron. The head, about 10 inches long, is set through a hole into the knob of a stout handle. The cutting edge is never more than 2 inches broad, but it is wonderful what huge trees the men can fell with this narrow implement. The axe is essential to the hunter for cutting up the animal, and will chop through the bones of the larger beasts. It is also used for cutting down the necessary carrying-poles (*imitembo*) and for stripping off the bark (*ulushishi*) used for tying up. A Lamba proverb has it that *Uli nekatemo emwine wanama*, "He who has the axe is the owner of the meat." The owner of the axe needed to cut up an animal will claim his share of the meat even if he took no part in the killing.

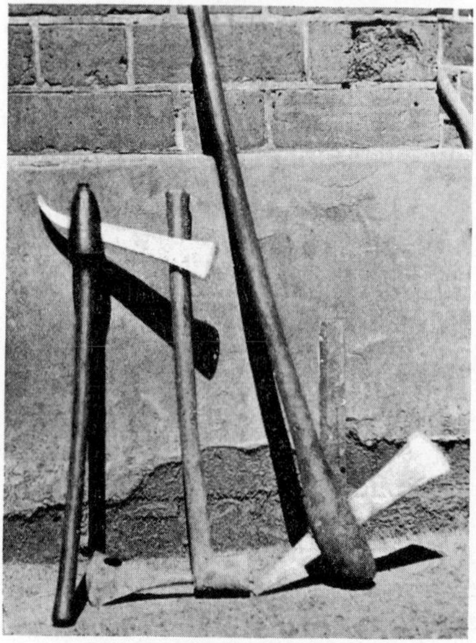

FIG. 93. LAMBA AXES
Photo by C. M. Doke

The Hunt

In Lambaland the best times for hunting are just after sunrise and just before sunset. The hunter prefers the early morning, as he has the day before him should he wound an animal. Often he will set out, sometimes alone, sometimes with one or two other men, long before sunrise, so as to reach the spot where he expects to find the game as soon as it is light enough to see. The best part of the year for hunting is toward the end of the dry season, when there is still a certain amount of long grass about for cover, and yet burnt patches in which the new shoots attract the game.

The Lambas are very good trackers of the spoor, and I have known some who could follow a trail almost as quickly as a Bushman. Should the hunter come upon fresh spoor before reaching his destination, he will examine it carefully to see how recent it is. The freshness of a bit of broken grass, the amount of spring in grass or leaves trodden on, the state of the sand on the edges of the footprint all tell whether it is minutes or hours since the buck passed, and whether it will be worth while following.

334

If he decides to follow, the hunter's first concern is to determine the direction of the *kaŵeshya*, for even when all seems still there is likely to be a slight drifting tendency of the air in some direction. A little sand is picked up in the hand, and dropped in order to show the direction. This will determine the amount of caution

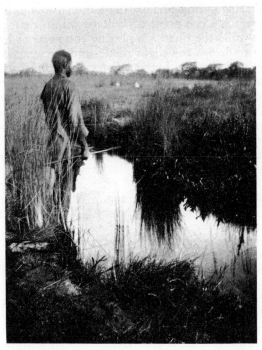

FIG. 94. ON THE LOOK-OUT FOR GAME AT A WATER-HOLE
Photo by C. M. Doke

necessary in following any trail. From the spoor the hunter knows at once whether it is sable, hartebeest, roan, waterbuck, eland, or any other large buck he is following. If he is following sable he can tell whether he is following a bull or a cow not from the footprint so much as from watching for the sudden scratch across the trail which the sable bull repeatedly makes with his hoof.

After careful following of the spoor the quick eyes of the huntsman may catch a glimpse of his unsuspecting quarry. Instantly he sinks to the ground, once more tests the direction of the air, and begins to stalk, taking advantage of every bit of

335

cover, bush, grass tuft, or ant-heap. He watches his quarry. The buck becomes uneasy, looks up from his feeding with ears erect—maybe looks straight in the direction of danger, sniffing the air. The hunter stands rigid, perhaps within full sight of the animal, but so still that he is mistaken for a tree-stump or an ant-heap. After a while the buck lowers his head once more to continue grazing. Immediately the hunter resumes his cautious stalking to reach some point of vantage within easy range. He knows that while the quarry is grazing the noise of his chewing is sufficient to drown any slight rustle, and the scent of the grass so near his nostrils dulls his sense of smell. But he knows also that the nearer the ground the head of the animal, the better he hears any foot thud that the hunter may make. Then, without any further warning, the arrow is released; the noble beast rears up with an arrow fast in his flank, and goes off at lightning speed.

The hunter is satisfied. He sits down, kindles a fire, takes out his pipe for a smoke, calls up his friends, who have remained some distance back in hiding. After a rest they all leisurely take up the spoor, to come upon the animal after a few miles, lying dead from the effects of the virulent poison. The lump of meat around the arrow is cut out and thrown away. The rest is cut up and conveyed to the village.

Lamba hunters at times train dogs to pull down small animals when wounded, though they usually depend upon their own speed in following badly wounded game and their skill with the spear to dispatch them.

The animals most feared by the native hunter are the elephant, the buffalo, and the sable. Of the buffalo they say, *Lambwe munongo, mukaŵanda mulume muŵyo,* "Buffalo bull when in the pot, but on the veld he is your rival!" They dare not mention the buffalo bull by his name, *lambwe,* except when he is in the pot being cooked; when he is in the veld he is as fierce as a man who has been despoiled of his wife. The sable bull, *kantanta,* has been credited with standing at a ford and preventing people from crossing. It is believed, too, that should a young man make the sable his first kill he would be lost and never return to his village. Similar wizardry is believed of the eland.

With the Lambas the eland is royal game. If killed, the animal has to be taken to the paramount chief. If distance makes this impossible, the skin, horns, and tail have to be taken to him.

The death of an elephant is the signal for the gathering of villagers from far and near like vultures to feast on the carcass. The Lambas say, *Umuntu ninsofu, ukwafwa takuluŵikwa,* "A man is an elephant; where he dies is not forgotten." That is, neither the death of a man nor the death of an elephant can be hidden.

The habits of the wild game are well known to every Lamba hunter. Advantage is taken of the innate curiosity of the roan. The hunter, after approaching as closely as possible to his quarry, will sit down behind a bush and wave a piece of rag above it on the end of a stick. The curiosity of the roan is aroused,

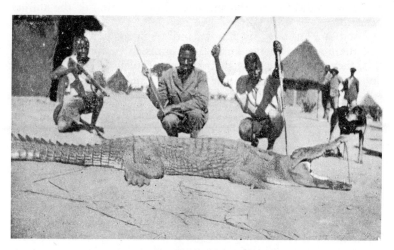

FIG. 95. A MAN-EATER AT KAFULAFUTA MISSION
Photo by the Rev. A. J. Cross

and nearer and nearer he will come to see this wonder. When he is near enough the shot will be fired.

For duiker-hunting a 'duiker pipe'[1] is made. Often this is the slit stem of a pumpkin leaf. When this is blown a shrill note is sounded, resembling the cry of a young duiker. This attracts any old duiker near, which will run up to find out the reason for the cry. The concealed hunter has his advantage. To add insult to injury duiker pipes are sometimes constructed from a portion of duiker horn itself, the wide part of which is covered with thick cobweb (*lembalemba*). The narrow end is blown across in the same way as the mouth of a bottle to produce a shrill sound.

In certain parts of Lambaland there are adventurous hippo-potamus-hunters who, armed with a barbed harpoon (*ichiŵingu*), attack the animals from boats in the water. The harpoon is

[1] See Fig. 92.

ingeniously constructed with a reed shaft for throwing, but is so arranged that when it strikes the shaft breaks off, leaving the short, heavy iron, attached to a long rope, embedded in the animal. These ropes are sometimes fixed to trees on the river-bank; and with several harpoons in their quarry the hunters will exhaust and eventually dispatch the hippo. Usually, how-ever, the reed shaft is also attached to the rope at a little distance from the metal, so that when detached the reed will float up and act as an indicator, on the surface, of the position of the animal beneath.

Ant-bear hunting in Lambaland demands special courage, and there are not many ant-bear hunters to be found. Despite this, they are regarded by the natives as foolish persons, for they are sometimes blocked in the holes by the animals and buried.

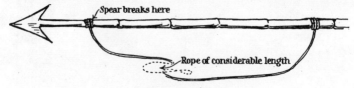

Spear breaks here

Rope of considerable length

FIG. 96. ICHIWINGU

The hunter (*umupalu wampendwa*) usually goes with two com-panions to where ant-bears (*impendwa*) have been found at work. By examining the state of the ground thrown up and any spoor there may be the hunter determines which hole the ant-bear has last entered ; and he too enters, with his spear. Fearlessly he goes down the narrow burrow until he finds the animal asleep, or else drives it to the end of the tunnel, where he spears it. The hunter then shouts and shouts until those above locate his position, and dig down to him, for the ant-bear cannot be dragged out through the narrow, tortuous passage. When an ant-bear hunter goes hunting his wife has to observe certain taboos. She must not close tightly her door at night, nor must she closely shut her door by day if she leaves the house, for if she should do this the ant-bear would shut in her husband, and he would lose his life.

In the Lambaland forest the honey-guide (*inguni*), the joy of the hungry traveller, is the bane of the *umupalu*. Directly this curious little bird sees a human being it begins to chatter in order to attract his attention. The traveller wanting honey will follow the honey-guide as it flies from tree to tree until it reaches the hive, for this bird hopes for the young bees scattered about when the honey is cut out. But the hunter's anger is roused when he hears the honey-guide chattering, and he pelts it with stones to drive it away, for the noise it makes warns the animals that people are about.

Trapping

As we have already observed, trappers and fishers belong to quite a different category from hunters. They are looked upon as ordinary folk, and their calling not as a profession. This is mainly due to the fact that, in the ordinary way, no *ubwanga* is used in the pursuit of their occupations. As a matter of fact, fishers are often derided and called *aŵatwa*, swamp-dwellers.

Aŵamyando

Nevertheless, trappers of a certain type do use *ubwanga* in preparation for their work. These are men who set certain rope-traps. They are called *aŵamyando*, people of the ropes, or even by courtesy *aŵapalu ŵamyando*, hunters of the ropes; they also have *ifipanda*, but these are differentiated from those of the proper *aŵapalu* by the name of *ifipanda fyamyando*, shrines of the ropes. Such a trapper plaits a long, strong rope, and when it is completed takes it and hangs it upon his *ichipanda*. He then collects a quantity of leaves of a certain tree which constitutes his peculiar *umusamu*, makes a heap of them beneath the *ichipanda*, and sets fire to the heap so that the rope is thoroughly smoked. In the morning he takes his rope and goes to set his trap. A long branch of an *umwenje*-tree, having a diameter of about 5 inches, is cut down. A hole is dug, and the pole planted in it. The pole is then bent over and connected to the rope-trap, which has been carefully concealed in a path along which the animals come. When the animal treads on the concealed trap the pole is released, and, springing up with tremendous force, catches the animal by its leg. This type of trap is called *ichinsala*, and small buck, such as grysbok, stembok, duiker, and even at times reed-buck and gazelle, are caught in it.

Ubwanga is not employed with any other type of traps, nor are any of the animals killed in these other traps ever offered at an *ichipanda*; but the trapper may say, *Imipashi yanji yampela*, "My spirit has given it to me," in this way praising and acknowledging the spirit for whose welfare he is responsible. The real *umupalu* digs no game-pit and sets no spring-trap; his trust is in his weapons and the *ubwanga* of which he has control.

Small animals and birds of various species are caught by

several kinds of spring-traps. It is said that the turtle-dove coos this mournful refrain:

> *Akatembo kaŵi kakampelanya,*
> *Kakampampala panshi !*
> *Ichifu chiliwȇme kachimpumpula kumutwi,*
> *Kamfwa, kanduŵa-ko !*
>
> " The bad bird-trap swings me to and fro,
> And dashes me down !
> The trap that is good hits me on the head—
> I die and forget ! "

Ichifu

Under this name the two main types of bird-trap are alluded to. Little boys are fond of setting traps for small birds and mice by means of a poised slab of stone or a piece of ant-heap. Bait is placed beneath—corn or maybe caterpillars to attract the thrushes—and when they peck at this the little sticks which support the weight are touched and bring it down.

Umwando

Nooses of plaited string are set in the grass runways which guinea-fowl are wont to use. The birds catch their heads in these and are strangled. Similar nooses, called *akatembo* or *ingoloŵola*, are set near corn-heads for doves and parrots, while a special type of string-trap is set at the mouth of prickly cucumbers (*ifitungusa*), and is exceptionally successful in catching the *pwele*, or African thrush. A larger type of string-trap, called *ichinkoloto*, is baited with dead mice, maize, etc., and used to catch mungooses, monkeys, genets, and other such small animals.

Yet another type of trap, the *inkola*, is constructed of a tube of hard bark with string fixed thereto. This is inserted in the tunnels of mice and moles. It is said that the mole will snap the string at one end, but that the one at the other will for that reason hold him all the more tightly.

Uŵuchinga

It is evident that the successful trapper has to study the habits of each species of animal he desires to catch. Big game is usually caught by means of the game-pit (*uŵuchinga*). At times the villagers construct rude fences of poles and branches, maybe extending for a couple of miles through a tract of forest. At intervals gaps are left, and in these gaps the game-pits are dug. Herds of animals, trekking across the country, come upon the fences, and skirt along them until they find an opening; thus some unwary ones are caught. Natives state that the reed-buck (*impoyo*) is never caught in such a trap. He suspiciously moves along the fence at a distance in the long grass until he reaches the end of it.

Usually, however, the Lamba trapper watches the favourite haunts of certain animals and sets the game-pit there. Some of the large anthills contain an amount of salt, and the game in places have licked large hollows in them. It is in the game path at such a place that a game-pit will be dug. The pit is usually about eight feet in length and some six feet deep; it may be four feet wide at the top, tapering down, V-shaped, to less than a foot at the bottom. Very light sticks and branches are placed over the pit; these are covered by grass, which is plentiful, with earth above the grass.

So cleverly are the pits covered that it takes a watchful eye to see them. On two occasions a carrier gripped my arm and saved me from stepping into one of these pitfalls. This type of game-pit is called *uŵuchinga bwalutando*. I have not observed the Lambas using stakes at the bottom of such a pit. They depend upon the shape of the pit to hold the game which falls in, for the more an animal, especially one of the larger ones, struggles, the more firmly do its legs become wedged. The trapper visits his game-pit every day, and with his spear dispatches any animal he may find therein. After the animal has been removed the pit is covered again as before.

For trapping hippo the Lambas dig circular pits, about five feet in diameter and from seven to eight feet in depth, in the paths frequented by these animals. This type of pitfall is called *uŵuchinga bwachinu* or *uŵuchinga bwanchili*. It is covered in the same way as the ordinary game-pit, but sometimes sharpened stakes are fixed upright in the bottom. Should a hippo fall into one of these holes, even though he be ten feet in length, it would be impossible for him to get out, on account of his enormous weight.

Etiquette

In trap-setting and examining there is an etiquette which most Lambas rigidly observe. They say, "The trap one sets in the presence of a child one also examines with the child present." If anyone were present at the setting of the trap, even though he be but a youngster, he must be called to share in whatever is caught.

THE LAMBAS OF NORTHERN RHODESIA

Sense

The Lambas avoid anything in the way of lion-hunting. A man who kills a lion is not called *umupalu*, but is designated by the term *umukali*, a fierce person. They often, however, set traps for leopards if these have been worrying their dogs or goats. Should a leopard catch a dog, the villagers will follow the trail in the morning, and in all probability will find a portion of the dead animal not consumed. This they will take back to the village and place in a small, hastily constructed hutch of poles. In this hutch-trap, which they call *sense*, are two compartments, the one where the carcass is having no opening apart from the interstices between the poles, the other having a narrow doorway. A large log is poised in an upright position above this opening, and kept in place by a contrivance of sticks and ropes within.

That night the leopard will return to eat the rest of his kill, follow the trail back to the village, and locate the hutch with the remains of the carcass within. After trying every other way to get at the meat he will enter the narrow doorway. Directly he treads on one of the poles on the floor within the poised log will be released, fall down, and block up the entrance. In their excitement at such a capture the natives usually rush out and pierce the leopard through and through with their spears, the spaces between the poles giving them this opportunity. In this way they more often than not completely spoil the skin. At times a live dog or a live goat is confined in the closed compartment to attract leopards or hyenas. Lamba children trap cane-rats with a similar but smaller type of *sense*.

Catching Flying Ants

The Lambas have a curious way of catching flying ants, one of those little delicacies of which they are so fond in the rainy season. They dig a small hole at the ant-heap where the ants have been coming out, build a little imitation house over the hole to darken it, and pour in water. The insects, thinking that it is night and raining, emerge in great numbers, and are caught and collected into pots.

Fishing

In Lambaland fishing is very clearly divided as follows into:

(1) *Ukuloŵa*, to fish with line and hook.
(2) *Ukwikashya*, to fish with net.

(3) *Ukwalila*, to fish with weir-trap.
(4) *Ukutwila*, to fish by poison.
(5) *Ukupila*, to fish by bailing.
(6) *Ukusasa*, to fish by treading.
(7) *Ukusumba*, to fish by spearing.

Fishing is distinctly the work of the men, but there is one type of fishing, that by bailing, which is performed by the women. Most of the rivers of Lambaland, especially the Lufuŵu, the Luswishi, and the Lunga, abound in fish, particularly the barbel and the bream. Practically everybody takes part in fishing of one sort or another, and the art is not so restricted to professionals as is that of hunting. Nevertheless, there are men and communities specially skilled in fishing who make it a trade, dried fish being bartered for meal and other commodities or sold to obtain tax money.

(1) *Ukuloŵa*. Lamba boys amuse themselves by catching tiny fish, much like sprats, with small, barbless hooks (*indoŵo*) attached to native twine. Barbed hooks have only been used since the Europeans came into the country. The boys attach the string to a reed, watch the fish, and whip up the hook if one bites at the bait. Skilful fishers land a fish at almost every whip. The bait used is *inshima* porridge. For barbel night lines are usually set with a barbed hook and, if possible, the entrails of a fowl for bait. Often grasshoppers (*ŵatete*) or worms (*ifinashi*) are used. These lines are secured to a tree at the side of the pool or to reed floats. Women sometimes fish with worms (*ifyambo*) threaded on to the end of a piece of bark string (*ulushishi*) which is fixed to a stick. When the fish attempts to swallow the worm it is suddenly jerked out into a basket.

(2) *Ukwikashya*. Native nets of string work, called *utombe*, are dragged across ponds and up streams when the water is subsiding. Sometimes the fish are driven into hidden nets by beating the water or throwing stones into it. This type of fishing is sometimes done by means of the *ulwando*, a long fence of *imisengelo* mats weighted with stones, and built across a marsh. Many people go behind this fence and continually push it forward, driving the fish into the shallows. Then the obstruction is fastened at the ends, and the people enter the fish-filled shallows and kill with *imyondo* (fish-spears).

(3) *Ukwalila*. Early in the rainy season, when the rivers begin to rise and flood on to the plains, and principally at the end of the rains, when the plains begin to drain off and the rivers to subside,

343

THE LAMBAS OF NORTHERN RHODESIA

Lamba fishermen construct weirs (*ifipanda*) of poles, sods, and grass across the entrances to plains and across the smaller streams. These weirs dam back the water, which is forced through specially made openings. In these openings are placed funnel-shaped fish-traps; into these the fish either are forced by the strength of the current, or force their own entrance in their desire to proceed upstream or downstream, according to whether the waters are rising or subsiding.

The simplest form of fish-trap is the *umono*, a large funnel of split bamboos woven with bark, having a very wide open end and a narrow end closed and tightly secured with bark string. This type of trap is only used where the current is strong, or where there is a considerable fall in the water dammed up, so that the fish cannot get out against the force of the water. Other names for these traps, according to their size, are *umunsala* and *mumanga*. The *mumanga*, however, is usually accompanied by what is called the *ichifubwilo*, a container attached to the narrow end, which in this case is left open. When the container is filled with fish it is detached; the end of the trap is then tied up, and the container is taken to the village to be emptied and returned again.

The most cunningly made fish-trap, however, is the *imfwambi*, a smaller type of which is called the *akafwambimono*. In shape the *imfwambi* resembles the *umono*, but it has the addition of an inside guard of stiff grass or reed. This grass gives way as the fish pushes in, but it is impossible for the fish to get out again, as the sharp ends of the grass point inward.

By means of these traps vast quantities of fish are caught every season. The larger fish are disembowelled and smoke-dried; the smaller fish are dried as they are caught, and provide a stock of relish (*ifyakutoŵela*) for many months.

(4) *Ukutwila.* The bark of various trees, such as the *umuneŋene*, the *ichimamba*, the *akanchyense*, and the *umulombe*, as well as the roots of the *uŵuŵa* shrub, are used by the Lambas for poisoning fish. The *uŵuŵa*, a plant which grows about a foot in height, is the most commonly used poison. The roots are dug up, pounded, and thrown into a pond, or into a pool in the river where the stream is not too strong. The fish are in some cases killed outright, and float to the surface, but usually the effect of this poison is to stupify the fish, which float on the water until the rays of the sun revive them. For this reason the poison is usually introduced in the evening, and all the villagers turn out at earliest dawn to fill their baskets with fish before the sun revives them.

344

When a quantity of *uŵuŵa* has been set stranded fish are found for miles down the stream, and many more people benefit than those who set the poison.

(5) *Ukupila.* This type of fishing is engaged in by the women. When the plains are drying up the women construct banks across the pools. On these banks they place fish-baskets (*iŋwanga*), and proceed to bail out the small ponds with little baskets, throwing the water into the bigger fish-baskets. The *iŋwanga*

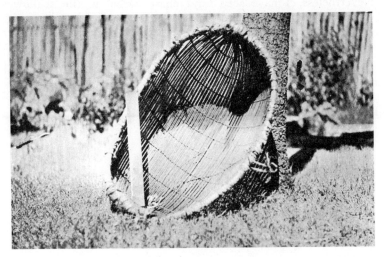

FIG. 97. THE FISH-BAILING BASKET
Photo by C. M. Doke

are constructed from the strong runners of a shrub called *ulusokoti*, bound together with bark. Sufficient space is left between the runners for the fish-basket to act as a sieve. The water runs through and drains away. When the pool is bailed out numbers of small fish are either left in the mud at the bottom or stranded in the fish-baskets.

(6) *Ukusasa.* In the more or less shallow runnels of water (*ifisapa*) draining off from the plains the natives congregate in numbers and tread about in order to stir up the mud. The fish become practically drunk, and rise to the surface to try to get clean water, when they are pierced by *imyondo*. A few naturally get trodden on and killed in that way.

(7) *Ukusumba.* The Lamba fish-spear, *umondo* or *umusumbo*, is long, slender, and light. To a long reed haft is attached a narrow,

345

needle-like iron spike. In most cases this spike is four-sided or
three-sided, tapering to a sharp point, each side at its thickest
being about half an inch across. The best fish-spears are rough-
ened, to resemble very coarse rasps, with small pieces of the metal
protruding, so that if a fish is speared it does not slip off the spear
when it is pulled back. It is seldom that the natives watch for
the fish. They usually prod at random along the dark banks of
the river, getting their fish, usually barbel, merely by chance.
Nevertheless, I have seen boys chase barbel in the shallower
water on the plains, where they have gone to feed on the young
grass shoots, and spear them as they tried to return to the deeper
water.

CHAPTER XXI

UŴUFUSHI—THE PROFESSION OF SMITH

A PROFESSION which is fast disappearing in Lambaland is that of the blacksmith, smelter or metal-worker, *umufushi*. Now that imported implements are so easily obtained there is practically no demand for his services, and men who have the art of *uŵufushi* (smithing) are becoming increasingly difficult to find. In the olden days, however, when the metal had to be won from the earth by primitive methods, the man who knew the secret, and could produce hoes, axes, and spears, was not only certain of amassing a certain amount of wealth, but commanded considerable influence in the community, and was regarded with a respect not second to that accorded to the *umupalu* (professional hunter). *Umufushi* is a word derived from the verb *fula*, meaning to work metal.

The art is learnt during a period of apprenticeship with a master-smith. The learner goes to live with his teacher, watches how he makes axes and hoes, and helps him by making the fire and working the bellows. He assists him when building the *ichintengwa* (smelting-house), and when he has gone through all the menial parts of the work he begins himself to forge axes. From that he goes on to the making of spears, and then to hoes. When his period of apprenticeship and probation is over he sets up his own smithing establishment. His payment to the master-smith is very small, maybe a gift of about two shillings' worth of beads, for while learning he is also helping his teacher; furthermore, he supplies his own raw materials at first, and the finished articles which he makes during his apprenticeship belong to the master, who sells them for himself.

Ichintengwa

When smelting is about to take place the *umufushi* has to observe an important *umushiliko* (prohibition). He may not have intercourse with his wife on the night before his work begins. It is feared that, should he break this taboo, the metal would remain soft and never harden. This prohibition does not apply to those who help him. This is man's work, and women may not enter a smelting-room, but they are permitted to bring food to the smelters outside the room.

The *umufushi* calls a number of helpers to go with him to dig up *umutapo*, the iron ore. In his wanderings the smith has seen near some stream indications of the presence of iron ore beneath the surface of the ground. They all go to the spot, and, digging down, find detached nodules of ore, which they break up into

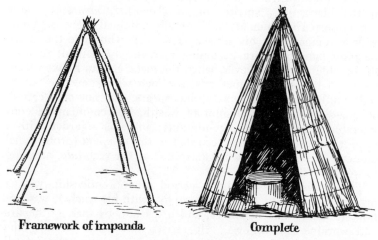

Framework of impanda   Complete

FIG. 98. ICHINTENGWA

stones the size of one's fist. These are then gathered into bundles of grass (*imisantu*), and carried and deposited in a heap at a chosen spot in the bush. When a large quantity has been gathered in this way some of the people go off to cut dry boughs of the *umukoso*-tree. When this is burnt it does not form ash, but charcoal (*amashimbi*), which is required for the smelting. Meanwhile the others set about erecting the *ichintengwa*, the house for smelting. Four very long forked poles (*impanda*) are procured, and set up in the form of a tall *inkunka*. These four main poles are tightly secured, and then other long poles are cut and leant against them to complete the house. Grass is then thatched over and bound with *ulushishi* (bark rope) to the poles. No *imango* (withies) are used at all. *Imango* on an *inkunka* are but to strengthen it against lions.

When this roof is finished a big hole about three feet deep is

dug in the centre of the floor. All round the edge of this circular hole a mud wall about a foot in height is built; in this wall
are left six openings (*ifilyangwa*), for the insertion of the bellows
(*imyuŵa*).

Amashimbi* are now put at the bottom of the hole, and on top
of them a layer of *umutapo*; then another layer of *amashimbi* and
again a layer of *umu-*
tapo*; and so on until
the hole is filled. Fire
is then set to the char-
coal, and six men work
the six bellows which
are inserted in the *ifi-*
lyangwa*. The bellows

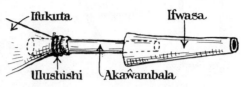

FIG. 99. NOZZLE OF BELLOWS

are made of puku, reed-buck, or bush-buck skins sewn up. At
one end there is a hole into which is inserted a hollow piece of
wood, which they call the *akaŵambala*. This is secured by a
bond of bark rope (*ulushishi*). The nose of the *akaŵambala* is
in turn inserted into a nozzle-shaped piece of ant-heap (*ifwasa*),

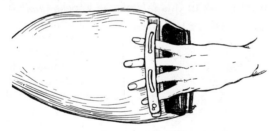

FIG. 100. HOW THE BELLOWS ARE HELD

which enters the *ichilyangwa*. In the olden days the *akaŵambala*
was composed of beautifully made burnt clay. The *umuuŵa* is
gripped at the base by one foot; at the opening at the top are
fixed two pieces of wood with slots made with leather and thongs
for the insertion of the four fingers in front and the thumb behind. In this way the bellows are worked up and down and
the air forced out through the nozzle.

The six men keep the bellows going, and as the mass within the
ichintengwa subsides more *amashimbi* and *umutapo* are added above.
Whenever the blowing of the bellows is so strong that the flames
rise high there is boisterous shouting (*ingwele*) at the smelting-hut.
This is kept up until late in the day. Then the workers leave.
The master-smith himself remains to knock away the clay wall

and inspect the metal that is at the bottom of the hole. Taking
green wood poles that will not burn, he prods it out; when he gets
it out of the hole he rolls it to a safe place, and himself retires
to the village to sleep.

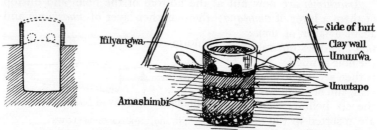

FIG. 101. DIAGRAM OF THE INTERIOR OF AN ICHINTENGWA

In the morning the *umufushi* comes with his helpers and brings
with him an *inkunko yachyela*. This is a ball of metal partly
encased in a piece of grysbok skin, which is sewn on when wet,
and allowed to dry hard. Skin handles are fixed to this for the
operator to grip. With this *inkunko* he knocks (*kunka*) the metal
lump, breaking off the
dross and slag (*ifinya-
nchyela*) from round the
true metal. He then pro-
ceeds to break up the
mass of metal left, for
this is all cracked and
seamed where the dross
has been knocked out.
The pieces of clean metal
thus broken off are called
inkama. They are taken to the village and stored away. From
them the various implements are later made by the *umufushi*.

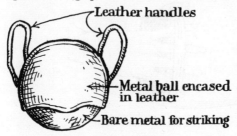

FIG. 102. INKUNKO

The smith may have as many as ten men to help him in the
collecting of the ore and the charcoal. These he pays for their
services. To each unmarried man he gives an axe-head and to
each married man an axe-head and a hoe.

The men who work the bellows for the smith are not paid for
their help. They come in numbers from far and near for the
enjoyment of it, and for the conversational time they have.
There seems to be a general social gathering when it is heard that
the *umufushi* is going to smelt metal. The men work at the
bellows in relays, and keep the fire going at a constant heat.

350

Forging

For the purposes of forging hoes, axes, etc., from the *inkama* which he has already smelted the smith uses a smaller *ichintengwa* (smithy). He chooses a place where there is a big, strong stone, upon which he can hammer the *inkama*. Over this he erects a shelter of branches like an *umutanda*. In his work he usually has two assistants, and if these are not learners he will pay them for their services. A fire of charcoal is made in a hole in the ground, and one of the men works the bellows. When a lump of *inkama* is red hot the smith takes it with a piece of green bark for tongs (*ichimanto*) and sets it on the stone. His other assistant now takes the *inkunko* and hammers the mass of metal, the *umufushi* meanwhile pointing out to him where he wants him to strike. When it cools the metal is put back again on to the fire, and when hot is worked once more, until the shape needed is attained. Now it is the work of the master-smith himself to straighten and finish off the implement. This he does with the aid of two metal hammers. The one, of solid, heavy metal, is called *inondo*, and in the olden days was equivalent in value to a slave or a gun. The other is the *mukoma*, with metal head and wooden handle, very much like an ordinary hammer.

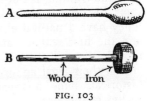

Wood   Iron

FIG. 103

A, *inondo*; B, *mukoma*.

Small smithies are often erected in the villages. These are built of a few upright poles surmounted by a thatched roof, like an *insaka* or summer-house, and are only used for sharpening, mending, or straightening (*tentula*) axes, hoes, and spears. *Inkama* is never dealt with in these.

So great was the esteem in which the *umufushi* was held that a great number of chiefs learnt the profession. The old chief Nsensa, brother to Shiŵata, was a well-known smith, and from him Makwati learnt the art. Besides making the larger implements and weapons, Lamba smiths do a lot of more delicate work; and since there is metal in the construction of the *akalimba*, or hand-piano, the *aŵafushi* are the manufacturers of these.

There is evident among the Lambas the remains of a guild of smiths, for there is to be noticed between them a bond of friendship. One smith coming to a village and hearing that there is a smith there will at once go to him and be well received. In the same way with hunters, one *umupalu* receives and entertains another *umupalu*.

CHAPTER XXII

FOLKLORE AND MUSIC

THOUGH the written literature of any of the Bantu peoples, other than the Swahili, is but in its infancy, the Bantu have their poets, their historians, their legal expositors, and their story-tellers. They have a natural eloquence; every man is a public speaker, and the first real literature of the native peoples of Africa will include the collection of their songs, their poems of praise to the chiefs, their legal aphorisms, and their vast oral tradition, some historical, some mythical, and much belonging strictly to the realms of folklore.

Among the Lambas we have already noticed a firm belief in the real existence of *ifiŵanda* (demons) and *ifinkuwaila* (goblins). In their folklore they include another weird being, the *shishimwe* or *shishimunkulu*, which corresponds to our ogre, sometimes with two heads or three heads, always fearsome and monstrous; then there is the *akachyekulu* or *kandyanga*, a kind of gnome of the forest, renowned for its one long tooth, blood-red and sharp, with which it kills its victims.

Among their genuine beliefs which we must relegate to the realm of myth are two which should be mentioned here—the *ichisonga* and the *funkwe*. They say that the *ichisonga* is a water animal which resembles a rhinoceros, having a horn on its forehead. It is said to inhabit the Kafue river. When it hears the hippo in a pool it comes out of the river, lest it be scented, and goes along the bank. When it reaches the pool it enters the water again, chooses the biggest bull hippo it can see, and stabs it with its horn. It does not eat the hippo, but merely kills it. It eats grass. The Lambas say, further, that when people kill an elephant near by the *ichisonga* roars and drives the people away. It then comes and remains near the dead animal, maybe for several days, until the people get tired of waiting and the dead animal rots. This creature is said to be prompted by *uŵulwishya*, jealousy.

The *funkwe* is said to be a huge snake, its length being anything up to eighty miles—from the source of the Kafulafuta river to

352

its junction with the Kafue. It has a tail like that of a fish. These creatures are said to live at the source of the Kafulafuta and at that of the Itabwa. They coil themselves up in a hole deep down beneath the source of the river. When one of them desires the fish to be plentiful in the river it comes out and goes downstream, and swarms of fish follow it. By the time its head has reached the Kafue its tail is still at the source of the tributary. On its return from the great river it brings with it the big fish.

Almost every Lamba can tell a folk-tale, and tell it well, but there are several well-known *raconteurs* among the people. I well remember listening spellbound to the recitals of a man named Mulekelela, who was known as the best story-teller of the Lamba people; in fact, on one day this man reeled off to me 750 Lamba proverbs with-

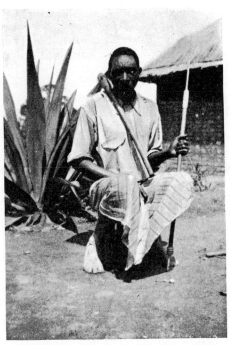

FIG. 104. MULEKELELA, THE STORY-TELLER OF
THE LAMBAS
Photo by Miss O. C. Doke

out any pauses except those caused by the cramp in my arm as I tried to keep pace with him in writing them down. Mule-kelela told me that it is the women who are the chief repository of folklore; it is they who pass on the tales to their children. As to the origins of these tales, he could tell me nothing—"They have been passed down from mother to child from time imme-morial." The underlying unity of Bantu folklore proclaims great age for many of these tales. Some, however, I have recently found to be of very modern origin.

At various times I have gathered numbers of folk-tales, and gathered them in different ways. Some I have taken down

353

from dictation, others have been written out for me by boys who could write, and latterly I have recorded still others on the dictaphone. The last method is the best for preserving the flow of language and inflexion of voice, though it too is far from being a perfect method of recording the wonders of the tale, which one can only get by watching and listening to the teller in his native setting.

I have never heard folk-tales told with such life and reality as when I have been on trek with my carriers, and have camped in the heart of the forest. When the long day's tramp is over, the stockade for protection built, the evening meal cooked and eaten, the tired yet satisfied carriers will be lying or sitting around the numerous camp-fires within the stockade. It is then that the true atmosphere for an *ichishimichishyo*, as it is called, is found. Above is the inky-black sky, studded with bright stars; the firelight is playing on the leaves and branches of the trees overhead, and lighting up from time to time the faces of the men. The only sounds are the constant gurgle of the water in the calabash pipe as it is passed round from friend to friend, the cheerful chirping of one tree lizard to another, or the sharp cries of the galagos as they jump from branch to branch. And then one of the men will commence his tale, *Kambi kasuŵa . . .*, "On a certain day . . ." Instantly all ears are intent, and as he warms up to his theme men leave the more distant fires and crowd round him; the pipe is forgotten, and every word is caught with the utmost avidity. In some of these tales choric songs appear, and it is not long before the eager listeners have caught the refrain and join in the chorus whenever the time for it comes round. The full eloquence of the story can only be realized as one watches the speaker; the startling inflexions of his voice are accompanied by most expressive gesticulation and a changing expression of the face which can be read even by one who cannot understand his speech. The wonderful wealth of onomatopœia used is most ably supplemented by gesture, flashing of the eyes, or contortions.

Lamba folk-tales may be divided into three groups. First, there are stories of animals (which are usually personified and can speak), of which the greater proportion centre in the cunning of the little hare. Then, secondly, there are numerous stories of domestic life, and it is in these that the mother-in-law is so often held up to ridicule. Lastly, there are tales in which ogres, gnomes, and fairy princesses play the important part; and these are the tales which remind one of much in European lore, and much that every one of us has read in Grimm. Most of these folk-tales point some moral, condemning greed, cowardice, stupidity, disobedience; and in them cunning is often extolled and shown to be superior to brute strength. In the stories of Mr Little-hare, as he is called, are found the pure fountains of the Brer Rabbit tales, which come back to us from the negroes of America. Here is one—a short one:

The countryside was being decimated by the ravages of a lion; people were in terror, and at last Ŵulambe, the chief's son, was caught and killed. Ŵulambe's sister was a beautiful maiden, and many were her suitors. Her mother announced that whoever should avenge Ŵulambe and kill the lion would thereby win the hand of Ŵulambe's sister. Suitor after suitor set out, only to share Ŵulambe's fate, until no one dared to go. One day Little-hare arrived at the village with a big sack, and made known his intention of marrying Ŵulambe's sister. "First kill the lion!" said the girl's mother. He agreed to the conditions, and off he went with his sack. He had not gone far in the forest before he heard a honey-guide twittering. He followed the bird from tree to tree till he reached a place where many weapons were lying about; he knew then that he had come to the place where the other suitors had met their fate. Then he saw the lion coming. Putting down his sack, he bowed low and said, "Greeting, O master!" The lion said, "Greeting!" Then Little-hare asked, "Where is your home, sir? Let me go with you and have a smoke." Away they went to the lion's lair. When they had finished smoking Little-hare said, "Sir, I have a wonderful trick I could show you. Come to where my sack is." He then entered the sack, and said to the lion, "See if you can lift me up." As the lion was about to lift the sack Little-hare caught a strong root through the bottom of the sack. The lion strained, but could not lift him. Out came Little-hare, and said, "Now you go in, and Mrs Lion and the children, and I will lift you all up." They all went into the sack. Little-hare started to tie up the mouth of the sack with a tremendous rope. The lion objected, but Little-hare said it was just to have something to hold on to. When, however, he had secured the sack he began to vilify and threaten the lion for his stupidity. Then he got a great stick and began to flog them through the sack, beating and beating until every movement from within had ceased. Then off he went to the village to call the men. At first they would not believe him, but in the end they accompanied him, and found the lions dead in the sack. They cut a pile of firewood and burnt

355

them as witches. When they returned to the village Little-hare married Wulambe's sister.

There are many of these tales, and some of them are very long and full of intricate plot. Much laughter usually greets the numerous stories in which the mother-in-law figures. Here is one representative of this type of folk-tale:

A man had not been married many days before his mother-in-law said to him, "If you are a true son-in-law you will catch for me a scavenger eagle." The son-in-law was thunderstruck on hearing that, but still out he went to perform the practically impossible task. He killed a buck, took the skin, and on reaching the plain lay down and covered himself with it. An eagle spied what he thought was a dead animal, and swooped down to get some meat. When he settled on the skin the man caught him. Home he went, and gave the eagle to his wife to take to her mother. His mother-in-law was amazed at the skill of her son-in-law. After some days he determined on his revenge, and said, "Mother-in-law, if you love me, bring me water from a place without frogs." She took her pot and went to the river. "Are there frogs in this river?" she asked. A chorus of croaks greeted her. On she went to the next stream, with the same result. On and on she went; frogs were in every stream, and at length she died of sheer exhaustion. At the village the son-in-law was arrested and taken before the chief. The man defended his case, and said, "It was my mother-in-law who started to make my life miserable by telling me to catch a scavenger eagle for her; but I did it. Now this task I set her to do she has brought upon herself through her attitude to me." And the chief said, "He is not guilty! Rise, and go to your home!"

Ordinary folk-tales are called by the Lambas *ifishimichishyo*, but there are certain others generally called *utushimi*, which we might translate as 'choric stories.' These tales are interspersed with verses which are sung, and as soon as the listeners have memorized the verses they join in the choruses with gusto whenever the appropriate moment comes.

One of the best tales of this type which I have heard is called *Ulushimi lwashishimunkulu*, "The Choric Story of the Ogre." In this story an ogre visits a village when the people are away hoeing, gives back strength to a girl whom he had previously 'broken up,' and gets her to dance. After the dance he 'breaks her up' again, and leaves her in the hut. But during the dancing various creatures take part, and sing as they dance. First, the cock beating the drum, the hen dances and sings:

FOLKLORE AND MUSIC

> *Kombolwe lishye'ngoma !*
> *Kombolwe lishye'ngoma !*
> *Uku nindume, uku mulume,*
> *Kombolwe lishye'ngoma !*
>
> " Cock beat the drum !
> Cock beat the drum !
> Here a brother, here a husband,[1]
> Cock beat the drum ! "

Then the cock dances and sings in answer:

> *Chyechyo chyatula-ko'mwine !*
> *Chyechyo chyatula-ko'mwine !*
>
> " That she has published herself !
> That she has published herself ! "

Then an old piece of elephant-hide takes itself down from the wall of the hut, where it has been hung against a famine time, and with heavy, loud rhythmic beating dances and sings:

> *Ndi chikanda, ndi chikanda,*
> *Ŵanjipike mu chinongo chyaŵo !*
> *Ndi chikanda, ndi chikanda !*
>
> " I am a hide, I am a hide.
> Let them cook me in their big pot !
> I am a hide, I am a hide ! "

When the old hide has hung itself up again down comes a little galago, and, with light and frisking step, dances and sings:

> *Ŵanchyele'mala, kanchyenda,*
> *Neluŵalaŵala, nelunchyanchya !*
> *Ŵanchyele'mala, kanchyenda,*
> *Neluŵalaŵala, nelunchyanchya !*
>
> " They've scooped out my entrails, and I still walk,
> I the hopper, I the dancer !
> They've scooped out my entrails, and I still walk,
> I the hopper, I the dancer ! "

The goat sings:

> *Memetu, memetu !*
> *Kamwangufyo'kuchinda, memetu, memetu !*
> *Ŵene-mbushi ŵaisa, memetu, memetu !*
>
> " Grazer, grazer,
> Hasten to dance, grazer, grazer !
> The goat clan has come, grazer, grazer ! "

The signs of scuffling and dancing on the courtyard soon made the villagers suspicious, and, waiting in hiding one day, the

[1] The cock is the hen's brother as well as husband.

357

relatives of the afflicted girl slew the ogre before he was able to 'break her up,' and she was thus restored to health and strength.

Music

Even the most primitive or most decadent of races are imbued with the love of music in some form or other.   The Bushmen of the Kalahari indulge in the revels of all-night dancing, accompanied by chanting and songs which, to the European ear, at first seem weird and grotesque; but as one becomes accustomed to this foreign music the melody of it gradually appears and grows upon one.   Musical instruments too are not unknown to such people, and when they are carefully examined their construction often shows a remarkable technique.

In music and musical technique too the Bantu peoples as a whole are in a relatively advanced stage, and the Lambas are quite representative of the Bantu.

Most of the Lamba music centres in the dance.   Practically every dance is carried out to the accompaniment of the drum, and so in common parlance the terms *ingoma* (drum) and *amashya* (dance) are almost synonymous.   Dancing takes place at night, and usually continues until dawn.   The common drum consists of a large, hollowed log of wood with a piece of hide, sometimes of iguana-skin, stretched tightly across the larger end.   The drum rests on its side, and the drummer sits astraddle, beating with his hands on the hide in front of him.   Professional drummers go from village to village to play at the various mourning or initiation dances.   While camping in a native village recently I was able (being kept awake most of the night by the noise) to listen somewhat closely to the constant changing in the rhythmic methods of the drumming.   The women—or the men, as the case might be—would start up a song, and the drummers would listen for a bar or two to catch the rhythm, and then would join in; presently the drum would predominate, and the dancing would be in full swing, the singing dropping almost into a secondary place as a chorus.   Then, when that dance was over, another song would be started, necessitating quite a different method of drumming, which would quickly be grasped by the drummers and would take possession of the dance.

The Dances

The most important of the Lamba dances are the following:

(1) *Amaombe*, or *ingoma shyamaombe*.   This dance is held only

358

in honour of a girl initiate (*pakuwishyo'mwane'chisungu*). The dancing is normal, not being in imitation of anything. One or two accomplished old women dance alone, with dancing skirts (*uŵuyombo*) of grass beads and rattles (*insangwa*). All and sundry watch, and all join in the singing. One man beats *ingoma yamambwa-kuŵili*, the ancient double-faced drum. He stands with the drum tied to his waist. Two men beat *imikunto* (ordinary drums), standing with them tied to their waists, while yet another man sits down and beats one *ilinkuŵala* (sounding boat) with two sticks (*imishimpo*). The dancers and beaters are usually paid by the father of the initiate. The songs sung are all of the variety called *ichimbwasa*.

(2) *Ichimbwasa*, or *ulwimbo lwachisungu*. Danced in honour of a girl initiate. Three ordinary drums are used. One or two old women dance. The people sit round and sing. At times a few *ŵamukamwami* may dance for payment. The dancing is normal.

(3) *Ichinsengwe*. Professional hunters (*aŵapalu*) dance one at a time, and ordinary men also take their turn. *Aŵayambo* are paid to lead this dance. Women may look on, but never take any part. The dance is held in honour of Kaaluwe, the guardian spirit of the game herds; but when *aŵayambo* dance they do so in honour of the spirits of the Twa hunters which are believed to possess them. The dance is performed while the heart, ears, and meat of the head of the slain animal are being cooked. One *umukunto* and one large drum (about 4 feet high) are used, while sometimes an *imbila*, calabash and hide drum, is used. In the dancing there is imitation of hunting, of stalking and wounding animals, also imitation of the gait of animals and of their movements when wounded and dying.

This dance is also employed during beer-drinking in honour of the *imipashi*, departed spirits, during mourning ceremonies (*amalilo*).

(4) *Umuchinko*, or *ichipelu*. One large drum is used and one *umukunto*. Danced in honour of initiates (*ifisungu*) and at *amalilo* in honour of the departed.[1] One man and one woman dance together at a time. They hold one another with arms round one another's shoulders, much as Europeans do when dancing. The spectators, men and women, form practically a close circle round the dancers all the time. This dancing is supposed to be confined to *aŵashichye* (unmarried people), but when his wife is at a distance a married man will often take part.

---

[1] The term *imipashi* is not used here.

359

A married woman may dance thus with men well known to her (*aŵeneshi*), especially an *umulamu* (brother-in-law) or *umufyala* (cross-cousin); she will never dance with an *indume* (brother or cousin of the same clan), a *mwinshyo* (maternal uncle), husband, or father-in-law, and she should not with any other man. If the elders are present none will dare to catch hold of the women; they merely dance round and round one another. When alone the men at times catch the women by the breasts, and lustful passions are roused.

(5) *Akasela* (also called *akashimbo*, *umusakasa*, *ichila*, and *shiŵoyongo*). One large drum and one small one are used in this dance. It is held in honour of the departed (*ŵalashyanino' fwile*) and in honour of an initiate. A line of women faces a distant line of men. One from each line goes out to dance in the space between. If the elders are present they merely dance round one another, but in the absence of the elders the dance may become immoral.

(6) *Akaŵale*. One large drum is used. An *umulaye* (doctor) starts the songs (*ukutatula*), or, in his absence, one of the elders. The drummer is in the midst, and all the people, men and women mixed indiscriminately, dance in a rank around him, going in one direction, maybe four deep. They sing, *Kankonkwa, kuno kwesu ŵalukutwa'kaŵale!* "*Tock!* Here at our home they are stamping the *akaŵale* root!" The *umulaye* brews beer for the people, and they all dance in honour of *imipashi yakwe* (his spirits). This dance is usually held in the daytime.

(7) *Amambalakata*. This dance was introduced long ago from the Kaonde and Mbwela people, but is now regarded as a Lamba dance. Two *imikunto* and one large drum are used. One man dances at a time. He may be an *umupalu* (hunter) or a man without a profession. The dancer wears two *inchyema* (serval) skins, one in front and one behind, hanging from a waist-band. Two other skins, of galago, wild-cat, or genet, are worn at the sides. In his hand he carries a dancing axe (*ichiŵanga*), and when dancing keeps far from the drums. He imitates the elephant in its gait, the way it looks round, its anger, etc. The people standing round sing. An *umupalu* dancing this does so in honour of Mwishyaŋombe (the guardian of the herds); when an ordinary man dances it he does so in honour of the hunter.

(8) *Ichilaila*, or *ichinsenseŵele*. Women only dance, while men may look on. No drum is used, but the rhythm is preserved by hand-clapping. This dance is performed merely for enjoyment, and not in honour of any person or event. One of the women

acts as *umutatwishi*, to start the refrains, and the others dance round and round (*ukushinguluka*). This kind of dancing is sometimes called *ichishyaneshyane*, a dancing anyhow or dancing irregularly.

(9) *Ŵumoŵa.* Danced by male and female *ŵamoŵa* in honour of the *ifinkuwaila* which possess them. Three *imikunto* are used, while the dancers perform singly or two at a time. They do this for payment, and the dance is practically the same as the *ichimbwasa.*

(10) *Amalimba.* Women or men dance to the rhythm of the gourd piano, *amalimba.* This dance has no significance; it is performed purely for enjoyment.

(11) *Ichiŵitiku.* Women dance one at a time to the accompaniment of one large drum and hand-clapping (*amakuku*). This is danced when an *umulaye* has brewed beer, and is in honour of his spirit.

Drummers (*aŵalishi ŵangoma*) and the starters and leaders of the songs (*aŵatatwishi ŵakasela*) are held in considerable respect, and are in demand at *amalilo* and *ifisungu.* They will not assist in an honorary capacity at friendly dances, but only when paid. For two to four nights of this work they were in the old days paid in calico and fowls; now the payment is about five shillings each. Ntambika was skilled in both departments; Sepete is an *umulishi*, and Muŋomba an *umutatwishi.*

Lamba songs are divided in type according to the dance with which they are used. We have already noticed a number of typical songs in connexion with initiation and mourning ceremonies, and in the cults of the *aŵayambo*, *ŵamoŵa*, and *ŵamukamwami.*[1]

Here is one refrain, sung by a man at the initiation ceremonies as he rushes into the circle to dance a solo part:

> *Mamafyala, mamafyala,*
> *Kamufunda-po umwana wenu,*
> *Alandaŵishya !*
>
> " Mother-in-law, mother-in-law,
> Instruct your daughter;
> She reviles me ! "

Musical Instruments

Lamba musical instruments make an interesting study. The best-known instrument is the *akalimba*, or small hand-piano,

[1] Ninety-five songs are given in my *Lamba Folk-lore*—see pp. 527–545.

consisting of thirteen iron slips fixed over a carved wooden sounding-board. Usually a small calabash is attached beneath to act as a resonator. The whole instrument is easily held in the two hands, while the two thumbs play over the notes. This instrument, modified in one way or another, is found among the Bantu tribes practically from the east coast of Africa to the west. Among the Lambas there are several distinct types of *akalimba*. The small instrument called *akankoŵele*, which has more players than any of the others, has a small circular hole in the middle of the sounding-board, which is covered with stiff

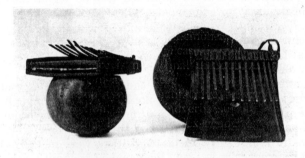

FIG. 105. COMMON AKALIMBA (HAND-PIANO) AND AKALIMBA KAMASWAO
(SHOWING MOVABLE BITS OF METAL)
Photo by W. Paff

cobweb (*lembalemba*). The large type of this instrument is called *indimba*. Then there is the *akalimba kamaswao*, which has a hollowed sounding-board, in which are set movable pieces of metal, which rattle as the instrument is played. Yet another rare type is the *ichintimbwa*, a very large instrument with a wooden sounding-box the size of a native stool. On this are cross slats of wood; the notes are made from bamboo. Very few men can play this instrument, but Lunsala (father of Mulekelela), Nsonkomona, and Chilyobwe (father of Longwani) were known to be players. The instrument is played by night in the house. The *aŵaŵashishi ŵakalimba*, makers of these instruments, are held in considerable renown throughout the country; they are smiths (*aŵafushi*) with special skill. Makwati of Nsensa's and Lufumpa, the present Ntenke, are skilled in this way. *Aŵalishi ŵakalimba*, the players of these instruments, are not very numerous; it is not every man who can play the *akalimba*, but no particular merit is attached to the accomplishment. Never-

362

theless, some Lambas are very skilful players on the *akalimba*, and there is a proverb which states, "A borrowed *akalimba* doesn't finish a tune"—so wedded to his instrument is the player that he never lends it long enough.

The *ilimba*, usually called by the plural term *amalimba*, is a huge instrument about 4 feet in length, composed of carved wooden notes strung together upon a frame over calabashes, which act as resonators. This instrument is very rare in Ilamba. Known players were Nselenje (the Congo Lambaland paramount chief), Masombwe, and Mushili (who died in 1917). The players, *aŵalishi ŵamalimba*, and the makers, *aŵafii-chishi ŵamalimba*, are the same: it is the player who carves and builds his own instrument. Nselenje is at present the only man in Ilamba who plays the *amalimba*. He is an itinerant player.

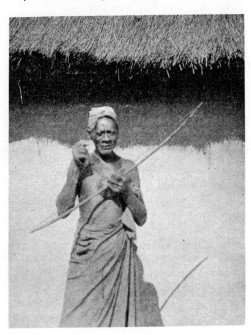

FIG. 106. PLAYING THE AKANKOTO
Photo by C. M. Doke

He travels through the country with his two wives, who dance to his playing. He begins the songs, and they act as chorus. I heard him at Kafulafuta Mission in 1916, and his skill in manipulating the two sticks was wonderful. His playing is greatly esteemed by the Lambas, and I understand that he now plays before Europeans in Elisabethville. The *amalimba* also has a wide range over Bantu Africa. The Chopi people are renowned for their orchestras of *timbila*, as they call these instruments.

Another instrument, used widely, is the *umunkoto*, or *akankoto*. This is really a two-stringed instrument, the one string being unevenly divided by a piece of gut attaching it to the centre of the bow and to the calabash resonator. The strings are tapped by a piece of grass stalk, and are damped down by the fingers to alter the note.

The *isese* is an instrument which was commonly played by every young man of the last generation. It is composed of a piece of wood at the end of which is half a calabash and beneath which are stretched two strings.

A less commonly found instrument, the use of which seems to

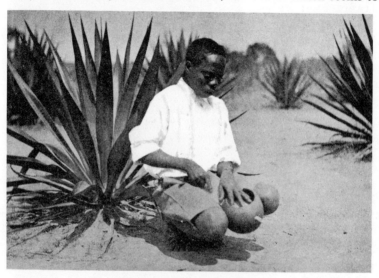

FIG. 107. PLAYING THE UBWESELA
Photo by C. M. Doke

be dying out among the Lambas, is the *ubwesela*. This is a type of six-stringed harp, as the accompanying photograph shows. The strings are stretched across a flat piece of board, two pieces of wood inserted beneath the strings serving to raise them. The method of tuning is extremely interesting. One long string is threaded through the holes to make up the six strings, and when any one string is out of tune the whole six have to be readjusted for tuning. Again the calabash resonator is used. From the picture it will be seen that the fingers are used for altering the pitches, as is the case with the playing of the violin.

Lamba boys are quite clever at making and playing a species of flute called the *ichiloli, umuloli,* or *umusembe,* which is cut from a piece of reed. Apart from the hole for blowing, there are two

holes not very far from the end of the instrument. The flute has
to be soaked in water before it can be played, and then very
pleasing notes are produced on it.

One further type of instrument must be mentioned here.
This is the *ilinkuŵala* (plural, *amankuŵala*), or sounding boat.
Two small, heavy pieces of wood are hollowed out almost to the
shape of dug-out canoes. These are laid on their sides, and,
when struck with stout sticks, give forth loud and resonant
notes. A variation of the notes is obtained by striking different
parts of any one *ilinkuŵala*. These instruments are mostly

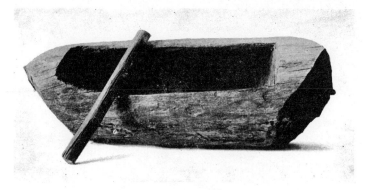

FIG. 108. ILINKUŴALA
Photo by W. Paff

used for bird-scaring. On the top of a high anthill in the gardens
the player will sit striking his 'liquid' notes on the *amankuŵala*,
and chanting some such song as this:

> *Iminina, nkupele chiŵa,*
> *Chiŵa wamena'maŵele !*

> " Stand still, and let me give you a dove,
> The dove has grown breasts."

The following are the different kinds of drums used by the
Lambas:

(1) *Ingoma yamambwa-kuŵili*, or *iyamaombe*, the large double-
faced drum used at initiations.

(2) *Intambangoma*, the friction drum. This was associated
with the chief, and particularly with his war affairs. Unlike
that of the ordinary drum, the diaphragm at the end was pierced,
and through the hole was inserted a piece of reed with a wad at
the end to prevent its slipping out. To sound this type of drum

the wet hand is worked up and down the reed, when a loud, booming noise is produced. The Lambas call this drum *ingoma yaŵukali*, the drum of fierceness, and it could not be used for any trivial matter. When it was heard they knew that there was an important matter on at the chief's village.

The *intambangoma* was used on the following occasions:

(*a*) On killing a man. A. is sent by the chief to such-and-such

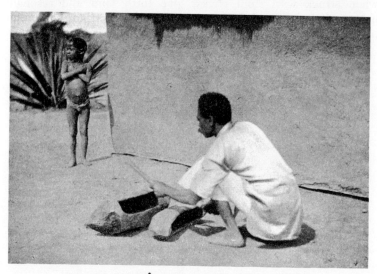

FIG. 109. SANDAŴUNGA PLAYING THE AMANKUŴALA
Photo by C. M. Doke

a village to kill B., who has committed an offence. On A.'s return to the chief's village the villagers sound the *intambangoma*, and A. performs his dance of triumph (*ukwanga*). The women sound their shrill *lululu*-ing (*ukulisyo'lumpundu*), while the man leaps about with his spears and bow and arrows. At times he shouts, "It is I who killed him, and if the chief sends me to slay another man I'll slay him too!" He then rushes to his companions, shouting, *Chiweleni!* "Shout ye!" and they all shout and sound the *intambangoma*.

(*b*) When the chief sets out on the war-path he does so with one *intambangoma* ahead and another behind the caravan.

(*c*) When an *umulenda* is being erected in honour of the spirit of a departed chief, and when light beer is being drunk as a similar honour, the friction drum is used.

366

These drums used to be held in great respect, and were only found at the village of the paramount chief, but in these days they are made and used by anyone.

The term *intambangoma* is also applied to the *lendya*, or bull-roarer, the bulb of the gladiolus plant twirled on string. But among the Lambas the bull-roarer is but a child's plaything, and has no further significance.

(3) *Umukunto*, the ordinary drum.

(4) *Imangu*, a large drum struck not with the hand, but with

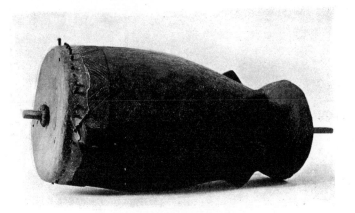

FIG. 110. INTAMBANGOMA
Photo by W. Paff

imishimpo, and used in time of war or on the death of a man. It remains in the village because it is too heavy to carry.

(5) *Umutungu*, a large calabash drum used by women.

Women use rattles made from calabashes or wild oranges and called *insai*. *Insangwa* rattles are worn on the legs at all dances. The *awalaye* use hand rattles called *imisewe*, and similar ones are used by people at *ichinsengwe* dances.

Hunters make a 'pipe' for calling duiker. This is called *ichinyenye*, and consists of a cut piece of horn with a piece of hard cobweb stretched over one end. The breath is blown across the open end, as children do with empty cartridge cases.

The *ulusengo*, a 5-foot elephant tusk, was the property of a great chief. It was blown as a horn, and was sounded to announce the death of a chief and also to call the people together to a war council. In these days the one in Mushili's village is blown by Mwewela, and is taken to the chief's gardens to help in the bird-scaring. It is thought that the birds should fear, because the *ulusengo* is *imfumu*, of the importance of a chief.

Whistling (*ukulishyo'munsu*) has no ceremonial significance: it is *ichilishyelishye*, done on any occasion. *Amakuku*, the clapping of hands, accompanies *ichilaila* and *ichinsengwe* dances and those in connexion with the *ichisungu* ceremonies. *Ulumpundu*, the shrill *lululu*-ing of the women, accompanied by the tapping of the lips, is used at initiation ceremonies, the *ichinsengwe* dances, and on occasions of joy (*ukusemba*), triumph (*ukwanga*), and the death of an elephant.

CHAPTER XXIII

LANGUAGE

In concluding this monograph on the Lamba people it will be well to say something about their language. Lamba belongs to the Central Group of the Bantu language family. It is generally conceded, by those who know anything of them, that the Bantu languages show high cultural development and an extremely advanced inflexional system. Their system of grammatical agreement, while in many respects parallel to that in Latin, is one of prefixal concord, while the latter is one of suffixal concord. Latin is one of the sex-gender languages, while the Bantu family is composed of class-gender languages.

Phonetics [1]

The Bantu field as a whole has proved a happy hunting-ground for the phonetician, but the Lamba language is singularly free from special phonetic phenomena. We find it to be typically Bantu in its possession of a simple seven-vowel system, which for ordinary purposes can be well indicated by the five vowels *i, e, a, o*, and *u*. Lamba also adheres to the rule that each syllable either is, or ends with, a vowel. Of more or less special sounds the following are the chief:

The Bilabial Fricative. It has been stated that in many Central Bantu languages the sounds *b, v*, and *w* are interchangeable. This is a mistaken idea. These languages employ a fricative sound made with the lips much in the position for *b* or *w*, and having the acoustic effect on the untrained ear of a *v*. This is the bilabial voiced fricative, indicated in the script of the International Phonetic Association by *β* and in the orthography of the Lambaland missionaries by *ŵ*.

The Flapped Lateral. Central and other Bantu languages also provide the riddle of the so-called interchangeable *l-d-r*. Here, again, the attempt to associate an entirely new sound, "the flapped *l*," with the known in European phonetics has led

[1] This I have analysed in " A Study in Lamba Phonetics " (*Bantu Studies*, vol. iii, No. 1, July, 1927).

to some people hearing *l*, others *d*, and others *r* for an entirely new sound, one which resembles *r* to a certain extent, but has only a single flap instead of a rolling, and of which the first air-escape is lateral.

Palatal Sounds. Lamba uses the palatal explosives *c* and *ɟ* (represented in this book by *ch*, *chy*, and *j*). *c* is pronounced with the centre of the tongue against the roof of the mouth, almost like a very forward *k* or *ky*, but not with the blade of the tongue as is the English *ch* (phonetic *tʃ*). *ɟ* is the corresponding voiced sound. There is also a palatal nasal *ɲ* very like the French sound in *rɛɲ* (*règne*) ; but in Lamba this has rigorously to be differentiated from *ny*, which also occurs, much like the sound in English 'onion.' In Lamba the palatal fricative corresponding to the English *ʃ* in 'ship' has a succeeding *y*-glide, which is indicated in this book by *shy*. In Lamba *s* and *sh* belong to the same phoneme —*i.e.*, they are mutually exclusive in their choice of environment. *s* occurs before *e*, *a*, *o*, *u*, and *w*, while *sh* occurs before *i* and *y*. In the Mission orthography the symbol *s* serves for both *s* and *sh*, so that *si* and *sy* are always read as *shi* and *shy*.

The Velar Nasal. In addition to the combination *ng*, Lamba uses the sound *ŋ* (as in English 'song') quite frequently—e.g., *liŋwiŋwishya* (murmur).

The Voiced Explosives. Except in the case of *bw*, the sounds *b*, *d*, *ɟ*, and *g* do not occur apart from their homorganic nasals in the combinations *mb*, *nd*, *nj*, and *ng*.

In any analysis of Lamba phonetics it is necessary to differentiate between the normal grammatical phonetics and the extra-normal phonetics, in which onomatopœia plays so large a part. We cannot here consider the many interesting phonetic phenomena which come into the extra-normal phonetics.

Lamba shares with some other Bantu languages the phenomenon of semantic length; that is to say, the change in the length of a vowel may involve an entire change of meaning in the word. In this work I have followed the suggestion of the International Institute of African Languages and Culture in indicating the length of a vowel by doubling it. It must be remembered, then, that when two like vowels are written together one long vowel is indicated. Examples of semantic length :

lela (nurse)	*leela* (fade)
posa (weave)	*poosa* (throw)
ŵuka (divine)	*ŵuuka* (awake)
ukupa (to give)	*ukuupa* (to marry)
amala (intestines)	*amaala* (nails).

Lamba may further be described as a tone language, one in which the musical pitch of a syllable is a significant factor. But its tone system, when compared to those of Zulu, Sotho, Kongo, and many other Bantu languages, is very simple, and consists mainly in 'peaks' of tone, which appear at certain intervals and upon certain syllables. Nevertheless, tone is seen to be semantic in a number of cases in Lamba, as, for instance, *akaṇndṵ* (quail) and *akaundṵ* (jigger-flea).

The stress in Lamba is normally on the penultimate syllable of each word, and in this way is to a great extent the determining factor in word division. The Bantu rule that "each word has one and only one main stress" is adhered to in Lamba word-division. The present Mission orthography [1] is most inaccurate in this respect, and it is to be hoped that this important improvement—nay, rectification—will soon be effected.

Grammar

The present state of Bantu grammatical treatment and classification is extremely unsatisfactory. Hitherto [2] practically no serious thought has been given to the possibility of Bantu grammar demanding a different treatment from that of English, French, German, or Latin. A French investigator presses his Bantu language into a French mould, a classical scholar squeezes his into a classical mould, a German missionary forces his into a Teutonic mould, and the English field-worker twists and bends the Bantu verb to fit an English mould! They all recognize noun classes, verbal derivatives, concordial agreement, and other such *obvious* divergences from their own systems, but they discuss seriously case, comparison of adjectives, participles, aorists, prepositions, and many another phenomenon *which does not occur in Bantu languages*. If the French investigator, the classical scholar, the German missionary, and the English field-worker each produce a different classification of the same language, can they each be right? Such preconceptions as are going to hamper an impartial investigation and classification must be put aside, and the spirit and conception behind the Bantu grammatical forms must be sought for. [3] We must look through Bantu eyes.

[1] For which I was to a certain extent responsible.

[2] See my *Grammar of the Lamba Language* (Kegan Paul, 1922), wherein I have committed three great faults, an ultra-disjunctive method of writing and classification, the old method of grammatical treatment, and an attempt at a case and declension system.

[3] I have attempted this in my recently published *Text-book of Zulu Grammar* (1st ed., University of the Witwatersrand Press, 1927; 2nd ed., Longmans, Green, 1931).

THE LAMBAS OF NORTHERN RHODESIA

The following are the principles upon which I would base the classification:

(1) First determine the correct word-division—the natural minimum of syllables which the native can use in isolating a word. Here the stress rule is all-important, as is accurate ear-work.

(2) Next, each word, not each portion or formative syllable of the word, must be taken to comprise a part of speech.

(3) Each part of speech must be classified, firstly according to the work it does in the sentence, and secondly according to its form and special signification.

The investigation of the Lamba sentence reveals the fact that, unless it is an interjection, each sentence must be or must contain a predicate. The sentence may be composed merely of a predicate; e.g., *Twaisa*, "We have come," *Muntu*, "It is a person." The noun, then, is not the most important part of the Bantu sentence, as it is commonly stated to be. Next to the predicate, however, the noun is of extreme importance in the sentence, for the changing prefixes of the nouns are the basis of the alliterative concord, which is one of the features of Bantu sentence-structure.

In order that the reader may understand the sentence-structure in Lamba I take the following as a typical sentence and analyse it:

Aŵantu ŵesu aŵakulu ŵalishibwene inama ishyo shyonse pachinika mailo.

Our big people saw all those animals on the plain yesterday.

Analysis
Subject: *aŵantu* (noun).
Enlargement of subject: (1) *ŵesu* (possessive);
(2) *aŵakulu* (adjective).
Predicate: *ŵalishibwene* (verb).
Object: *inama* (noun).
Enlargement of object: (1) *ishyo* (demonstrative pronoun);
(2) *shyonse* (enumerative pronoun).
Extension of predicate: (1) *pachinika* (locative adverb);
(2) *mailo* (time).

Parsing
aŵantu: substantive, noun, Class 1, plural, subject of predicate *ŵalishibwene*.

ŵesu: qualificative, possessive, 1st person plural, stem *-isu*, with 1st class plural possessive concord *ŵa-*, agreeing with *aŵantu*.

372

aŵakulu: qualificative, adjective, root *-kulu*, with 1st class plural adjectival concord *aŵa-*, agreeing with *aŵantu.*

ŵalishibwene: predicative, verb, principal [1] positive, indicative,[2] simple,[3] perfect,[4] remote past,[5] 3rd person, 1st class, plural of *ŵona* (with 3rd person, Class 5, plural object concord agreeing with the object *inama*). (Note that *ŵalishibwene* standing alone is a complete sentence, meaning "They saw them.")

inama: substantive, noun, Class 5, plural, object of predicate *ŵalishibwene.*

ishyo: substantive, pronoun, 3rd demonstrative, Class 5, plural, in apposition to *inama.*

shyonse: substantive, pronoun, enumerative, root *-nse*, with pronominal concord *shyo-* of Class 5, plural, in apposition to *inama.*

pachinika: descriptive, adverb, locative, formed with Class 11 locative prefixal formative *pa-*, inflecting *ichinika*, noun of Class 3 singular, extending the predicate.

mailo: descriptive, adverb of time, extending the predicate.

According to the present word-division *ŵalishibwene* is written *ŵa li shi bwene* and treated as follows:

ŵa: nominative personal pronoun, Class 1, plural.

li: verbal auxiliary.

shi: accusative pronoun of Class 5, plural.

bwene: verb, perfect.

From this it is seen that the grammatical classification is all dependent upon the method of word-division.

Our analysis of Lamba grammar gives the following six main parts of speech:

(1) *Substantive*, a word signifying anything concrete or abstract.

(2) *Qualificative*, a word which qualifies a substantive.

(3) *Predicative*, a word which signifies an action connected with a substantive or the state in which a substantive is.

(4) *Descriptive*, a word which describes a qualificative, predicative, or other descriptive.

(5) *Conjunction*, a word which introduces sentences or links up words or sentences.

(6) *Interjection*, an isolated word or group of words which have no grammatical or concordial bearing upon the rest of the sentence.

These six basic parts of speech, when examined according to the form in which they appear and according to their special

[1] Conjugation. [2] Mood. [3] Implication.
[4] Manner—i.e., *-bwene* is the perfect stem of *ŵona*. [5] Tense.

373

signification, have certain subdivisions, which we may consider the real Lamba parts of speech.

I. Substantive:	(a)	noun.	(1)
	(b)	pronoun.	(2)
II. Qualificative:	(a)	adjective.	(3)
	(b)	relative.	(4)
	(c)	numeral.	(5)
	(d)	possessive.	(6)
III. Predicative:	(a)	verb.	(7)
	(b)	copulative.	(8)
IV. Descriptive:	(a)	adverb.	(9)
	(b)	radical.	(10)
V. Conjunction			(11)
VI. Interjection			(12)

Lamba is a Bantu language with the feature of dissyllabic noun prefixes, and with the additional feature of pre-prefixes, which are invariably monosyllabic. Among the pre-prefixes must be reckoned the three locative prefixes of Classes XI, XII, and XIII.

In Lamba the substantive is divided into the two main parts of speech, the noun and the pronoun. We may define the noun as a word which signifies the name of anything concrete or abstract, and the pronoun, in contrast, as a word which signifies anything concrete or abstract without being its name.

The Noun

The feature of the noun in Lamba is that it is (with rare exceptions) composed of two formatives, stem and prefix. The stem of the noun is the constant element, while the prefix changes in many cases to form the plural, and varies according to the class to which the noun belongs. The noun prefix is of extreme importance, for it determines the form of the pronouns representing the noun and of the concords used in forming the adjectives, relatives, numerals, possessives, and verbs brought into relationship therewith.

Following is a list of the thirteen noun classes in Lamba, showing the distinction of the full dissyllabic prefixes from the pre-prefixes:

Class		Full Prefixes		Pre-prefixes
I.	Singular	umu-	(1)	—
	Plural	aŵa-	(2)	ŵa-
II.	Singular	umu-	(3)	—
	Plural	imi-	(4)	—

LANGUAGE

Class		Full Prefixes		Pre-prefixes
III.	Singular	ichi-	(7)	chi-
	Plural	ifi-	(8)	fi-
IV.	Singular	aka-	(13)	ka-
	Plural	utu-	(12)	tu-
V.	Singular	in-[1]	(9)	—
	Plural	in-[1]	(10)	—
	Quantitative plural	ama-	(6)	—
VI.	Singular	ulu-	(11)	—
	Plural	in-[1]	(10)	—
	Quantitative plural	ama-	(6)	—
VII.	Singular	uŵu-	(14)	ŵu-
	Plural	ama-	(6)	—
VIII.	Singular	ili-, i-	(5)	li-
	Plural	ama-	(6)	—
IX.	Singular	uku-	(17)	—
	Plural	ama-	(6)	—
X.		uku-	(15)	—
XI.		—	(17)	ku-
XII.		—	(18)	mu-
XIII.		—	(16)	pa-

The numbers in brackets correspond to Meinhof's system of classification of Ur-Bantu for comparative purposes.

It is seen that each full prefix begins with a vowel, whereas each pre-prefix begins with a consonant. The presence or absence of the initial vowel is very important. For instance, *umuntu* (I, singular) may have its diminutive from either column in Class IV, singular—viz., *akantu* or *kamuntu* (where the pre-prefix, *ka-*, is placed before the shortened form of the original prefix *umu-*). Now, taking the two words *akantu* and *kamuntu*, the copulatives are *kantu* and *nikamuntu* and the locatives *kukantu* and *kulikamuntu*; and the forms of these inflexions generally depend upon whether there is an initial vowel or not.

In Class V the singular and plural prefixes are the same, but the concords used with the singular differ from those used with the plural; e.g., *Imfumu yanji iyo yaisa* ("That chief of mine has come"), *Imfumu shyanji ishyo shyaisa* ("Those chiefs of mine have come"). The prefix *ama-* is often used to denote a quantitative plural; *e.g.*,

> *Inkalamu imo*, one lion.
> *Inkalamu shitatu*, three lions.
> *Amakalamu aenji*, many lions.

Class IX contains only four words, which indicate parts of the

[1] This prefix varies in the form of the nasal, which is assimilated to the form of the initial 'phone' of the stem, and appears as *im-, iŋ-, ing-, inj-*, etc.

375

body. They cannot be treated as belonging to Class X, as they all take plurals in *ama-*, nor can they be treated with the locative, Class XI (as Meinhof would have them), for their prefix is dissyllabic and may also take the locative pre-prefix—e.g., *kukulu*, to the leg.

The existence of Classes XI, XII, and XIII is typically Central Bantu. These are locative classes, and syntactically all words in them may be treated both as nouns and as adverbs. In addition to their indicating adverbial location (*Fiŵike pachipuna*, " Put them on the stool "), they may be used as subject or object of a predicate, with possessives, adjectives, verbs, etc., in concordial agreement (*Apa pachipuna panji apaweme palikosele*, "Here on my fine stool it is hard"—*i.e.*, "The top of my fine stool here is hard").

The Pronoun

There are four main types of pronouns in Lamba, the absolute, the demonstrative, the enumerative, and the qualificative. The pronouns must be distinguished rigidly from the verbal concords, whether subjectival or objectival. In Bantu generally the pronouns, in addition to their use as subject or object of the predicate, are often used in apposition to another substantive.

The **absolute pronouns** merely indicate the substantives, in no way limiting or qualifying them, but they may also be used for purposes of contrast. The forms for the 1st and 2nd persons are dissyllabic—viz., *neŵo, fweŵo, weŵo, mweŵo*—but those of the various classes of the 3rd person are monosyllabic—viz., *ye, ŵo, chyo, fyo, shyo*, etc.

The **demonstrative pronouns** indicate four positions, for which there are forms for each class of nouns. These positions are:

(1) This, *uyu, aŵa, ichi, ifi*, etc.
(2) This here (within view), *uno, ŵano, chino, fino*, etc.
(3) That, *uyo, aŵo, ichyo, ifyo*, etc.
(4) That yonder (within view), *ulya, ŵalya, chilya, filya*, etc.

The demonstrative pronoun may stand alone or in apposition to a substantive, when it may succeed or precede the substantive. When the demonstrative precedes a noun the initial vowel of the noun is elided, and one word-group results; e.g., *uyo, umuntu uyo*, or *uyomuntu* (that person).

In the formation of adverbs, copulatives, and locative predicative forms definite inflexions of the demonstratives take place; *e.g.*,

376

uyu (this person), *aŵa* (these persons).

Locative adverbs: *kuliwuyu, kuliŵaŵa* (" To . . .").

Copulatives: *niwuyu, niŵaŵa* ("It is . . .").

Locative predicates: *ngu* ("Here he is"), *mba* ("Here they are").

The Enumerative Pronouns. Besides the definite numeral forms for 'both,' 'all three,' 'all four,' etc.—viz., the stems *-ŵilo, -tatu, -nane, -sanu*, giving the forms *fweŵilo* (both of us), *mwetatu* (all three of you), *shyonane* (all four *animals*), *fyosanu* (all five *birds*), etc.—Lamba has three special enumerative pronominal stems—viz., *-nse* (all—e.g., *fwense, ŵonse*, etc.), *-enka* (only—e.g., *fwenka, ŵenka*, etc.), and *-pele* (the same, not having distinctive forms for the 1st and 2nd persons—e.g., *ŵopele, chyopele, popele*, etc.).

The Qualificative Pronouns. These are formed from qualificatives. In Lamba the qualificative succeeds the substantive, and if for any reason it is used either before the substantive or instead of it it ceases syntactically to be a qualificative, and becomes a pronoun, either in apposition to or instead of the substantive. Adjectives and numerals suffer *no change of form* when becoming pronouns; e.g., *Umuntu umukulu waisa* or *umukulu waisa* ("An elder has come"), *Aŵantu ŵaŵili ŵaisa* or *ŵaŵili ŵaisa* ("Two people have come"). In the case of relatives, there is a change in the concord of the singular of Class I; e.g., *Umuntu ufiitile wafwa* or *umufiitile wafwa* ("A black person is dead"). Possessives are regularly inflected by prefixing the typical vowel of the noun prefix to form pronouns; e.g., *wanji* becomes *uwanji, chyesu* becomes *ichyesu, ŵamano* becomes *aŵamano*, etc.

The Qualificative

As has just been hinted, in Lamba there are four different qualifying parts of speech covered by the term qualificative. The important distinction between these four parts of speech is that each one has its own particular set of concords. The four qualificatives are (1) adjective, (2) relative, (3) numeral, and (4) possessive. The adjectival concord is used with a very limited number of stems, such as *-kulu* (big), *-chye* (small), *-ipi* (short), etc. There are about twenty adjectival stems in Lamba.

The relative concord is not used in Lamba with distinctive relative stems as it is in Zulu, but it forms relative clauses with various portions of verbs, especially the perfect stems; for

377

THE LAMBAS OF NORTHERN RHODESIA

example, *umuntu uweme*, a fine person (*-weme* being the perfect
stem of *wama*), *ichintu ichikashichile*, a red thing (*-kashichile* being
the perfect stem of *kashika*).

In Lamba the numerals 1 to 5 have a special set of concords,
which are shared with the root *-mbi*, other. The numerals
10 and 100 are nouns used in apposition. 6 to 9 are compound
numerals, since the Lamba system of counting is quinary.

The possessive concords are used with pronominal possessive
stems, and also with nouns shorn of their initial vowel. The
shortened prefix of the singular of Class VIII is not elided, but
coalesces with the final vowel of the possessive concord. Examples: *uŵukulu bwanji* (my size), *uŵukulu bwamfumu* (the size
of the chief), *uŵukulu bwesana* (the size of the egg); in the case
of *imfumu* the initial vowel is elided; in that of *isana* coalescence
of *a + i* to *e* takes place.

The following are the lists of the qualificative concords:

Class		Adjective	Relative	Numeral	Possessive
I.	Singular	umu-	u-	u-	wa-
	Plural	aŵa-	aŵa-	ŵa-	ŵa-
II.	Singular	u-	u-	u-	wa-
	Plural	i-	i-	i-	ya-
III.	Singular	ichi-	ichi-	chi-	chya-
	Plural	ifi-	ifi-	fi-	fya-
IV.	Singular	aka-	aka-	ka-	ka-
	Plural	utu-	utu-	tu-	twa-
V.	Singular	i-	i-	i-	ya-
	Plural	ishi-	ishi-	shi-	shya-
	Quantitative plural	a-	a-	a-	a-
VI.	Singular	ulu-	ulu-	lu-	lwa-
	Plural	ishi-	ishi-	shi-	shya-
	Quantitative plural	a-	a-	a-	a-
VII.	Singular	uŵu-	uŵu-	ŵu-	bwa-
	Plural	a-	a-	a-	a-
VIII.	Singular	ili-	ili-	li-	lya-
	Plural	a-	a-	a-	a-
IX.	Singular	uku-	uku-	ku-	kwa-
	Plural	a-	a-	a-	a-
X.		uku-	uku-	ku-	kwa-
XI.		uku-	uku-	ku-	kwa-
XII.		umu-	umu-	mu-	mwa-
XIII.		apa-	apa-	pa-	pa-

It is seen that in Lamba the relative concord differs from the
adjectival concord only in the singular of Class I.

The following examples illustrate the use of the four types of
concord with the singular and plural of Class I:

378

(1) Adjective: *umuntu umukulu*, a big person;
aŵantu aŵakulu, big people.
(2) Relative: *umuntu uweme*, a good person;
aŵantu aŵaweme, good people.
(3) Numeral: *umuntu umo*, one person;
aŵantu ŵaŵili, two people.
(4) Possessive: *umuntu wamfumu*, servant of the chief;
aŵantu ŵamfumu, servants of the chief.

The Predicative

This, the essential part of each Lamba sentence, may be of two kinds, the verb or the copulative. Except in the imperative and infinitive moods, the verb in Lamba is composed of at least two parts, the subjectival verb concord and the verb stem. The verb stem may undergo certain inflexions, particularly in the formation of the perfect. The verb subjectival concord has hitherto been regarded as a pronoun, but it is not in itself a word; it is merely a formative. Various auxiliaries are brought in to assist in forming the tenses, and these are placed some before, some after, the subjectival concord.

There are three conjugations in Lamba: (1) principal positive, (2) relative positive, and (3) negative (the same for both principal and relative constructions).

There are five moods:

(1) Infinitive, which has the prefix *uku-* and is in reality a noun of Class X. In Lamba there is no negative infinitive, but three forms of the positive: the indefinite, the continuous, and the perfect; e.g., *ukukaka* (to tie), *ukulukukaka* (to be tying), *ukulukwichyele* (to be seated)—used only of stative verbs.

(2) Imperative; e.g., *kaka* ("Tie!"), *kakeni* ("Tie ye!").

(3) Indicative.

(4) Dependent;. e.g., *nkake* ("Let me tie!" or "That I may tie"). There is also a future dependent; e.g., *nkakake*.

(5) Conditional; e.g., *ningakaka* ("I should bind," "I would have bound"), etc.

In the indicative mood are found three implications:

(1) The simple; e.g., *ndukukaka* ("I am tying"), *nshilukukaka* ("I am not tying").

(2) The progressive; e.g., *nchikaka* ("I still tie"), used in the positive conjugations only.

(3) The exclusive; e.g., *nshingakaka* ("I have not yet tied"), used in the negative conjugation only.

THE LAMBAS OF NORTHERN RHODESIA

In addition to the distinctions of mood and implication there is the triple distinction of manner which was observed in the infinitive—viz.,

(1) Indefinite; e.g., *naikala* ("I sat").
(2) Continuous; e.g., *nalukwikala* ("I used to sit").
(3) Perfect; e.g., *nalukwichyele* ("I was seated").

It must be observed that in the present tense there is no indefinite form; what has been taken to be such is a tense belonging to the relative conjugation.

The tense divisions—*i.e.*, the determinations of time significance—are very exact in Lamba. They are remote past, immediate past, present, immediate future, and remote future. The dividing line for the remote and immediate tenses is the coming midnight for the future and the past midnight for the past. The following examples of the tenses are of the simple implication, indefinite manner, in each case 1st person singular:

Remote past: *nalikachile*, "I tied" (yesterday or before).
Immediate past: *nakaka*, "I tied" (to-day).
Present: *ndukukaka*, "I am tying." [1]
Immediate future: *nakukaka*, "I shall tie" (to-day).
Remote future: *nkakaka*, "I shall tie" (to-morrow or later).

The above are naturally but representatives of the tenses in the indicative mood. Each complete tense has forms for 1st and 2nd persons, and for each class of the third person. As an example of a full tense I give the negative habitual tense of *ukuŵepa*, to tell lies.

1st pers. sing. :	*nshiŵepa*, " I do not lie."
plur. :	*tatuŵepa*.
2nd pers. sing. :	*toŵepa*.
plur. :	*tamuŵepa*.
3rd pers. Cl. I, sing. :	*taaŵepa*.
plur. :	*taŵaŵepa*.
II, sing. :	*toŵepa* or *tauŵepa*.
plur. :	*teŵepa* or *taiŵepa*.
III, sing. :	*tachiŵepa*.
plur. :	*tafiŵepa*.
IV, sing. :	*takaŵepa*.
plur. :	*tatuŵepa*.
V, sing. :	*teŵepa* or *taiŵepa*.
plur. :	*tashiŵepa*.
quant. plur. :	*taaŵepa*.

---

[1] It has already been observed that there is no indefinite manner in the present : this is continuous in form.

3rd pers. Cl. VI, sing. :		*taluŵepa.*
	plur. :	*tashiŵepa.*
	quant. plur. :	*taaŵepa.*
VII, sing. :		*taŵuŵepa.*
	plur. :	*taaŵepa.*
VIII, sing. :		*taliŵepa.*
	plur. :	*taaŵepa.*
IX, sing. :		*takuŵepa.*
	plur. :	*taaŵepa.*
X :		*takuŵepa.*
XI :		*takuŵepa.*
XII :		*tamuŵepa.*
XIII :		*tapaŵepa.*

When the object of a verb is definite (such as would be indicated by 'the' in English) an objectival verb concord is used, and this is invariably placed immediately before the verb stem within the verb. In Lamba the subjectival and objectival concords are the same with the exception of (1) those of the 2nd person singular, which has *u-* for the subjectival and *ku-* for the objectival concord, (2) 2nd person plural, which has *mu-* for the subjectival and *mu-* . . . *-ini* for the objectival concord, and (3) the 1st Class singular of the 3rd person, which has *a-* for the subjectival and *mu-* for the objectival concord. Examples: *ndukuŵono'muntu* ("I see a person"), *ndukumuŵono'muntu* ("I see the person"), *mulukumbona* ("You see me"), *ndukumuŵoneni* ("I see you").

An examination of the stem of the Lamba verb reveals the following classification:

(1) **Regular dissyllabic verbs,** ending in the vowel *-a* in their simplest form; e.g., *ŵona* (see), *fwaya* (want), *pama* (strike).

(2) **Monosyllabic verb stems,** limited in number, but indicating such common actions as *lya* (eat), *nwa* (drink), *pa* (give), and including the defective forms *ti* (say) and *li* (be).

(3) **Vowel verbs**—*i.e.,* verbs commencing in vowels; e.g., *enda* (travel), *upa* (marry), *iŵa* (steal).

(4) **Derived verbs**—*i.e.,* verbs not primitive in form. These are of three types:

(*a*) *Verbal derivatives*—*i.e.,* verbs derived from a simple verb by suffix formation; of these more in a moment.

(*b*) *Radical derivatives*—*i.e.,* verbs derived from radicals by suffixing, generally *-ka* (intransitive), *-la* (transitive), and *-shya* (causative); *e.g.,* from *aŵu* (of taking or coming out of water or across water) are formed *aŵuka* (cross a stream), *aŵula* (pull out of water), *aŵushya* (take across a stream), etc.

(*c*) *Adjectival derivatives*—*i.e.,* verbs formed from adjectival

381

roots by suffixing *-pa* or *-mpa*; e.g., *-ŵi* (bad) > *ŵipa* (be bad), *-tali* (long) > *talimpa* (be long), etc.

Verbal Derivatives

Lamba is exceptionally rich in this method of verb-formation, which closely resembles that in Hebrew and other Semitic languages, and is also a feature of the Hamitic family of languages in Africa, of which Nama Hottentot is an extant example in South Africa. I cannot go into any detail of these here, but would refer to Chapter IX of my *Grammar of the Lamba Language*, where a fairly full survey is given. In regular formation Lamba has the following verbal derivatives:

(1) The passive in *-wa, -iwa*.
(2) The neuter in *-ika, -eka*.
(3) The applied in *-ila, -ela, -ina, -ena*.
(4) The intensive in *-ishya, -eshya*.
(5) The causative in *-ya, -ishya, -eshya*.
(6) The perfective in *-ilila, -elela, -inina, -enena*.
(7) The reciprocal in *-ana, -anshyanya*.
(8) The associative in *-akana, -ankana*.
(9) The reversive in *-uluka* (intransitive), *-ulula* (transitive), *-ulushya* (causative), also *-unuka, -onoka, -oloka, -ununa, -onona, -olola*, etc.
(10) The extensive in *-ala* or *-aula* (transitive), *-aka* or *-auka* (intransitive), *-ashya* or *aushya* (causative).

There are certain other forms, frequently but not regularly found, which include the following:

(1) Stative in *-ama*; e.g., *fisama* (be in hiding).
(2) Contactive in *-ata*; e.g., *fumbata* (grasp).
(3) Excessive in *-ashika*; e.g., *pemashika* (pant).

As an example of derivative formation let us take the verb *kaka* (tie).

Passive: *kakwa*, be tied.
Neuter: *kakika*, get tied, be tieable.
Applied: *kakila*, tie for.
Intensive: *kakishya*, tie tightly.
Causative: seldom used in Lamba with transitive verbs, but note *wama* (be good) > *wamya* (make good).
Perfective: *kakilila*, tie once for all, tie for good.
Reciprocal: *kakana*, tie one another; *kakanshyanya*, tie each other.

Associative: *kakankana*, be tied to one another.
Reversive: *kakulula*, untie; *kakuluka*, come untied.
Extensive: *kakala*, tie extensively.

The Copulative

The verb is not the only type of predicative in Lamba. Predicatives are also formed by inflecting other parts of speech, such as nouns, pronouns, and qualificatives; such predicatives I call copulatives. In the conjugation of certain copulative tenses the auxiliary verb *li* is used.

Formation from Nouns. Nouns with dissyllabic prefix drop the initial vowel and generally raise the tone on the remaining syllable of the prefix; e.g., *umuntu* (a person) > *mùntu* ("It is a person"). Nouns with no prefix, with pre-prefix, or with the monosyllabic prefix of Class V (singular and plural) and Class VI (plural) preplace *ni-*; e.g., *tata* (my father) > *nitata* ("It is my father"); *fimenso* (large eyes) > *nifimenso* ("They are large eyes"); *inkalamu* (lion) > *ninkalamu* ("It is a lion"). Nouns of Class VIII (singular) with the short prefix *i-* revert to the full form *ili-* and are treated as nouns with dissyllabic prefix; e.g., *itaŵa* (maize) > *lìtaŵa* ("It is maize").

Formation from Pronouns. To absolute pronouns *ni-* is preplaced; e.g., *nineŵo* ("It is I"), *niŵo* ("It is they"), etc. The same formative is preplaced to modified forms of the demonstrative; e.g., *uyu* > *niwuyu*, *ichyo* > *nichichyo*, *palya* > *nipapalya*, etc. Copulatives are not formed from enumerative pronouns, but the copulative formed from the corresponding absolute pronoun is used; e.g., *ŵenka* (they only) > *niŵo ŵenka* ("It is they only").

Formation from Adjectives. Adjectives with dissyllabic concord drop the initial vowel and raise the tone on the remaining syllable of the concord; e.g., *aŵantu aŵatali* (tall people) > *aŵantu ŵàtali* ("The people are tall"), *pantu apatali* (at a distant place) > *apopantu pàtali* ("That place is distant"). Adjectives with monosyllabic concord merely raise the tone on that concord; e.g., *imiti ikulu* (big trees) > *imiti ìkulu* ("The trees are big"). A similar tonal inflexion takes place with possessives; e.g., *ifintu fyanji* (my things) > *ifintu fyànji* ("The things are mine").

It is a noteworthy feature of Bantu languages that inflexion is the basic principle in the formation of predicates from other parts of speech. The verb 'to be' or 'to become' is only brought in in an auxiliary capacity as tense-former.

THE LAMBAS OF NORTHERN RHODESIA

The Adverb

In Lamba there is a very close connexion between the noun and the adverb. The same word in many cases may be used syntactically as a noun and as an adverb. The best instance of this is found in noun classes XI, XII, and XIII. The following sentences will illustrate:

(1) Noun: *Muŋanda mwakwe umukulu mùfiitile*, " Inside his big hut is dark."

(2) Adverb: *Ŵalilele muŋanda*, " They are sleeping in the hut."

(3) Noun: *Pamenso pamwanakashi uyu pàweme ukwakuti*, " The face of this woman is very comely."

(4) Adverb: *Ampama pamenso*, " He struck me in the face."

In the same way other nouns may have two syntactical significances; e.g., *uluŵilo* (speed, quickly), *uluchyelo* (morning, in the morning), *umukome* (slow gait, slowly), *ichiine* (truth, indeed), etc. There are also certain words which may only be used adverbially.

The Radical

Of parallel use to the adverb is the other descriptive, the radical. This constitutes a part of speech, as such, unknown to European languages. While the adverb describes a predicate, qualificative, or other adverb in respect of time, place, and manner, the radical describes in respect of manner, colour, sound, and action. In my " Study in Lamba Phonetics " I found it necessary to divide the subject into (1) "Normal Grammatical Phonetics," excluding phenomena which have their origin in onomatopœia or interjection, and (2) "Extra-normal Phonetics," dealing with the specialized phonetics of onomatopœia. In Bantu languages the division is not always easy to make, for onomatopœia and other extra-normal phones are introduced through the radical into the normal grammatical construction of verbs and nouns. The radical breaks through the normal rules of stress, length, and tone which apply to Lamba; ultimate and ante-penultimate stresses occur; while the normal tone shape of the Lamba sentence, with more or less regular peaks of tone, is interrupted with rising and falling tones and extremes of height and depth.

The term 'radical' which I have used to indicate this part of speech is plainly applicable to Zulu, where the vast majority of the examples are definitely the roots (*radices*) from which verbs are formed, and there is no indication that the radicals are derived from anything more primitive. In Lamba, however, the term is

384

not quite so satisfactory. In many cases verbs *are* formed from radicals; e.g., *Kumfwa umwando putu!* "And the string went snap!" or *Penka umwando waputuka!* "Then the string snapped!" where *putu* is obviously the root from which *putuka* is formed by suffixing *-ka*. On the other hand, in Lamba some radicals are as obviously formed from verbs. For example, from the simple form *fisa* (hide) are formed the regular reversives *fisuluka* (come out of hiding) and *fisulula* (reveal). Now there are accompanying radicals to each of these forms—viz., *ukufisuluka fisuluku* and *ukufisulula fisululu*. From this we can only conclude that these radicals are derived from the verbs in each case. From the knowledge we have at present it seems that in Bantu the radical is the more primitive form, and the term a correct one to use for this part of speech; but in Lamba and some other Bantu languages secondary later forms have been derived to accompany certain verbal derivatives or to be used as their equivalents.

The radicals in Lamba follow a more or less natural classification, the one which I have adopted for Zulu.[1] There are (1) monosyllabic radicals, such as *weee*[2] (of light flashing), *tooo* (of firmness), *twiii* (of anger); (2) dissyllabic radicals, such as *fundu* (of mixing up), *kono* (of snapping), *tusu* (of stone striking); (3) trisyllabic radicals, such as *ndùkutu* (of quick pace), *pakatu* (of buffalo running), *pengele* (of swimming); (4) quadrisyllabic radicals, such as *mpolompompi* (helter-skelter), *kolokoso* (gait of tortoise), *piliwili* (of swift entrance).

These radicals may be repeated for purposes of emotion, thus:

na na na na (of a boy running).
nge nge nge (of bell ringing).
shyeŵu shyeŵu shyeŵu (of nibbling).
pompoto pompoto pompoto (of lion running).
kalakasa kalakasa (of tortoise walking).

In the case of the dissyllabic radicals it is the regular rule that a single radical is used with the simple form of the verb derived therefrom, but if an extensive form of the verb be used, then the radical is reduplicated; for instance, *ukusokoka soko*, to get knocked out, *ukusokaka soko soko*, to get knocked out wholesale.

In Zulu further divisions of the radicals are made according to the tone sequences, but the complete difference of the tone system of Lamba does not seem to make this feasible in the latter

---

[1] See my *Text-book of Zulu Grammar*, Chapter XIV.
[2] Prolonged length indicated by three like vowels.

language. It may be possible to make the subdivisions in Lamba dependent upon the characteristic vowel of the radical, but more research upon this interesting question is necessary.

Conclusion

Conjunctions and interjections do not need any special treatment here, except to observe that all so-called vocatives are but interjections, and should be so treated.

There is no place in Bantu grammar for prepositions. The so-called prepositions are either (1) adverbial formatives or noun-class prefixes, such as *ku-*, *mu-*, and *pa-*, or (2) possessive concords, such as *wa-*, *kwa-*, *fya-*, etc. There is also no place for the article in Bantu: its lack is supplied by the demonstrative pronouns and the objectival concord. Further, case is not a grammatical feature of Bantu. There is no formal distinction of a substantive as subject or object of a sentence. There is no genitive case, the possessive, a separate type of qualificative, being used. The vocative is an interjection, and the adverbs supply the need for oblique cases felt in other languages. Sex-gender is never a grammatical feature in Bantu languages; class-gender of nouns is the hall-mark of Bantu. Among the Bantu languages Lamba is peculiarly rich in the number of noun classes it employs, and in the suffixal verbal derivatives it is one of the most prolific.

Naturally in the space at my disposal in this chapter I am able to give but a brief survey of the wonderfully inflexional language which the Lambas speak with such grammatical exactitude. For further details I must refer the reader to my *Grammar*, to which reference has already been made. This unfortunately has been treated in the old method, but the details are there ready for use in the Bantu mould which I have endeavoured to cast in this chapter.

BIBLIOGRAPHY

DOKE, C. M.: "A Specimen of the Folk-lore of the Lamba People of Northern Rhodesia," a paper contributed to *Bantu Studies* (vol. i, No. 3, October, 1922, pp. 1–5).

—— "A Study in Lamba Phonetics," a paper contributed to *Bantu Studies* (vol. iii, No. 1, July, 1927, pp. 5–47).

—— *Lamba Folk-lore* (American Folk-lore Society Memoir, No. XX, 1927). This contains 159 folk-tales, 1695 aphorisms and proverbs, 95 songs, and 144 riddles in Lamba text, with English translation and annotation.

—— *Text-book of Zulu Grammar* (2nd ed., Longmans, Green, London, 1931).

—— *Grammar of the Lamba Language* (Kegan Paul, 1922).

JUNOD, H. A.: *The Life of a South African Tribe* (2nd ed., Macmillan, London, 1927).

LACERDA: *The Lands of Cazembe: Lacerda's Journey to Cazembe in 1798*, translated by R. F. Burton (John Murray, London, 1873).

MADAN, A. C.: *Lala-Lamba Handbook* (Clarendon Press, Oxford, 1908).

—— *Lala-Lamba-Wisa Dictionary* (Clarendon Press, Oxford, 1913).

—— *Lenje Handbook* (Clarendon Press, Oxford, 1908).

MEINHOF, C.: *Grundzüge einer vergleichenden Grammatik der Bantu-sprachen* (Dietrich Reimer, Berlin, 1906).

MELLAND, F. H.: *In Witch-bound Africa* (Seeley, Service, London, 1923).

MOUBRAY, J. M.: *In South Central Africa* (Constable, London, 1912).

SMITH, E. W., and DALE, A. M.: *The Ila-speaking Peoples of Northern Rhodesia* (Macmillan, London, 1920).

THOMSON, J.: "To Lake Bangweolo and the Unexplored Region of British Central Africa," a paper in the *Geographical Journal* (November, 1892).

TORREND, J.: *Specimens of Bantu Folk-lore from Northern Rhodesia* (Kegan Paul, London, 1921).

Lambaland, quarterly missionary record.

GLOSSARY

The following glossary of native terms used in the foregoing pages is exclusive of words used on pages 107–118 (list of foodstuffs), pages 254–259 (kinship terms), and in Chapter XXIII on the language. Words are not entered under stems, but as they appear in the book, and where both singular and plural forms occur the meaning is given under the singular, reference being made thereto under the plural. If only the plural has been used the meaning is given thereunder.

akabwangala, top of the skull.
akachyekulu, a type of gnome.
akafunga, (1) miscarriage ; (2) still-born babe.
akafwambimono, species of small fish-trap.
akakuŵo, a Lamba moon.
akakwa, small bark dish.
akalembwe-lukasu, a famine food.
akalimba, hand-piano.
akalimba kamaswao, rattling hand-piano.
akalindi, small hole.
akalonde, old, worn-out hoe.
akalongelo, small hole.
akalukwa, small basket.
akalulu, hare.
akalunguti, species of tree.
akalusafya-manika, a Lamba moon.
akaluŵi, doll, figure of person.
akampabwa, lying flat on the back.
akampeshimpeshi, lightning.
akanchyense, species of tree.
akanichye akamukoa, youngster with a navel-string.
akankoto, two-stringed musical instrument.
akankoŵele, small hand-piano.
akansokolwa, leaf funnel.
akaŋanda kambuluŵulu, small circular hut without an opening.
akapafu, stomach.
akapafu peulu, stomach upward.
akapalala, a Lamba moon.
akapeshi, (1) spirit hut of renowned chief ; (2) grass basket of *muka-mwami.*
akapeshi kaŵami, grass basket of *mukamwami.*

akapingwe, platform.
akapinisansa, species of adder.
akapofwe, plant used for soap.
akapokoshi, Kafir-pox.
akapolobwe, species of cane-rat.
akapondo, murderer.
akapoopo, disease consequent on irregular birth.
akapota, species of tree.
akapyantoto, a Lamba moon.
akasabwa, species of tree.
akasakanenga, species of mungoose.
akasako, (1) staff ; (2) feather.
akasako kanduŵa, a Lamba moon.
akasansa, small strip of cloth.
akasela, type of dance.
akasembe, tsetse-fly.
akasemo, shout of triumph.
akasenshimbeŵa, baby born with teeth.
akashimbo, type of dance.
akasuŵa, (1) sun ; (2) day.
akasuŵa-kachye, a Lamba moon.
akatembo, noose trap.
akatemo, axe.
akatete, sorghum beer.
akatiŵi, breast of an animal.
akatundu, large grain basket.
akatuutwa, species of small bird.
akaŵale, type of dance.
akaŵambala, wooden tube connecting nozzle to bellows.
akaŵengele-ntanga, a Lamba moon.
akaŵeshi, small knife.
akaŵungo, house of deceased chief.
akayeŵela, small fabulous animal said to be used by witches.
akayinga, small potsherd.
akeshiŵilo kaŵuleme, sign of honour.

amabwe, pl. of *ibwe*.
amafinje, cursing.
amafwasa, pl. of *ifwasa*.
amaila, Lenje for *amasaka*.
amakandi, testicles.
amakonkola, species of fruit.
amakoosa, armlets.
amakowela muntiŵi, severe pains in the chest.
amakuku, hand-clapping.
amalilo, mourning rites.
amalimba, pl. of *ilimba*.
amaluko, young of bees.
amalya, omens of coming food.
amamba akwe Lesa, mica ("scales of God").
amambalakata, pl. of *ilimbalakata*.
amamena, sprouting grain, malt.
amamfutenuma, walking backward.
amanata, leprosy.
amankamba, complete teeth.
amankulukwapa, hair of the armpits.
amankumanya, goods of reconciliation for meeting.
amankunamwa, state of cutting upper teeth first.
amankuŵala, pl. of *ilinkuŵala*.
amansangwa, pl. of *insangwa*.
amansanshi, children's miniature play-huts.
amansanshi ambuli, play-huts of girls.
amansanshi atwanichye, play-huts of little children.
amansanshi aŵalalume, play-huts of boys.
amantabwa, edible famine-time roots.
amaŋanda antanda, walled houses.
amaombe, initiation dance.
amapasa, twins of unlike sex.
amapundi, Ngoni from Nyasaland.
amasafwa, species of fruit.
amasaka, sorghum.
amasasa, pl. of *isasa*.
amasasa ampoolo, mats of soft grass.
amasengo, horns.
amashiko, hearths, firesides.
amashilampindwe, intersections of paths.
amashimbi, charcoal.
amashya, dance.
amashyashya, Mbwela for *ifisako*.
amashyaŵe, persons possessed by a dancing spirit.
amaso, pubic hair.
amasonje, filed or chipped teeth.
amasuku, species of fruit.
amata, pl. of *uŵuta*.
amatala, grain-houses.
amatete, pl. of *itete*.

amateŵe, pl. of *iteŵe*.
amatuka, filthy reviling.
amatwi, ears.
amawo, red millet.
amaŵoni, pl. of *uŵuŵoni*.
amaŵula afiŵanda, leaves efficacious against demons.
amaŵumba aŵakulu, assemblies of the elders.
anika, (to) spread out to dry.
aŵachyete, pl. of *umuchyete*.
aŵafiichishi ŵamalimba, makers of gourd-pianos.
aŵafu, dead people.
aŵafushi, pl. of *umufushi*.
aŵafyala, pl. of *umufyala*.
aŵako, sons-in-law.
aŵakoleshi ŵamfula, pl. of *umukoleshi wamfula*.
aŵakulu, pl. of *umukulu*.
aŵalamu, pl. of *umulamu*.
aŵalaye, pl. of *umulaye*.
aŵalaye ŵakankwese, doctors of the circling of the axe-handle.
aŵalembo, pl. of *umulembo*.
aŵalishi ŵakalimba, players of the hand-piano.
aŵalishi ŵamalimba, players of the gourd-piano.
aŵalishi ŵangoma, drummers.
aŵalomweshi, pl. of *umulomweshi*.
aŵalonga, fish clan people.
aŵalongo, clan opposites.
aŵalukoso, persons of no consequence, unrelated.
aŵalunda, pl. of *umulunda*.
aŵamankunamwa, pl. of *uwamankunamwa*.
aŵamano, clever people.
aŵamfwi, grey-headed persons.
aŵami, pl. of *umwami*.
aŵamyando, trappers by rope traps.
aŵanaŵankashi, brethren.
aŵanichye, pl. of *umwanichye*.
aŵantu, people.
aŵantu ŵamilimo, servants.
aŵantunshi, human beings.
aŵanyama, meat clan people.
aŵapalu, pl. of *umupalu*.
aŵapalù ŵamyando, trappers.
aŵapanga, favourite attendants.
aŵapupa, pl. of *umupupa*.
aŵapupwishi, dew-dryers.
aŵasanu, chief's wives.
aŵaseesa, pl. of *umuseesa*.
aŵashichye, pl. of *umushichye*.
aŵashishi, bark rope people.
aŵatatwishi ŵakasela, leaders in dance songs.

aŵaŵashishi ŵakalimba, hand-piano makers.
aŵaŵashishi ŵamato, boat-builders.
aŵaŵashishi ŵameno, teeth-chippers.
aŵayamba, pl. of *uŵayamba*.
aŵayambo, pl. of *umuyambo*.
aŵayembe, Kaonde for *ŵamoŵa*.
aŵenachyela, metal clan people.
aŵenachyoŵa, pl. of *umŵinachyoŵa*.
aŵenachyulu, pl. of *umŵinachyulu*.
aŵenakaloŵa, soil clan people.
aŵenakalungu, bead clan people.
aŵenakani, grass clan people.
aŵenakashimu, bee clan people.
aŵenakasonga, scorpion-sting clan people.
aŵenakauluŵe, river-hog clan people.
aŵenakaŵundi, galago clan people.
aŵenakunda, pigeon clan people.
aŵenaluŵo, wind clan people.
aŵenamaila, pl. of *umŵinamaila*.
aŵenambeŵa, mouse clan people.
aŵenambulo, metal clan people.
aŵenambushi, pl. of *umŵinambushi*.
aŵenambwa, pl. of *umŵinambwa*.
aŵenamfula, rain clan people.
aŵenamilenda, pl. of *umŵinamulenda*.
aŵenamishishi, pl. of *umŵinamishishi*.
aŵenampumpi, wild dog clan people.
aŵenamulilo, fire clan people.
aŵenamumba, clay clan people.
aŵenamusamba, bark rope clan people.
aŵenanama, meat clan people.
aŵenango, scorpion clan people.
aŵenanguluŵe, river-hog clan people.
aŵenanguni, pl. of *umŵinanguni*.
aŵenankalamu, lion clan people.
aŵenankulimba, pigeon clan people.
aŵenankuwa, dog clan people.
aŵenansanje, blue monkey clan people.
aŵenansofu, pl. of *umŵinansofu*.
aŵenansoka, snake clan people.
aŵenansumbi, fowl clan people.
aŵenanswi, pl. of *umŵinanswi*.
aŵenanyendwa, needle clan people.
aŵenaŋandu, crocodile clan people.
aŵenaŋanga, doctor clan people.
aŵenatembo, pl. of *umŵinatembo*.
aŵenaŵesa, plain clan people.
aŵenaŵuko, wife's relatives.
aŵene ŵamupashi, pl. of *umŵine ŵamupashi*.
aŵeneshi, people well known to one.
aŵenshikulu, pl. of *umŵinshikulu*.
aŵensu, visitors, strangers.
aŵepwa, pl. of *umŵipwa*.
aŵika, (to) soak.
aŵofi ŵaŵyaŵo, their brothers-in-law —*i.e.*, men who have married sisters.

aŵongwa, lawless persons, persons of low morals.

bwela, (to) return.

chichile'shiŵyakwe, (to) keep back his mates.
chikankati, species of salt grass.
chikasole, reed-buck horn of buffalo medicine.
chikukulu, species of salt grass.
chikuto, child born with membranous covering over him.
chilangalume, species of shrub.
chilele, blind-worm.
chimulonda, sable antelope horn of medicinal power used to detect thieves.
china, (to) foment.
chindika, (to) honour.
chipishyamenda, woman slave attendant.
chipyaila, servant of *mukamwami*.
chite'chipa, (to) cast lots, conjure.
chiŵangalume, species of salt grass.
chyembe, (1) species of grass ; (2) salty encrustation.
chyenjela, (to) be intelligent, cunning.
chyesa, (to) cut corn heads, etc.
chyochyo, paddle of spear.

fiso'ŵulishi, (to) hide its crying.
fula, (to) work metal.
funda, (to) instruct.
fundika, (to) confine.
funku, sorghum beer.
funkwe, mythical monstrous water-snake.
fwaka, tobacco.
fyashya, (to) assist in giving birth.

ibwe, stone, nether grindstone.
ichibwela-mushi, a Lamba moon.
ichifu, trap of poised weight.
ichifubwilo, container of funnel fish-trap.
ichifuŵa, cough.
ichikondo, bark canoe.
ichikwa, large bark trough.
ichila, type of dance.
ichilaila, women's dance.
ichilambe, muddy water, morass.
ichilambu, a big gift, large payment.
ichilapo, oath.
ichilende, hole dug for grave.
ichileŵeleŵe, species of medicine.
ichilindi, hole.
ichilishyelishye, a sounding of no significance.

ichiloli, type of flute.
ichilolo, headman not of chief's rank.
ichilonda, sore, ulcer.
ichilukwa, grass meal basket.
ichilundo, four-yard strip of calico.
ichilundu, cowrie-shell.
ichiluŵulantumbe, initial crop cultivated by a man for his wife's
relatives.
ichimabwe, communal grinding-house.
ichimamba, species of tree.
ichimanto, tongs.
ichimbela, woman past child-bearing,
midwife.
ichimbushi, red blanket, red calico.
ichimbwasa, type of initiation dance.
ichimfwembe, large-mouthed pot.
ichimo, small razor.
ichimpata, cattle or goat kraal.
ichinchyewa, species of bush.
ichingalangala, feather headdress.
ichingwali, smallpox.
ichinjishi, child before learning to talk.
ichinkoloto, large string trap.
ichinkuwaila, kind of goblin.
ichinkuŵu, species of wooden hammer
for bark cloth making.
ichinsala, rope trap.
ichinsengwe, hunting dance.
ichinshingwa, shadow, picture.
ichinsonta, sharp wooden stake.
ichintengwa, smelting-house.
ichintimbwa, large wood and bamboo
hand-piano.
ichinu, mortar, stamp-block.
ichinyenye, duiker pipe.
ichipa, lots.
ichipa chyabwanga, lots to detect
demon interference.
ichipa chyafiŵanda, lots to detect
demon interference.
ichipa chyakasuŵa, lot of the sun.
ichipa chyakwe sumba, green lizard lot.
ichipa chyamalya, lot to tell of food.
ichipa chyaminyeŋu, lot of the black ant.
ichipa chyapaŵuchyende, adultery lot.
ichipa chyaŵukulu, lot to detect the
biggest.
ichipa chyeshyamo, trial of ill-luck.
ichipaapo, carrying-cloth for babe.
ichipachilo, type of hairdressing.
ichipamba, hammering axe used in
bark cloth preparation.
ichipanda, (1) hunting shrine; (2)
weir.
ichipanta, strip of cloth.
ichipantu, lower fire-stick.
ichipeela, leaf charm to prevent rain.
ichipelu, species of dance.

ichipembe, screen.
ichipembwe, village of an *umwinamulenda*.
ichiponje, ornamented neck-band.
ichipoosela, state of longing in pregnancy.
ichipuna, stool.
ichipyolo, wooden knife used in pot-
making.
ichisanji, relish pot.
ichisanshilo, pot for brewing beer.
ichisekele, maize beer.
ichiseleŵele, women's dance.
ichishika, a Lamba moon.
ichishimichishyo, folk-tale.
ichishyala, bag containing diviner's
outfit.
ichishyaneshyane, aimless dancing.
ichisoko, bag containing diviner's
outfit.
ichisolo, native 'draughts' game.
ichisonga, mythical water animal resembling rhinoceros.
ichisongola, demon.
ichisoshi, locusts (Lenje).
ichisumiko, beer-strainer.
ichisungu, (1) girl initiate; (2) initiation.
ichitashi, tree with salt-producing
leaves.
ichite, child late in learning to walk.
ichitenje chyaŵuufi, marriage-feast.
ichitenje chyesoŵololo, court of justice.
ichitondo, medicine given by *mukamwami*.
ichitupa, shelf or loft in house.
ichituuka, house of deceased person.
ichityoneko, riddle, myth.
ichiwa, features.
ichiŵakeŵake, building without plan.
ichiŵanda, demon.
ichiŵanga, ceremonial dancing axe.
ichiŵango, circular bond for hut-roof.
ichiŵansa, large courtyard.
ichiŵansa chyamfwa, the court of
death.
ichiŵi, door.
ichiŵimbili, blind-worm.
ichiŵinda, professional hunter.
ichiŵingu, harpoon.
ichiŵitiku, women's dance.
ichiŵoŵo, species of tree.
ichiyaŵafu, abode of the dead.
ichiyinga, potsherd, cracked pot.
ichyambawilo, meeting-house.
ichyandaŋombe, tug-of-war.
ichyanga, charm.
ichyangama, long delay in the rains.
ichyani, grass.

GLOSSARY

ichyeso, (1) halved calabash container ; (2) salt percolator.
ichyonde, Lenje for *umulenda*.
ichyulu, anthill.
ichyumbo, pall used at initiations.
ichyungwa, lawless person.
ichyupo, marriage pledge.
ififiitishi, mamba snakes.
ififufu, stacks of corn-heads, corn stands.
ififumbe, species of caterpillar.
ifilaila, pl. of *ichilaila*.
ifilolo, pl. of *ichilolo*.
ifilukwa, pl. of *ichilukwa*.
ifilundo, pl. of *ichilundo*.
ifilyangwa, openings.
ifimbela, pl. of *ichimbela*.
ifimbolo, hyenas.
ifimbwasa, pl. of *ichimbwasa*.
ifimpelampela, miracles.
ifimpwampwa, cakes of tobacco, etc.
ifinani, meat.
ifinashi, worms.
ifinjishi, pl. of *ichinjishi*.
ifinkuwaila, pl. of *ichinkuwaila*.
ifinsangwe, after-birth.
ifinsengwe, pl. of *ichinsengwe*.
ifinsonta, pl. of *ichinsonta*.
ifinu, pl. of *ichinu*.
ifinyanchyela, dross, slag.
ifipa, pl. of *ichipa*.
ifipa fyamalya, pl. of *ichipa chyamalya*.
ifipanda, pl. of *ichipanda*.
ifipanda fyamyando, shrines of the ropes.
ifipapwa, shells, outer bark.
ifipembwe, pl. of *ichipembwe*.
ifipuna, pl. of *ichipuna*.
ifipupu, combs.
ifisako, small branches with twigs and leaves.
ifisapa, drainage channels in marshes.
ifisele, shallow bamboo baskets.
ifishimba, medicine enclosed in horns.
ifishimu, caterpillars.
ifisompe, patches of rank grass.
ifisukuŵya, species of caterpillar.
ifisumiko, pl. of *ichisumiko*.
ifisunga, non-intoxicating Kafir beer.
ifisungu, pl. of *ichisungu*.
ifita, fighters, band of raiders.
ifiteme, piled timber for burning in gardens.
ifiti, poles.
ifiti fyachipembe, poles for the screen.
ifitumbo, the outskirts of the village.
ifitungusa, prickly cucumbers.
ifiŵanda, pl. of *ichiŵanda*.
ifiŵaya, drinking gourds.

ifukuta, bag of the bellows, etc.
ifumo, spear.
ifunama, (to) turn over, back upward.
ifwasa, nodule ant-heap.
ifyakulunga, condiments.
ifyakutoŵela, relish.
ifyambo, worms.
ifyamushimu, good omens.
ifyanga, pl. of *ichyanga*.
ifyeso, pl. of *ichyeso*.
ifyuni, birds.
ikanga, guinea-fowl.
ikata, (to) catch.
ikondyo lyafwaka, nicotine.
ikungulu, a Lamba moon.
ikungulu lyamitondo, a Lamba moon.
ikwikwi, hornless owl, a bird of ill-omen.
Ilamba, the country of the Lamba people.
ilambo, death-place.
ililila, (to) go away for good.
ilimba, gourd-piano.
ilimbalakata, elephant-hunting dance.
ilinkuŵala, hollow wooden sounding boat.
ilonga, eating trough.
iloŵa, soil.
imango, withies.
imangu, large gourd drum struck with sticks.
imbafi, ornamental axe.
imbafuta, white calico.
imbeŵa, mouse, rat, etc. (generic term).
imbifi, sinner, immoral person.
imbiko, omen, ill-omen.
imbila, calabash and hide drum.
imbile, working party.
imbilichila, species of kernel.
imbishi, zebra.
imbokoma, calabash pipe.
imboo, buffalo.
imbote, honey beer.
imbu, salt lick in anthill.
imbuli, immature girl.
imbushi, (1) goat ; (2) water-beetle.
imbushi yapamenda, water-beetle.
imfula, rain.
imfuma, grass beer basket.
imfumbe, species of mouse.
imfumu, chief.
imfumu yaŵuleme, prominent chief.
imfundanga, gunpowder.
imfungo, species of fruit.
imfupo, payment to dancers, etc.
imfuti, gun.
imfuulu, bark container.
imfwa, (1) death ; (2) dead body.

393

THE LAMBAS OF NORTHERN RHODESIA

imfwambi, species of fish-trap.
imfwiti, witch, wizard, warlock.
imfwiti yankumbu, a merciful witch.
imichishi, apparitions, ghostly forms.
imichyeka, pl. of *umuchyeka*.
imifwi, arrows.
imikoka, pl. of *umukoka*.
imikoshi yamabwe, large Mbundu beads.
imikunko, flat boards for bark-beating.
imikunto, pl. of *umukunto*.
imilala, raised garden beds.
imilambu, pl. of *umulambu*.
imilandu, pl. of *umulandu*.
imilao, instructions of a dying man.
imilenda, pl. of *umulenda*.
imilombe, pl. of *umulombe*.
imiloto, dreams.
imilyashi, pl. of *umulyashi*.
imimpe, mice tunnels, rays of the sun.
iminkonka, bracelets.
imintimpa, season of the end of the rains.
iminyeŋu, black biting ants.
imipashi, pl. of *umupashi*.
imipashi yakwe, his spirits.
imipashi yaŵamoŵa, spirits of professional dancers.
imipishi, apparitions, ghostly forms.
imisamba, pl. of *umusamba*.
imisamu, pl. of *umusamu*.
imisanse, clumps of grass.
imisantu, pl. of *umusantu*.
imiseeŵa, bier.
imisengelo, pl. of *umusengelo*.
imiseŵe, pl. of *umuseŵe*.
imishi, pl. of *umushi*.
imishiliko, pl. of *umushiliko*.
imishiliko yaŵalaye, prohibitions of the doctor.
imishimpo, sticks for beating *amankuŵala*.
imishishi, hair of the human head.
imishyangalala, pl. of *umushyangalala*.
imisuku, pl. of *umusuku*.
imita, pl. of *umuta*.
imitala, near-by villages.
imitanda, pl. of *umutanda*.
imitanti, pl. of *umutanti*.
imitembo, pl. of *umutembo*.
imitima, (1) pl. of *umutima* ; (2) vitals.
imitima nematwi, the vitals and ears.
imiŵanga, pl. of *umuŵanga*.
imiŵela, pl. of *umuŵela*.
impali, wife of polygynist.
impanda, pl. of *ulupanda*.
impande, valuable shell ornament.
impasa, mat of split reeds.

impele, the itch.
impelo, upper grindstone.
impemba, councillor.
impendwa, ant-bear.
impilipili, chilies.
impindo, pl. of *ulupindo*.
impindo shyamulemu, charm sticks of red protea.
impinga shyandale, charm sticks of *ndale* wood.
impoli, pipe.
impompwe, ornamental axe.
impoyo, reed-buck.
impula, solid metal spear.
impundu, (1) species of fruit ; (2) pl. of *ulumpundu*.
impyani, heir.
imyele, knives.
imyondo, pl. of *umondo*.
imyumbu, pl. of *umumbu*.
imyuŵa, pl. of *umuuŵa*.
inama, animal, game, meat.
inama shyabwanga, meat of the charm.
inchyema, white-tailed mungoose.
indale, species of tree.
indili, hole.
indimba, large hand-piano.
indoŵo, fish-hook.
indume, brother (of female).
inembo, incisions, tattooing.
ingoloŵola, noose trap.
ingoma, drum.
ingoma shyamaombe, initiation dance.
ingoma yamambwa-kuŵili, ancient double-faced drum.
ingoma yaŵukali, drum of fierceness.
inguni, honey-guide.
inguŵo, cloth.
inguŵo yamafuta, oil-softened bark cloth.
ingwele, shouting, cheering.
injelekela, a Lamba moon.
inkaka, (1) armadillo shell ; (2) charm therefrom.
inkalamu, lion.
inkama, piece of metal broken from the forged lump.
inkamfi, pl. of *ulukamfi*.
inkashi, sister (of male).
inkofwa, snail shell.
inkola, trap for moles made of bark tube.
inkole, hostage.
inkombe, (1) present as sign of submission ; (2) messenger.
inkombo, pl. of *ulukombo*.
inkombo shyamusoolo, long-handled calabashes.
inkomfwa, species of fruit.

inkoshyanya, grass support for pot on head.

inkoshyanya yachisansa, cloth support for pot on head.

inkoti, vertebræ of an animal's neck.

inkuku, girl's bead headdress.

inkumbu, pity, compassion.

inkuni, heavy firewood.

inkunka, lean-to hut.

inkunko ⎱ ball of metal used
inkunko yachyela ⎰ as hammer.

inkusu, (1) species of tree ; (2) kernel of fruit of this tree.

inkuule, roughly hoed soil.

inkuŵo, a Lamba moon.

inkuŵonkulu, a Lamba moon.

inkwa, pl. of *ulukwa*.

inondo, (1) teetotum ; (2) solid metal hammer.

inongo, pot.

insai, rattle of wild orange.

insaka, summer-house.

insala, hunger, famine.

insalamu, ring.

insama, bird-scaring or other shelter.

insambo, wire bracelets.

insamfu, kindling wood.

insanguni, fabulous monster, half fish, half man.

insangwa, seed rattles.

insasamyenje, rays of the sun.

insengo, pl. of *ulusengo*.

insengo shyanshya, duiker horns.

insense, veranda.

insenshi, cane-rat.

inshima, thick porridge.

inshingwa, whip top.

inshinko, stopper.

inshiŵo, powdered clay for moulding.

insoni, sorrow, bashfulness.

insono, sharpening stone.

insonta, forked roofing-poles.

insukuso, pot for finger-washing.

insumbi, domestic fowl.

insungo, calabash.

intafu, ball.

intalo, pot for *inshima*.

intambangoma, friction drum.

intanda, (1) Venus ; (2) hut with upright walls.

intelele, species of plant.

intende, grass stalks.

intetele, species of wild snapdragon.

intongo, sorghum beer.

intumbe, beer basket.

intuntu, pipe-bowl.

inuma, the back.

inununshi, mud wasp.

inyemba, cloth girdle.

inyenda, needle.

inyimbo shyachinsengwe, songs of the chase.

inyimbo shyaŵamoŵa, songs of the *ŵamoŵa*.

iŋanda, house, hut.

iŋande'kulu, the great house, the house of the principal wife.

iŋande'nini, the small house, the house of the inferior wife.

iŋanga, (1) doctor, diviner ; (2) species of bird.

iŋanga yakwe shiwakota, species of bird.

iŋumba, barren woman.

iŋwanga, pl. of *uluwanga*.

ipike'chinsengwe, (to) cook for the hunting dance.

ipike'limbalakata, (to) cook for the elephant dance.

ipupwe, ceremonial offering.

isa, (to) come.

isambwe, bark bowl for medicine.

isasa, mat of marsh grass.

isaŵi, fish.

ise, hoe.

isese, type of musical instrument.

ishiku, incest.

ishilu, madman.

ishitumpile, foolish (animals).

ishyala, ash-heap, midden.

ishyamo, ill-luck.

ishyaŵamoŵa, dances of the *ŵamoŵa*.

ishyula, support beneath grass basket.

isongwe, demon.

isoŵololo lyamulandu, discussion of a case.

itembo, wasp.

itete, reed.

iteŵe, chief's stool.

iŵamba, species of cutting grass.

iŵengele, a Lamba moon.

iŵengele-likulu, a Lamba moon.

iŵengele-linini, a Lamba moon.

iŵofu, goitre.

iŵumba, clay for moulding.

iŵushya-nama, dawn star, rouser of the buck.

iyakochya, grilled (fowl).

iyakwipika, boiled (fowl).

iyamaombe, double-faced drum.

Kaaluwe, the guardian of the animals.

kakwele, rhinoceros.

kalama, attendant.

kalume, male slave.

kamalekano-nalesa, a Lamba moon.

kamunkomene, hired assassin, one acting for another in evil.

395

kandyanga, kind of gnome.
kanga, (to) baffle.
kankasa, top bond on house-wall.
kansai, strong tobacco.
kanshya, girl assistant at initiation.
kantanta, sable bull.
kaŋumba, (1) demon ; (2) wind.
kapa, grandparent.
kasabwa, a Lamba moon.
kasaŵo, edible veld root.
katungu, (1) charm to ensure easy birth ; (2) child born after treatment by *mukamwami* or *umulaye*.
kaŵeshya, breeze, movement of air.
kaŵumbu, species of tree.
kokote'fupa, (to) gnaw bone.
kombolwe, cock.
kubwalo, to the chief's court.
kuchisompe, to the long grass (to relieve nature).
kuchiŵuula, at the place of instruction.
kumashilampindwe, at the cross-roads.
kumbo'bwalwa, (to) brew beer.
kunka, (to) knock.
kupala, (to) flick.
kwesa, (to) slice.
kwipanga, to the chief's abode.
kwiulu, above, in heaven.

lala, (to) sleep.
lalika, (to) have sexual intercourse.
lama, (to) protect.
lambila, (to) make obeisance, humble oneself.
lambwe, buffalo bull.
laŵishya, (to) upbraid.
laya, (to) promise, summon.
lelesa, (to) have tender compassion.
lembalemba, species of thick cobweb.
lembo'bwangà, (to) tattoo with a charm.
lendeŵuka, (to) split right down.
lendya, gladiolus bulb used as bullroarer.
Lesa, the usual name for the Deity.
lishya'kakoŵe, (to) hiss.
lishye'mpundu ⎱ (to) make a *lululu*-ing
lishyo'lumpundu ⎰ sound.
lishyo'lusota, (to) snap the fingers.
longela, (to) store corn.
lowa, (to) bewitch.
Luchyele, the name of the Deity as creator.
lukamfi, child born after treatment by doctor.
lukundula-fiŵunsa, a Lamba moon.
lukungwe, species of tree-snake.
lumbwe, consort.
luŵuka, (to) redeem oneself.

lwenshi, species of tree.
lwitaŵila, bird of ill-omen.
lya, (to) eat.
Lyulu, a name for the Deity.

mama, my mother.
masa, (to) plaster.
masombwe, stick insect.
moŵa, professional dancer.
moye, girl at the time of initiation.
muchitumbo, in the garden clearing.
muchyumbo, beneath the pall (of an initiate).
mufiŵafu, in the north and south.
mukamfwilwe, widow, widower.
mukamwami, spirit medium, prophet.
mukolo, principal wife of chief.
mukoma, hammer with wooden handle.
mukona, species of tree.
mukumulaya, in order to bid him farewell.
mukuta, species of bird.
mukutushishya-mo, in order to rest therein.
mukuŵuka, in order to divine.
mukwikato'mushili, in order to ' catch the soil.'
mulonda, watchman, attendant.
Mulungu, a name for the Deity.
mumanga, funnel fish-trap.
mumpanga, in the veld.
mutepa, younger wife of a chief.
mututungu, in the gardens.
mwami, Lenje and Ila for *umwami*.
Mwelaishyaŋombe ⎱ the guardian of the
Mwenshyaŋombe ⎰ herds.
mwika, child born with leg-presentation.
mwilole, in the chief's court.
mwinshyo, maternal uncle.
Mwishyaŋombe, the guardian of the herds.
mwitumbatumba, in the chief's court.

nanya, (to) stir.
nanye'nshima, (to) prepare porridge.
ndale, (1) species of tree ; (2) " Let me sleep."
nkombalume, elephant-hunter.
nkumbinkumbi, a Lamba moon.
ntenkentenke, a Lamba moon.
nteŵe, species of salt grass.
nwinshya, (to) administer a potion.
Nyambi, a name for the Deity.
nyina wabwanga, mother of the charm.
nyinachimbela, midwife.
nyinakulu, maternal grandmother.
nyinalochya, black salt.
nyina-mukulu, mother's elder sister.

GLOSSARY

nyina-mwanichye, mother's younger sister.

ofya, (to) entangle.

pala, (to) spit out chewed matter.
pamantila, (to) beat mud floor.
pamataŵa, when the maize ripens.
pambuka, (to) excrete.
pampa, (to) cut up meat.
pamutembo, on a carrying-pole.
pamuŵundo, at the time of the floods.
pamwela, during the dry season.
pata, (to) scold.
paŵama, (to) come down right side up.
peela, (to) swing to and fro.
peeshya, (to) try a fowl by ordeal poison.
pekawila, (to) fan.
pema, (to) breathe.
pesonde, outside.
pooso'ŵunga, (to) throw the meal for cleansing.
pupa ⎱ (to) make ceremonial of-
pupe'mipashi ⎰ fering to the spirits.
pupwe, species of tree.
pushya-mo, (to) penetrate.
puuta, (to) extend, cover, fill.
pwele, thrush.

saasa, (to) beg for pardon.
salulula, (to) choose.
samba, (to) bathe, wash.
sanshila, (to) ask questions in divining.
sanshile'miseŵe, (to) question the rattles.
sense, hutch-trap for leopard.
sesemuka, (to) hang over.
seŵa-pachyulu, a Lamba moon.
shikula, (to) exhume.
shikulu, lord, master.
shilika, (to) ward off.
shipila'mate mwiulu, (to) spit into the air.
shishimunkulu ⎱ ogre.
shishimwe ⎰
shiwakota, species of bird.
shiŵoyongo, type of dance.
Shyakapanga, a name for the Deity.
shyamawawa, impotent male.
solola ⎱ (to) talk over a case.
soŵolola ⎰
soŵongo, chronic ulcer.
sumba, species of large green lizard.
sumuna, (to) wipe.
sunsa, top capping to thatch.
sunsana, (to) shake hands (wrists).
sunsulula, (to) loosen.
suŵa, (to) smear oneself.

taata, (to) begin to speak (of a child).
taila, (to) bring offerings at a beer-drink.
tata, my father.
temangume, a Lamba moon.
tentula, (to) straighten metal implements.
teŵeta, (to) provide food.
teŵula, (to) cut down corn stalks.
teya, (to) set a trap.
teye'fipa, (to) cast lots.
tima, (to) breathe.
timbwa, fruit beer.
totaishya, (to) flatter.
tuka, (to) revile.
tula, (to) dig, dig up.

ubwalangwe, short cross-sticks.
ubwalwa, intoxicating Kafir beer.
ubwanga, charm, poison.
ubwanga bwachimbwembwe, charm for putting fear into enemy's hearts.
ubwanga bwakalwani, charm for chest troubles.
ubwanga bwakufyala, charm to procure easy birth.
ubwanga bwakulowa, witchcraft medicine.
ubwanga bwalukawo, charm for securing thieves in the gardens.
ubwanga bwalwela, charm for protection in fight.
ubwanga bwamboo, charm for hunting buffalo.
ubwanga bwamfula, charm for preventing rain.
ubwanga bwamfwiti, charm against witches.
ubwanga bwamutwi, charm for headache.
ubwanga bwanama, hunting charm.
ubwanga bwangwena, charm against crocodiles.
ubwanga bwankalamu, charm against lions.
ubwanga bwankatulo, charm against *utuyeŵela.*
ubwanga bwankondo, war charm.
ubwanga bwansofu, charm for hunting elephant.
ubwanga bwansoka, charm against snakes.
ubwanga bwashiŵuwungu, charm for garden protection.
ubwanga bwaŵulwele, charm against sickness.
ubwanga bwaŵupalu, hunting magic.
ubwanga bwaŵusuko, charm to prevent the rotting of pumpkins.

ubwanga bwayamba, charm for protection of foodstuffs.

ubwembya, whip.

ubwesela, type of musical instrument.

ubweya, type of axe.

ubwifutenuma, with the back turned.

ubwilangwe, mecklings.

ubwinga, the village of the husband.

ukochya, to burn.

ukubwa, to pop (of fish).

ukubwitaka, to twitch spasmodically.

ukuchindilo'mwanichye, to dance in honour of a new-born babe.

ukuchine'fishili, to foment the gums.

ukuchita'kampelwa, to swing.

ukuchito'tukonkola, to walk on stilts.

ukuchya, to dawn.

ukuchyesa, to cut corn heads.

ukufimba, to thatch.

ukufinga, to curse.

ukufishya kuŵulaye, to bring into the profession of a doctor.

ukufuka, to scratch out ground products.

ukufunda, to instruct.

ukufundika, to confine.

ukukando'wukala, to press the male organ.

ukukapa, to introduce into a new state.

ukukatika, to knead together.

ukukombole'nkwa, to strip soft bark from trees.

ukukosa, to be strong, hard.

ukukumba, to brew (beer).

ukukunga, to make headdress of beads.

ukukuula, to rough hoe.

ukukuya, to practise enlarging of the male organ.

ukukwamuno'lupaapi, to split down *ulupaapi* stick.

ukulala muŋanda, to sleep in the house.

ukulamba, to make obeisance.

ukulapa, to swear, take oath.

ukulaya, to take farewell, give parting instructions.

ukulima, to hoe, cultivate.

ukulishyo'lumpundu, to utter shrill whistling cries.

ukulishyo'munsu, to whistle.

ukuliteka, to enslave oneself.

ukulongela, to store grain.

ukulota, to dream.

ukulowa, to practise witchcraft.

ukuloŵa, to fish with line and hook.

ukulule'mfwa, to announce death indirectly.

ukululuma, to thunder.

ukumasa, to plaster.

ukunanya, to make porridge.

ukunonka, to seek wealth at a distance.

ukunwo'mufungo, to drink bitter fruit, to eat humble pie.

ukunyuke'fiseŵa, to soften skins.

ukupaapa, to carry pick-a-back.

ukupaapatila, to pray.

ukupakana, to shake hands.

ukupale'nkwa, to clean hard bark from soft.

ukupando'bwanga, to prepare charms.

ukupashila, to sew.

ukupeepeshya, to smoke with.

ukupela, to grind.

ukupeta, to fold up.

ukupila, to fish by bailing.

ukupooswo'ŵunga, to have meal ceremonially thrown on one.

ukuposa, to weave, intertwine, roll fibre, etc.

ukupose'filukwa, to weave baskets.

ukupota, to wring out.

ukupuma, to thresh.

ukupume'nkuule, to break up clods.

ukupupa ⎫ to make ceremonial offering to
ukupupe'mipashi ⎬ spirits.

ukupuupulula'ŵantu, to restore people to strength.

ukupyaila, to sweep.

ukupyata, to plait, roll in reverse.

ukusaasa, to beg for pardon.

ukusala ⎫ to hammer bark
ukusale'nguŵo ⎬ cloth.

ukusamba, to bathe, wash.

ukusanshike'fyaŵu, to construct bridges.

ukusanshila, to put questions during divination.

ukusasa, to fish by treading.

ukuseesa, to menstruate.

ukusema, to scare pigs or monkeys.

ukusemba, to rejoice.

ukusepa, to gather wild fruit or roots.

ukushilika, to ward off, prohibit.

ukushilika Kaaluwe, to counteract the guardian of the animals.

ukushilika ŵakolwe, to ward off monkeys.

ukushilike'chiŵanda, to ward off a demon.

ukushilike'fyuni, to ward off birds.

ukushilike'nguluŵe, to ward off wild pigs.

ukushingula, to smear with thin mud.

ukushinguluka, to go round.

ukusumba, to fish by spearing.
ukusumika, (1) to filter ; (2) to cup.
ukusumuna, to wean.
ukusunkana, to wrestle.
ukutala, to mark out a hut.
ukutando'tuuluka, to chase things that fly.
ukutane'ntafu, to play ball.
ukutatula, to start the songs.
ukutema, to fell trees.
ukutemwa, to be happy.
ukuteŵula, to cut down corn stalks.
ukuteye'chipa ⎫
ukuteye'fipa ⎭ to cast lots.
ukutinamina, to prefer, have longings.
ukutonda, to respect, hold in reverence, fear.
ukutongala ⎫
ukutukana ⎬ to revile.
ukutukana'matuka ⎭
ukutunta, to carry.
ukutwa, (1) to pound ; (2) to poison fish.
ukutwila, to fish by poison.
ukuuŵuluka, to shed skin.
ukuwe'chisungu, to undergo initiation.
ukuwela, to shout.
ukuwilwa, to become spirit possessed.
ukuŵanga, (1) to notch timber ; (2) to place building bonds.
ukuŵange'mango, to notch timber.
ukuŵansa, to take daily supply from corn-store.
ukuŵasa'masonje, to chip the teeth.
ukuŵimba, to twitch.
ukuŵomba, to bring gifts to avert disaster.
ukuŵombola, to claim a gift of clan relationship.
ukuŵuka, to divine.
ukuŵuka kumiseŵe, to divine by rattles.
ukuŵuka kumupini, to divine by axe-handle.
ukuyaŵa, to sing mourning songs.
ukwalila, to fish by weir trap.
ukwamina, to scare birds.
ukwanga, to triumph.
ukwanshika, to arrange (especially the bed).
ukwante'ntafu, to catch ball.
ukwaŵa, to portion out.
ukwela, to winnow.
ukwendelo'mushili, to prospect for good soil.
ukwikashya, to fish with net.
ukwiŵaka, to build.
ulufu, death.

ulukamfi, chewed leaves, etc.
ulukombo, drinking calabash.
ulukwa, soft inside bark.
ulumbashi, child who excretes at birth.
ulumombwe, species of caterpillar.
ulumpundu, shrill whistling cries of women.
ulunchindu, species of palm.
ulunyena, child who excretes at birth.
ulupaapi, species of small bush.
ulupako, cleft of tree.
ulupanda, forked pole.
ulupe, small winnowing basket.
ulupindo, piece of stick used as charm.
ulupinga, stick charm for snake-bite.
ulupopo, peg.
ulupumpu, centre pole of hut.
ulusanso, sieve.
ulusengo, (1) horn ; (2) ivory trumpet.
ulushiko, upper fire-stick.
ulushila, red ochre.
ulushishi, bark rope.
ulusokoti, species of shrub.
ulusonsolo, heavy double bell.
ulusuŵa, the hot season.
uluteeta, branch cut and bent over.
uluwanga, fish basket.
uluŵangula, hemp for smoking.
uluŵansa, court, courtyard.
uluŵeshi, spear-headed arrow.
uluŵya, relish pot.
ulwando, mat fence used in fishing.
ulwimbo, song.
ulwimbo lwachisungu, initiation song.
ulwimbo lwakuŵomba, song of the consultations.
ulwisonga, salt-producing plant, chickweed.
umfwe'nsoni, (to) feel shame.
umondo, fish spear.
umono, funnel of fish-trap.
umuchila, (1) tail ; (2) switch of zebra-tail.
umuchila wambishi, zebra's tail.
umuchinda, calabash water-container for pipe.
umuchinka, species of tree.
umuchinko, type of dance, often immoral.
umuchinshi, polite behaviour.
umuchyeka, palm-leaf mat.
umuchyenja, species of tree.
umuchyete, commoner.
umuchyeŵu, species of insect.
umuchyobwe, abuse, blasphemy.
umufolwa, trench.
umufushi, blacksmith.
umufuŵa, meal and water.
umufwi wamatwi, barbed arrow.

THE LAMBAS OF NORTHERN RHODESIA

umufyala, cross-cousin.
umukali, fierce person.
umukashi, wife.
umukashi-mukulu, principal wife.
umukashi-mwanichye, junior wife.
umukoka, clan.
umukokolo, species of tree.
umukole, (1) hostage ; (2) species of tree.
umukoleshi wamfula, driver away of rain.
umukopo, strip of cloth used as binder.
umukoso, species of tree.
umukulu, (1) elder brother of male ; (2) elder sister of female ; (3) village elder, old person.
umukunto, ordinary drum.
umukusa, sanseviera fibre plant.
umukuta, species of bird.
umukwa, bark plate.
umulalafuti, the Milky Way.
umulambu, offering of respect.
umulamu, (1) brother-in-law ; (2) sister-in-law.
umulandu, law, blame, case.
umulandu wamfwa, death-due.
umulaye, doctor, diviner.
umulaye umukulu, fully qualified doctor.
umulaye uwamipini, doctor of axe-handles, young doctor.
umulaye wachishyala, doctor of the instrument bag.
umulaye watuluŵi, ventriloquist doctor.
umulembeshi, tattooer.
umulembo, member of the bee clan.
umulembwe, greens.
umulenda, shrine, spirit hut.
umulenda waŵamoŵa, professional dancers' shrine.
umulishi, drummer, player of an instrument.
umulokashi, daughter-in-law.
umuloli, type of flute.
umulolo, species of shrub.
umulombe, (1) species of tree ; (2) fabulous witchcraft snake.
umulomweshi, inferior doctor.
umulomweshi wabwanga, charm doctor.
umulomweshi wansoka, snake-bite doctor.
umululu, species of tree.
umulunda, blood-brother.
umulyashi, burial-place.
umumbu, species of edible root.
umumfundwa, non-intoxicating honey beer.
umumpulumpumpi, species of shrub.
umuneŋene, species of tree.

umuninga, monkey-nuts.
umunkoto, two-stringed musical instrument.
umunsala, species of fish-trap.
umunshi, pestle.
umuntu umwine, the person himself.
umuntunshi, human being.
umunyanja, salt grass.
umupalu, professional hunter.
umupalu umukulu, great hunter.
umupalu wampendwa, ant-bear hunter.
umupapa, Rhodesian mahogany-tree.
umupashi, (1) spirit of deceased ; (2) good omen.
umupashi waŵulaye, spirit of divination.
umupini, handle of axe or hoe.
umupundu, species of fruit-tree.
umupupa, lawless person.
umuputu ⎫
umusaalya ⎬ species of tree.
umusafwa ⎭
umusakasa, type of dance.
umusako, demon which causes idiocy.
umusaku, boiled corn.
umusamba, species of tree.
umusamfu, convulsions.
umusamu, medicine.
umusamu wakulomona, medicine for treatment.
umusamu wamulombe, charm for witchcraft snake.
umusantu, grass bundle.
umusase, species of tree.
umusashi, double calabash for oil.
umuseesa, menstruating woman.
umusembe, type of flute.
umusengelo, split-reed mat.
umuseŵe, rattle.
umushi, village.
umushichye, person not in wedlock—bachelor, spinster, widow, widower, divorcee.
umushikalilo, species of bush.
umushiliko, prohibition, taboo.
umushitu, rank forest, grove of swamp trees.
umushya, female slave.
umushyakashi, woman slave attendant.
umushyala, orphan.
umushyangalala, piece of cinder, soot.
umusokolwe, new village site.
umusompo, bark cloth.
umusonko, tax.
umusuku, (1) species of fruit tree ; (2) cupping horn.
umusumbo, fish spear.
umusunga, ' leaven ' for beer-making.
umuswachi wameno, tooth-powder.

GLOSSARY

umuswema, species of snake.
umuta, barbel.
umutalu, medicine for exorcizing.
umutanda, zareba.
umutanti, cross-pole.
umutapo, iron ore.
umutatwishi, song-leader.
umutaŵa, species of tree.
umutembo, (1) carrying-pole ; (2) load.
umuti, (1) tree ; (2) medicine.
umutima, heart.
umutondo, large water-pot.
umutoŵo, species of tree.
umutungu, gourd drum.
umuuŵa, bellows.
umuŵanga, species of tree.
umuŵela, cowrie-shell.
umuŵili, body.
umuŵishi, premature birth.
umuŵundikwa, species of tree.
umuŵundo, flood season.
umuŵungo, rubber creeper.
umuyambo, professional h u n t i n g dancer.
umuyinga, professional hunter.
umwafi, (1) tree with poisonous bark ; (2) ordeal poison.
umwaka, year.
umwala wambishi, mane of zebra.
umwambwa, large cake of tobacco.
umwami, (1) spirit of Lenje chief ; (2) medium of Lenje chief.
umwana, child.
umwana umukulu-ŵantu, elder, eldest child.
umwana umwanichye-ŵantu, younger, youngest child.
umwana wabwanga, child of the charm.
umwana wanshiwa, orphan.
umwana waŵushichye, illegitimate child.
umwana-muŵyakwe, fellow-child.
umwanawaŵene, free man.
umwando, rope, noose trap.
umwandwalesa, species of shrub.
umwanichye, (1) y o u n g s t e r ; (2) y o u n g e r brother of male ; (3) younger sister of female.
umwefu, (1) beard ; (2) fresh green grass.
umwela, dry season.
umwenje, species of tree.
umwenshi, (1) moon ; (2) month.
umwenshi uŵulungene, full moon.
umwenye, a Lamba moon.
umwenye-masuku, a Lamba moon.
umweo, life.
umwinachyowa, member of mushroom clan.

umwinachyulu, member of anthill clan.
umwinamaila, member of sorghum clan.
umwinambushi, member of goat clan.
umwinambwa, member of dog clan.
umwinamishishi, member of human hair clan.
umwinamulenda, (1) keeper of shrine ; (2) undertaker.
umwinanguni, member of honey-guide clan.
umwinansofu, member of elephant clan.
umwinanswi, member of fish clan.
umwinatembo, member of wasp clan.
umwine wachisungu, bridegroom of an initiate.
umwine wamulume, owner of the husband.
umwine wamupashi, owner of the spirit.
umwine wamushi, village headman.
umwine waufwile, heir of the deceased.
umwine wayamba, owner of *yamba* charm.
umwinshikulu, grandchild.
umwipwa, (1) sister's child (of male) ; (2) brother's child (of female).
utombe, fishing nets.
utubwenje, small black stones used in witchcraft-divination.
utulindi, pl. of *akalindi*.
utulyamakumbi, little cloud-eaters, dwarfs.
utumimba, spirit huts of the crossroads.
utumwengwemwengwe, small stones used in witch-divination.
utunkolomwena, medium-sized Mbundu beads.
utupeshi, pl. of *akapeshi*.
utupingwe, pl. of *akapingwe*.
utupondo, pl. of *akapondo*.
utusamfu, kindling wood.
utusengo, little horns.
utuseŵa, sparrows.
utushimi, choric stories.
ututangu, Kaonde for *ŵamoŵa*.
ututi twafipa, small sticks for drawing lots.
ututundu, pl. of *akatundu*.
ututungu, garden shelters.
utuŵangaŵanga, stars.
utuyeŵela, pl. of *akayeŵela*.
uwamampandakanya, many-branched (tree).
uwamankunamwa, child who cuts upper teeth first.

uwayamba, doctor having power of *yamba* charm.
uŵowa, mushroom.
uŵuchi, honey.
uŵuchinga, game-pit.
uŵuchisa, relish (especially cooked leaves).
uŵuchyende, adultery.
uŵuchyonko, finches.
uŵufulu, chyme, stomach contents of animal.
uŵufushi, art of blacksmithing.
uŵufwiti, witchcraft.
uŵuko, village of the wife.
uŵukumbwaŋombe, species of bush.
uŵukushi, loin-strip.
uŵukwa, jealousy.
uŵulamba, Lamba language.
uŵulaye, craft of doctor or diviner.
uŵulembe, (1) species of creeper ; (2) arrow poison.
uŵuleme, glory.
uŵuleya, species of ground-nut.
uŵulunda, friendship.
uŵulwani, (1) ferocity ; (2) wild beast.
uŵulwishya, jealousy.
uŵunga, meal.
uŵungwa, roguishness.
uŵupalu, huntsmanship.
uŵusumfi, weevil.
uŵusunga, gruel.
uŵusunga bwamawo, red millet gruel.
uŵuta, (1) bow ; (2) weapon.
uŵutwa, old term for *umuyambo*.
uŵuŵa, shrub used for fish-poison.
uŵuŵoni, goods, wealth.
uŵuyombo, grass dancing skirt.

wila, (to) possess (of a spirit entering a person).
wilwa, (to) become possessed.
wishinkashi, father's sister.
ŵachiŵa, doves.
ŵachiwila, Lala for *ŵamoŵa*.

ŵachyandwe, parakeets.
Ŵakaaluwe, pl. of Kaaluwe.
ŵakapa, pl. of *kapa*.
ŵamoŵa, pl. of *moŵa*.
ŵamoye, pl. of *moye*.
ŵampundu, twins of like sex.
ŵamukamoŵa. See *ŵamoŵa*.
ŵamukamwami, pl. of *mukamwami*.
ŵamukumbe, maneless lions.
ŵamukupe, (1) apparitions ; (2) persons possessed by dancing spirit.
ŵamulonda, pl. of *mulonda*.
ŵamumpilwe, weird goblin-like beings.
ŵamwinshyo, pl. of *mwinshyo*.
ŵangashye, a Lamba moon.
ŵankonde, incisions between eyes and ears.
ŵanyinafimbela, pl. of *nyinachimbela*.
ŵanyinafyala, his mother-in-law.
ŵanyinakulu, pl. of *nyinakulu*.
ŵashiŵuwungu, persons able to transfer strength of crops.
ŵatete, grasshoppers.
ŵawishi, his father, his father's brother.
ŵawishifyala, his mother-in-law.
ŵila, (to) ferment.
ŵomba, (to) bring gifts to avert disaster.
ŵuka, (to) divine, exorcize.
ŵuka kumiseŵe, (to) divine by means of rattles.
ŵuka'mashilu, (to) exorcize demons of madness.
ŵumbe, species of meerkat.
ŵumoŵa, professional dancing in honour of the *ifinkuwaila*.
ŵunshya, (to) shake in water.

ya, (to) go.
yamba, charm (1) to prevent stealing food, (2) to prevent rain.
yamba wamulukombo, the charm in the calabash.

INDEX

ADULTERY, punishment for, 67–69
Afflatus of spirit, 241
Afterbirth, 132
Akalimba, 361–362
Akankoto, 363–364
Akapeshi (basket of *mukamwami*), 260–261
Akapeshi (spirit hut), 239–240
Amalimba, 361, 363
Amankunamwa, 138
Amankuŵala, 365
Amansanshi, 143–146
Animals, kinds eaten, 102–104; stories of, 354–356
Ant-bear hunting, 338
Arrest, wrongful, 74
Arrows, 332–333
Assassins, hired, 73
Aushi, 22–23
Aŵenamaswaka, 26
Aŵenambonshi, 26
Aŵenamilenda, 179, 180, 182 *et seq.*, 186, 187, 188, 189
Aŵenamukuni, 26
Axe, in hunting, 333–334; importance of, 96, 99
Axe-handle in divining, 271–272

BABIES, drowning of, 138
Ball, playing with, 142
Bark cloth, preparation of, 119–122
Bashfulness at marriage, 169
Baskets, making of, 118
Bathing, children fond of, 140–141
Beer, 107–108
Beer-drink, at mourning ceremony, 183–185; at shrine-building, 235–237
Behaviour, rules for, 208–210
Bellows, 349
Bier, 179
Bird-scaring, 112
Birds, of ill-omen, 250; kinds eaten, 103–104
Birth, 131–133; premature, 133; special cases of, 132–133; of twins, 133–134
Birth-prophet, 264
Blacksmith, 347–351
Borrowing, 75
Boundary disputes, 49–50

Bow and arrows, 331–333
Building of house, 88, 90–94
Burial, 180–182; of chief, 186–190; of children, 185; of lepers, 185; of pregnant woman, 184–185; preparation for, 178–179

CALENDAR of work, 94–96
Canoe, making of bark, 119; making of dug-out, 119
Carrying-cloth for baby, 136
Charm—see *Ubwanga*
Charm doctors, 279–280
Chief, group, 71–72; inheritance of, 60; installation of, 60–61; paramount, 50; territorial, 50
Chieftainship, origin of, 54–55
Chikoloma, 26
Chikundas, 38–39, 79
Chipimpi, 31–35
Chisumpa, 38
Chitina, 26
Chiwala, 44 *et seq.*
Choric stories, 356–358
Chyushi, 26
Clan customs, 198
Clan opposites, 197–198
Clan system, 193–207
Clans of chiefs, 197
Clapping of hands, 368
Clothing, 119–120; of baby, 137
Codrington, Captain, 47
Condiments, 105
Confinement, 134–135
Confinement at initiation, 153
Consort of woman-chief, 164
Cosmogony, 222 *et seq.*
Councillors, 57–59
Creditor, action of, 76
Crises of life, 148
Cross-cousin marriage, 162–163
Cupping, 126
Cursing, 77

DANCES: *akasela*, 152, 183, 184, 360; *akaŵale*, 360; to *amalimba*, 361; *amambalakata*, 328, 360; *amaombe*, 358–359; *ichilaila*, 360–361; *ichimbwasa*, 156–157, 359; *ichinsengwe*,

INDEX

INDEX

407

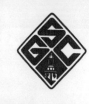

GLASSBORO STATE COLLEGE